# The International Handbook of Art Therapy in Palliative and Bereavement Care

T0341245

*The International Handbook of Art Therapy in Palliative and Bereavement Care* offers multicultural and international perspectives on how art therapy can be of help to individuals, groups, families, communities, and nations facing death and dying as well as grief and loss.

Over 50 art therapists from around the world write about the transforming power of art therapy in the lives of those facing terminal illness, dementia, loss, and grief. They offer practical descriptions and techniques for working with adults and children to guide professionals, including those new to using art therapy and creative approaches in end-of-life care services.

This international handbook is essential reading for art therapists, social workers, medical personnel, faith leaders, and psychologists interested in a collaborative and accessible approach to working with patients and families affected by loss.

**Michèle J.M. Wood BA (Hons), PGDip, MA, MClin. Res., SFHEA** is an HCPC Registered Art Psychotherapist with 30 years of experience as a practitioner, supervisor, educator and researcher. She is an international authority on art therapy in palliative care.

**Becky Jacobson LPC, ATR, LMT** has provided art therapy within hospice, bereavement, mental health, and community-based programmes locally and internationally. Her work focuses on combining psychotherapy, mindfulness, and creative self-expression.

**Hannah Cridford BA (Hons), MDes, MA** is an HCPC registered Art Psychotherapist, working in two hospices in the UK. She was awarded the Corinne Burton Memorial Trust Scholarship in 2010.

# The International Handbook of Art Therapy in Palliative and Bereavement Care

Edited by Michèle J.M. Wood,
Becky Jacobson, and Hannah Cridford

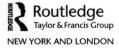

Routledge
Taylor & Francis Group

NEW YORK AND LONDON

First published 2019
by Routledge
52 Vanderbilt Avenue, New York, NY 10017

and by Routledge
2 Park Square, Milton Park, Abingdon, Oxon, OX14 4RN

*Routledge is an imprint of the Taylor & Francis Group, an informa business*

*Library of Congress Cataloging-in-Publication Data*
Names: Wood, Micháele J. M., 1960- editor. | Jacobson, Becky, editor. |
 Cridford, Hannah, editor.
Title: The international handbook of art therapy in palliative and bereavement care /
 edited by Micháele J.M. Wood, Becky Jacobson, and Hannah Cridford.
Description: New York, NY : Routledge, 2019. | Includes bibliographical
 references and index.
Identifiers: LCCN 2019005045 (print) | LCCN 2019005422 (ebook) |
 ISBN 9781315110530 (E-book) | ISBN 9781138087361 (hbk) |
 ISBN 9781138087330 (pbk) | ISBN 9781315110530 (ebk)
Subjects: | MESH: Art Therapy | Palliative Care | Hospice Care |
 Cross-Cultural Comparison
Classification: LCC RC489.A7 (ebook) | LCC RC489.A7 (print) | NLM WM 450.5.A8 |
 DDC 616.89/1656—dc23
LC record available at https://lccn.loc.gov/2019005045


ISBN: 978-1-138-08736-1 (hbk)
ISBN: 978-1-138-08733-0 (pbk)
ISBN: 978-1-315-11053-0 (ebk)


Typeset in Baskerville
by Apex CoVantage LLC.

# Contents

# Figures

# Tables

# Preface

This book has been conceived at a time when the Internet brings greater awareness of our shared humanity and opens up possibilities for global communication and connection. The relative ease of online communication has allowed its editors (MW, BJ and HC) to engage art therapists across the world to share accounts of their work within services providing hospice, palliative and bereavement care. Reaching out and gathering colleagues from around the world has been incredibly encouraging, and while some connections have not led to contributions to this volume, it is heartening to know that at a global level art therapy is alive and well. Art therapists (often operating as solo practitioners) are pioneering and researching innovative interventions, raising the profile of their profession within multi-professional teams, and supporting colleagues and communities to better manage the realities of terminal illnesses and death. The art therapist's work however, remains hidden away within the lives of their clients and the organisations they serve. Providing a bigger platform to share diverse art therapy approaches to adults and children facing physical illness, terminal illnesses and bereavement was a key factor motivating this book. Understanding different cultural perspectives is also important, especially since social migration for economic and political reasons has brought a range of people into art therapy services. There is one huge caveat to our gathering of the global art therapy community, and that is with language. Sadly, we have only been able to include texts in the English language; this is a considerable limitation and we are very grateful to those authors who have written their stories in a second language. Another limitation is our choice to limit the focus of this book to visual art therapy delivered by qualified art therapists. Nonetheless, art therapists are collaborators, and in this book, there are chapters co-authored with music therapists and psychologists. While we recognise the value of work by colleagues from other trainings (such as counselling, social work or nursing) who also make use of artistic and creative techniques, this book is aimed at promoting the benefits of the art therapy profession in all its diversity.

This has also been a time of global uncertainties, from climate change to political instability. Through images on television, newspapers and social media, we witness the effects of wars, economic disparities between citizens within our own countries and with other nations, and the senseless violence perpetrated by individuals against their own communities, such as seen in school shootings. These realities run alongside technological advancements that offer opportunities for people to live more happily, healthily and meaningfully. Thus, while life in the 21st century is complex, we continue to face the challenge of our own mortality. This is the backdrop to the themes and cases described here in the Handbook.

Corresponding with over 50 contributors has meant navigating the delays of life events, bridging gaps in time differences, clarifying cultural perspectives, and untangling the meanings and spellings for words used (we have decided to keep both US and UK spellings). However, it has been a great privilege to connect with new colleagues, to have our assumptions challenged, and to situate our own art therapy practices within a larger global picture. We are pleased that through our encouragement of new authors, we have brought to light innovative projects which build on existing knowledge of art therapy and palliative care. We hope readers gain a greater understanding of how we make a difference in prisons, in parks and in schools; and how our art therapy skills can help communities devastated by natural disasters, disease and acts of terror. We hope this book will be of benefit to everyone facing issues of mortality in their own lives and those of their clients.

Many thanks must go to our families and colleagues who have encouraged this project and supported us in ways too numerous to mention: Patrick, Madeleine and Benedict Wood; Emily Powis-Page; Yvonne Archdale; Jason Davidson; Jennifer Williams; Dan, Laurie and Vinnie Garbett for unerring support and tolerance; Meryl and Denzyll Garbett for extra childcare duties; Liz and Alan Cridford for provision of tranquility, a functioning computer and endless cups of tea; family Cridford Page for welcome distraction; Leslie and Lou Jacobson; Todd Stonnell for such valuable help with references; Derek and Phoebe Fowler for being such a supportive family, Chantea Cowan for the childcare she provided; Carol Olson for mentorship. Your encouragement and support have been vital. Our gratitude also goes to all the contributors for bearing with the lengthy process of bringing this book together.

Finally, thank you to all the patients who have generously consented to share their stories and artwork in these pages.

# Foreword

This delightful and insightful book takes us on a journey of discovery about art therapy and how it helps people facing advanced, progressive, life limiting illnesses, those who are close to them and those who care for them—throughout the experience of illness, loss, grief and bereavement. This is very timely as we face the challenge of increasing numbers of people living longer with more multiple conditions, but for whom, as for us all, dying and death are inevitable.

It helps practitioners of palliative and end of life care, and of bereavement services to understand and appreciate the immense contribution that art therapy and art psychotherapy can make. Reciprocally it helps art therapists to understand the practice and experience of palliative and end of life care, and of bereavement. In seeking to illuminate from both these aspects, this book provides a powerful opportunity for mutual learning and for fostering mutual respect for what each brings to our common goal of supporting and walking alongside people facing the last stage of their lives and families facing the prospect of this final separation.

The book is set out in three sections, taking us from considerations of how art therapy works with individuals to how it works with groups, families and communities. In the final section it moves to consideration of the wider issues of global and cultural challenges in this arena. The chapters often draw on examples of specific interventions and include some very personal narratives. The journey this book takes us on spans the continent of Europe, including the United Kingdom; Australasia; America and Asia. In bringing these wide-ranging contributions together, this book makes a rich contribution to the existing literature.

This is a gem of a book. I recommend it thoroughly to anyone who is interested in deepening their personal and professional understanding of the world of art therapy in the context of palliative and end of life care and bereavement, and is committed to enhancing their capability to help those in such a situation.

*Bee Wee*
*Consultant and Associate Professor in Palliative Medicine*
*Sir Michael Sobell House, Oxford University Hospitals NHS Foundation Trust, and*
*Harris Manchester College, University of Oxford*

# Introduction

This book is aimed at healthcare professionals working in hospices, nursing homes and other end-of-life care settings who may be curious to learn how art therapy can benefit their service users. It will also be of interest to art therapists seeking to know more about palliative, bereavement and end-of-life care. We particularly hope that it can be a resource for managers and commissioners with the responsibility of developing health and social care services for their citizens, and who may see the benefit of including art therapists in their interdisciplinary teams. Patients themselves may find this Handbook a valuable reference for learning about the range of support offered by art therapists.

In 2014 the World Health Assembly passed Resolution WHA67.19 (WHO, 2018a), in recognition of the increasing global burden of those who require access to palliative care. This Resolution urges nations to integrate the principles of palliative care at all levels of society, across all disease groups and for all ages. Its purpose is to promote quality of life, maintain human dignity and provide information and relief of suffering that is personally and culturally appropriate for those with incurable conditions. This is a collective endeavour between communities of lay and professional people and patients themselves. It requires compassion, innovation and the best scientific evidence available. The many examples described in this Handbook serve to illustrate these qualities in the work of art therapists, and we hope this collection will inspire services to draw upon the knowledge, skills and creativity of art therapists in their own parts of the world.

To orient our different readers, this introduction gives a brief overview of art therapy and palliative care, before outlining the key themes and structure of the book. A glossary of terms is provided to aid comprehension, and a list of art therapy associations around the world is offered as a resource for those wishing to learn more.

## Art Therapy

The profession of art therapy emerged from the work of artists, teachers and psychoanalysts in the UK and USA during the 1940s. Adrian Hill, an artist admitted into a sanatorium in the UK for tuberculosis, initiated art-making opportunities for his fellow patients. Hill's experiences, published in 'Art Versus Illness' (Hill, 1948), helped set the stage for another British artist, Edward Adamson, with whom Hill had worked, to offer similar art opportunities to patients within psychiatric hospitals. Adamson's approach was to create an environment within which patients could freely produce artworks without direction from him. Another influence on the development of the art therapy profession was the work of Gilbert and Irene Champernowne, who established Withymead, a residential therapeutic community informed by Jung's analytical psychology and credited as the first art therapy community in Britain (Hogan, 2000). Creative activities were central to the psychological care offered at Withymead, with many art therapists visiting it, including

Hill. Thus the relationship between physical and mental illness, and the belief in art making as a healing force, was forged in the shadow of World War II.

At the same time as art therapy was emerging as a profession in the UK, it was also forming within the USA. While many were inspired by the work of psychoanalysts and teachers using free and spontaneous art methods, two individuals in particular have been singled out as responsible for the development of art therapy in the USA: Edith Kramer and Margaret Naumburg (Rubin, 2010). Kramer, who worked largely with children in residential educational settings, placed her focus on the qualities integral to the art making process as an agent for healing in and of itself. Naumburg, however, considered art making to be a form of symbolic and metaphoric speech, emanating from the unconscious, to be interpreted by the artist themselves and analysed by the artist and therapist together. These two perspectives initiated the development of two distinct approaches which art therapists continue to utilise within their practice.

Since the 1940s art therapy, or art psychotherapy as it is also known, has become a recognised profession with a defined training, and in the UK the title 'Art Therapist' is protected by law. To become an art therapist in the UK and US requires two years full-time training (or equivalent) at postgraduate level. The training encompasses theories of psychology, models of psychotherapy, clinical work with clients, and ongoing engagement with artistic practice and personal psychotherapy. Once qualified, art therapists register with appropriate professional bodies (e.g. Health and Care Professions Council in the UK, while in the USA registration is done through the Art Therapy Credentials Board (ATCB) and licensing is done within individual states). They maintain their knowledge and skills through clinical supervision and ongoing independent learning. This model of postgraduate education for art therapists is not universal, although established trainings are beginning to offer satellite or franchised art therapy programmes; for example, US and Canadian art therapy training institutes validate programmes in Israel and Europe.

There are now over 37 international art therapy associations from Asia, Africa, Australia, Europe, the Middle East and the Americas (See Appendix at the end of the book for further details).

## Hospice, Palliative and End-of-Life Care

### Central Concepts

The modern hospice movement in the UK began with the pioneering work of Dame Cicely Saunders in the 1960s, who recognised that the needs of those with non-curable illnesses were being neglected. Acknowledging death as a part of life, she promoted healthcare that enhanced a person's life rather than prolonging it, advocating both compassion and the best scientific techniques to alleviate suffering. Saunders' concept of 'total pain' comprises physical, social, emotional and spiritual aspects and remains central to hospice care to this day. This holistic approach gained momentum with interest from colleagues across the world, including Florence Wald, who established the Connecticut Hospice in the USA in 1974, and Dr Balfour Mount, who set up Canada's first palliative care ward at Royal Victoria Hospital in Montreal, Quebec. In the UK, Palliative Medicine was recognised as a specialty in 1987, and there is an ongoing international movement to disseminate the core principles of interdisciplinary palliative care through education, service developments and research (Callaway et al, 2018).

By recognising suffering as an inevitable part of our humanity, and by highlighting the moral responsibility we have to alleviate our fellow humans' distress as far as we are able, palliative care draws out the deep meaning at the heart of the word 'hospice'—hospitality.

To receive palliative care is to feel welcomed by others, to feel understood for who you are, and be supported to find what you need to continue living well up to the end.

Thus, hospice and palliative care offers patients with advanced and terminal illness and their families the best quality of life by addressing their physical, psychological, social and spiritual distress. The nature and extent of individuals' distress will vary, but a palliative care approach recognises the following:

- Physical pain interferes with sleep, eating, thinking and social interactions
- Psychological symptoms are manifest as depression, anxiety and adjustment disorders
- Existential distress can be related to past, present and future concerns, giving rise to feelings of hopelessness, meaninglessness and disappointment
- Family dynamics are altered as financial and practical adjustments are made in light of the patient's changing health

By understanding and addressing patients' needs, and supporting them to cope with situations of adversity and suffering, good palliative care can also result in personal growth for everyone involved.

### Defining Terms: Supportive, Palliative and End-Of-Life Care

Scientific advancements in pharmacology and biomedicines have led to new treatments for the complications and symptoms of non-curative conditions, adding months and years to individuals' lifespans. For the patient it will mean living permanently with a heightened vigilance towards their health. While these changes are to be welcomed, the negative impact on economic productivity, social and cognitive functioning and psychological health is only now being recognised.

*Table 0.1* Significant Milestones in Palliative Care

| Year | Milestone event |
| --- | --- |
| 1967 | St Christopher's Hospice opens in London, England |
| 1974 | First Hospice programme in USA opens with Connecticut Hospice |
| 1976 | Royal Victoria Hospital Palliative Care Unit opens in Montreal, Canada |
| 1982 | Medicare funding is established for palliative care |
| 1988 | European Association for Palliative Care is formed |
| 1990s | International Association of Hospice and Palliative Care formed in USA |
| 1994 | South America Declaration of Florianopolis highlights lack of opioids |
| 2000 | Latin American Association of Palliative Care formed |
| 2001 | Asia Pacific Hospice Palliative Care Network |
| 2002 | Hospice Information Service established |
| 2003 | European Society for Medical Oncology recognises Palliative Care |
| 2005 | First World Hospice and Palliative Care Day |
| 2006 | EAPC Declaration of Venice to improve palliative care research in 'resource-poor' countries |
| 2009 | Worldwide Palliative Care Alliance constituted |
| 2011 | African Palliative Care Research Network formed |
| 2014 | Global Atlas of Palliative Care at the End of Life recognises extent of gaps in provision |
| 2015 | Publication of the Compassionate Cities Charter |
| 2015 | Ambitions for Palliative and End of Life Care published |

Source: Payne and Lynch (2015)

Three terms are commonly used to describe the treatment available to those who have been diagnosed with a life-threatening illness: Supportive care; palliative care; end-of-life care. All terms embrace the holistic needs of the patient and their families and take account of medical, emotional, spiritual and practical issues related to the illness. However, there are important distinctions.

'Supportive care' extends throughout all stages of life-threatening illness, including the period from diagnosis and treatment. 'Palliative care' focuses on the time when an individual's condition is understood to be non-curative. 'End-of-life care' narrows even further to the time when death is imminent, and in the UK and some other countries is generally understood as the last year of life. However, this term can also be used by some people when referring to care delivered in the patient's final days and hours.

### Variation in Palliative Care: A Multi-Professional Endeavour

This all-embracing approach requires a number of trained staff and volunteers, and consequently a key feature of palliative care is the multi-professional team. The composition of the team, the locations and the methods by which palliative care is delivered vary enormously between countries, and indeed between different settings within the same country. Doctors, nurses, psychosocial staff, faith leaders, pharmacists and others may engage with patients in a hospital ward, a dedicated hospice building, a community day centre, a residential or home setting, or a mobile clinic.

Healthcare professionals interacting at all points of the patient's trajectory of care will always need to consider the relationships with those close to the patient. Strong emotions and family dynamics can intensify as the patient draws closer to death, and support should be offered pre- and post-bereavement. The constellation of personnel offering palliative care and the levels at which they engage with each other and the patient and family can be summarised by two further descriptors of palliative care: generalist and specialist.

The generalist position is where any healthcare professional looking after patients can utilise the principles of palliative care to guide their interactions. Thus, General Practitioners, district nurses and hospital doctors can consult with and receive support from palliative care experts. Project ECHO, where specialists support staff in remote geographical locations through video consultations, is an example of this model being extended into the online environment (Zhou et al, 2016). Specialist services are provided to patients experiencing more complex situations, including admission to inpatient facilities. Higginson (Higginson, 2015) describes the three elements of specialist palliative care services: offering direction and education to generalist staff; offering direct care to highly complex patients and families; and engagement in research to benefit future patient care. In this book the reader will find examples of art therapists engaging in all three.

South African art therapists Berman and Woollett (Chapter 34) present their intervention for community workers delivering care to those living with HIV/AIDS in rural communities. Cooke et al (Chapter 35) describe their work in London, replicating the Indian model of the Neighbourhood Network in Palliative Care. Case studies from Wood, Yazdian Rubin, Orr, Jones et al, (Chapters 11, 19, 21, 23 respectively) illustrate a range of ways art therapists are integrated within specialist palliative care services. And very many contributors discuss how engagement in their own research is shaping new approaches to patient care.

### Bereavement Care

Grief is the feeling experienced in response to the loss of something that provided us with a sense of psychological security. This can be an object, place, animal or person.

Grief can be anticipated, as when recurrence of symptoms indicates disease progression, and preparations can be made for the inevitable bereavement. Or grief can be traumatic in situations where death is unexpected or characterised by stigma or brutality. An individual's experience of grief will be shaped by several factors, including the nature of the relationship and the time invested in it. Grief, and its outward expression of mourning, are socially and culturally determined, notably seen in rituals and religious practices. While informal support for those who are bereaved will come from family and friends, formal bereavement support is often a collaboration between community and specialist services. Pathological grief is where ongoing sorrow, a sustained desire for the deceased, and impaired social functioning continue in the individual for more than 12 months following the death. This will warrant a careful assessment and specialist support.

Different approaches to helping the bereaved have developed from observations of the process of grief and mourning. For example, Bowlby's Attachment Theory, which proposed that grief was the result of separation (Holmes, 1993); and the work of Kubler-Ross, who posited that grief progresses through a number of stages—denial, anger, bargaining, depression and acceptance (Kubler-Ross, 1969). Rather than progressing through stages, Worden (2010) proposed that grief has a number of tasks: breaking ties with the deceased; adjusting to a new environment without them; and developing connections with new people. Whilst acknowledging importance in these linear stage and task theories, recent developments suggest a different understanding of grief, including the Dual Process model (Stroebe & Schut, 2010), which describes an oscillation between focusing on and avoiding the loss; and Continuing Bonds (Steffen & Klass, 2017), which proposes that the work of grief is to find ways of maintaining a relationship with the dead through cultural practices and personal beliefs.

Bereavement support can be found in a wide variety of formats and settings. The accounts presented in this book demonstrate several modes of provision and ways art therapy is used to facilitate healthy grieving. For example, Bardot and McCaw's (chapter 20) describes a residential camp for bereaved children, and Kayleigh Orr presents an adolescent's request for bereavement support ten years after the death of her father, when she was only six years old (Chapter 21). Jacobson's vignette (24) gives an insight into her Mind Body art group for bereaved adults, the positive impact of which is beautifully described in Chapter 25, by Lynda Kachurek, a participant in this group. There are also other accounts of art therapists' own journeys of grief and self-care following personal bereavement.

### Challenges for Palliative Care in the 21st Century

The model for palliative care described so far, where a responsive, well-equipped and diverse interprofessional team delivers symptom relief to enhance quality of life activities and meaningful relationships for each individual, is not universally available. World Health Organisation figures indicate that only 14% of those who require palliative care receive it (WHO, 2018b). Low- to middle-income countries face the challenge of limited availability of medicines and trained personnel, and unstable political and social infrastructures (Connor & Bermedo, 2014). Additionally, the ethos of palliative care can clash with families' health beliefs, where accepting a terminal diagnosis is tantamount to giving up hope. In such situations patients may be shielded from the facts of their prognosis, and family members may invest all their resources in seeking treatments despite a clear lack of benefit, from a sense of 'duty'.

High-income countries like the UK and USA are not immune from the challenges of resource limitations. With an increasing ageing population and people living with co-morbidities and complex conditions, expectations for better services and the demand for palliative care are escalating. Costs of new treatments are placing a strain on health-care funding, raising concerns that palliative care may become marginalised in times of economic austerity. To mitigate this a strategic framework, 'Ambitions for Palliative and End of Life Care', was produced by an England-wide partnership of national organisations working in palliative and hospice care. Six ambitions boldly assert how the government's health and social care strategy for palliative and end of life care in England can be taken forward in the 21st century (National Palliative and End of Life Care Partnership, 2015). These are:

1.   Each person is seen as an individual
2.   Each person gets fair access to care
3.   Maximising comfort and wellbeing
4.   Care is coordinated
5.   All staff are prepared to care
6.   Each community is prepared to help

It is our hope that this Handbook indicates how art therapists already achieve these ambitions, and that their generic and specialist competencies make them a valuable resource for developing a workforce to meet palliative care needs in the 21st century.

## Aims of Art Therapy in Palliative Care

There are three broad aims of art therapy in palliative care: to facilitate the patient's process of adjustment following their diagnosis, treatment and ways in which illness has changed their life; to promote the process of rebuilding a new or renewed sense of 'self' for whatever time remains; and to develop in the patient and those around them the resources to cope.

This section will outline some of the available texts related to art therapy in palliative care, hospice care and bereavement, providing a backdrop for this Handbook and the contributions of the chapters within. The first collected essays on work in this area, *Art Therapy in Palliative Care: The Creative Response* (Pratt & Wood, 1998) presents a number of art therapists working in the UK and USA, who explore a range of settings, client groups and models of art therapy. In the same year, *Something Understood: Art Therapy in Cancer Care* (Connell, 1998) offered an in-depth case study of the art therapy service within a UK oncology service, with patients undergoing diagnosis and treatment for cancer or receiving news of a palliative condition. Since then, a number of publications have made valuable contributions to our understanding of the evolving range of art therapy practices with people living with incurable conditions, the dying and the bereaved: *Art Therapy and Cancer Care* (Waller & Sibbett, 2005); *Creative Arts in Palliative Care* (Hartley & Payne, 2008); a special issue of *Art Therapy* journal (2008); *End of Life Care: A Guide for Therapists, Artists and Arts Therapists* (Hartley, 2013); *Art Therapy with Physical Conditions* (Liebmann & Weston, 2015); *Complicated Grief, Attachment and Art Therapy* (MacWilliam, 2017).

The publication of academic papers on art therapy in hospice, bereavement and palliative care indicates an ongoing interest in this field. A summary of this literature points towards favourable outcomes for those accessing art therapy, broadly focusing on six main areas:

•   The effect of art therapy interventions for palliative care workers—clinical supervision, and promoting wellbeing and reduction in burnout

- Evaluations of art therapy interventions offered in specific areas of treatment—e.g. oncology, radiotherapy, chemotherapy, stem cell treatment
- Innovations in models of delivery
- Art therapy in paediatric palliative care settings
- In-depth case studies of client work
- The effect on the art therapist of working in end of life care and bereavement

Many papers seek to provide evidence of the benefits to patients, seemingly making a case for art therapy to be more widely recognised and offered within the sector (Wood et al, 2013). These papers focus on the positive effects of art making and creativity upon the patient, with particular emphasis on the relief of pain and physical symptoms (Lin et al, 2012; Lefèvre et al, 2016), relaxation of emotional state (Lin et al, 2012), promotion of post-traumatic growth (Collette, 2011), exploration of emotion (Buday, 2013; Meghani et al, 2018), communication and relief of distress (Holland et al, 2018), and creation of legacy and meaning making (Meghani et al, 2018). Art therapy with children also features within the literature, including a research study addressing anticipatory grief with children whose mother is diagnosed with life-threatening cancer (Holland et al, 2018), which reported better coping during treatment as well as improved preparation for parental bereavement.

Another area of particular focus is the examination of theoretical and practical frameworks underpinning the work (Hardy, 2013; Wood et al, 2013; Carr, 2014; Jones, 2007; Tjasink, 2010) and the evaluation of art therapy interventions at specific points along the cancer pathway (Agnese et al, 2012; Forzoni et al, 2010; Vianna et al, 2013; Lee et al, 2016). These papers offer a rich source of innovation for art therapists and their colleagues in palliative care, as do papers that offer in-depth accounts of work with patients (Furman, 2011; Safrai, 2013). Of particular interest is the exploration by art therapists into how work with seriously ill and dying patients affects them personally and professionally. Hardy examines how it is possible to sustain authentic engagement throughout repeated loss. By undertaking a literature review he reveals a reluctance to examine this aspect of the work, and offers ways to support both good practice and 'survival' (Hardy, 2001).

### *Impact of Caring for People at the End of Their Life on the Art Therapy and Healthcare Workforce*

Art therapy as a means of reducing stress for hospice staff, suggested decades ago by Belfiore (1994), continues to be explored. A study that combined art viewing and art making with hospice workers indicated positive impacts on wellbeing, communication, creativity and reduction of stress (Huet, 2017). Another recent study piloted art therapy groups for oncology and palliative care doctors with the aim of addressing the high rate of burnout (Tjasink & Soosaipillai, 2018). It also found favourable results, with statistically significant improvements in reducing emotional exhaustion and enhancing personal achievement in the participants. Outside of the UK, Potash and colleagues piloted art therapy-based supervision for end-of-life care workers in Hong Kong, finding it effective in developing increased emotional awareness, strengthening relationships and recognition of personal strengths, encouraging reflection on death and fostering meaning making, thereby reducing burnout (Potash et al, 2015).

The literature on art therapy in bereavement care is sparser, and hails largely from the USA. A recent systematic review of using visual modalities with bereaved people (Weiskittle & Gramling, 2018) covers 27 studies within the period 1981–2013, and signposts further opportunities for research. In *Complicated Grief, Attachment and Art Therapy*, several authors offer accounts of grief-specific applications of art therapy, with theoretical and personal perspectives of bereavement and how art making may help (MacWilliam, 2017).

This list is not exhaustive; individual chapters on working with cancer, serious illness, grief and death can also be found in books that have other leading foci in relationship to art therapy; for example in learning disability (Bull & O'Farrell, 2012), with older adults (Magniant, 2004), during assessment (Gilroy et al, 2012), wider healthcare settings (Malchiodi, 2013) and overarching texts such as the *Handbook of Art Therapy* (Gussak & Rosal, 2016) and *Grief and the Expressive Arts* (Thompson & Neimeyer, 2014). The blurring of borders between areas of specialty serve as a reminder that no person is immune to death and bereavement; it enters into every life and set of circumstances.

Additionally, there is crossover to be found in sister professions—the expressive arts, music therapy, dance/movement therapy, participatory arts projects, arts in health activity and spirituality. Art therapy intersects with these activities in differing ways, creating a rich landscape of arts-based interventions that may be of support to patients, family members, friends, staff and volunteers. It is important to locate this intersection within the multi-professional context of palliative care and the aforementioned concept of Total Pain (Saunders & Baines, 1989); no aspect of physical, social, emotional or spiritual pain exists in isolation, and there will be points of connection between the many professions that offer support to the patient and their family.

## Key Themes of This Book

### Mutability of Art Therapy Practices

The variety of approaches described within this book highlight the different conceptual models underpinning art therapy and art psychotherapy practices. Although all art therapists work within the ethical boundaries of a professional relationship established with their patients, their focus for addressing patients' needs inevitably varies. The trauma-informed approach described by Tripp (Chapter 8) builds on recent understandings from neuropsychology and recognises how the body's instinctual responses affect emotional regulation, memory and cognition. This perspective is implicit in other contributors' chapters too. Yazdian Rubin (Chapter 19) highlights how the creative and expressive aspects of art therapy push back the medicalisation of palliative care to keep Saunders' holistic view of 'Total Pain' central. The social value of arts practices is illustrated by Green's 'communitas-infused arts therapy' (Chapter 31). While many of the conceptual models described reflect the common approaches of UK and US art therapy trainings, the authors also demonstrate how practices are shaped by the ideas of the different locations within which art therapy is delivered. Art therapy in prisons, schools, community spaces, medical settings and delivered online as eHealth is a testament to the flexibility and mutability of the modality. Art therapy provides a language for physical and emotional pain in a way that words alone cannot, and it is available to be used across the entire lifespan, in childhood and old age. The ongoing developments in patient care through art therapists' innovations are also highlighted by authors' adoption of new technologies, novel research methodologies and by combining their skills with other interventions.

### Cultural Differences

The importance of cultural difference is another key theme in this book. Issues of gender, sexuality, religious belief and intercultural exchange are presented. Cultural awareness in art therapy is a hugely complex topic containing historical and current power injustices reflected in the discourses within the profession, the sources of art therapy pedagogies, and access to training by minority groups. There is a marked difference between Western countries and Asian, Middle Eastern and African nations when it comes to care for the ill and dying. In Western traditions the individual's right to self-determination is honoured over the wishes of their community or family. The person themself is informed of their prognosis, and is encouraged to make plans to direct their care, such as whether or not they wish to be resuscitated. This contrasts with those cultures whose values rest on the collective wellbeing of the family as a unit of society, and are manifest in the religious beliefs that guide communities' practices. When illness raises awareness of a person's mortality, the arts come to the fore in individual and collective rituals, and for existential and spiritual exploration. The value of art therapy to place a therapeutic relationship around this universal inclination towards the arts, in order to safely facilitate personal and collective sense-making, is clearly represented in the diverse cultural practices described in this book.

### Art Therapists Contribute to Staff Education and Support

Frequently there is only one art therapist within an organisation, often working on a part-time or sessional basis. As a consequence, art therapists face challenges of professional isolation and misunderstanding from colleagues about what they do. The art therapist will often have to deliver an ongoing programme of staff education to ensure colleagues understand the psychosocial as well as creative aspects of art therapy's contribution to care. Art therapists also use their therapeutic skills to supervise colleagues and facilitate staff support groups.

### Innovations and Research

Research plays an important part in enhancing our understanding of what works well for patients and their families, and in developing interventions to better address their needs. Being a young profession, art therapy research is still emerging. Nonetheless, research is a core theme in this book, with seven contributors explicitly presenting their research findings, and several others writing about how their research is informing their clinical practice. In her Snapshot of Practice (16), Dr Kaimal, in Philadelphia USA, offers insight into her outcomes research for caregivers of patients at the end of their lives, while Hilary Rapp's Snapshot (32) describes a pilot study into the effects of art therapy on anxiety and cancer-related fatigue in palliative patients in Singapore. Dr Carr's research (Chapter 9) has led to the development of a new intervention—portrait therapy—and she gives insights into how this has benefits pre- and post-bereavement. The importance of art therapy support for caregivers of relatives with dementia has been researched by a team of art therapists in Israel (Honig et al, Chapter 15) and suggests new interventions for this client group.

### Legacy

Understanding the importance of confidentiality is central to art therapists' ethical practise, and applies not only to what is spoken in therapy sessions but also to the artwork made. Discussions about who can view artwork and in which circumstances will be undertaken and documented. The issue of legacy is relevant here; deciding on who should have the patient's artwork after their death, and whether it can be used for the education of staff, is an important part of the art therapist's work. In this book consent from the artists/patients to include their art has been received. In several cases patients have wanted their *real* names to be mentioned. This connects with a deeply human desire not to be forgotten, and a wish to bequeath something of benefit to others.

## Overview of the Book

Recognising the ways in which terminal illnesses, death and bereavement influence all aspects of life, we have arranged the chapters in three sections: Art Therapy with Individuals; Art Therapy with Groups, Families and Communities; and Art Therapy for Cross-Cultural Encounters, National Tragedies and Disenfranchised Grief. These reflect the holistic focus of palliative care, where the needs of the individual patient, their family and their wider community are all considered. Within each section we have included short personal accounts to further illuminate the diversity of skills that art therapists bring to end of life and bereavement care. These eight 'Snapshots of Practice'—from Puerto Rico, United Arab Emirates, Singapore, England, Italy and the USA—demonstrate: Art therapists' engagement with the challenge of conducting research with palliative patients and their families; cross-cultural perceptions of artmaking, and how art media can promote embodied and existential experiences that are life enhancing for both children and adults. These snapshots provide insights into the motivations of art therapists working in this field and demonstrate how in the hands of a sensitive practitioner with or without years of experience, art therapy can transcend barriers of language, age and even blindness. For those new to art therapy in palliative care, reading these short contributions may be a good way to get started.

## References

Agnese, A., Lamparelli, T., Bacigalupo, A. & Luzzatto, P. (2012) Supportive care with art therapy, for patients in isolation during stem cell transplant. *Palliative & Supportive Care.* 10 pp. 91–98.

Belfiore, M. (1994) The group takes care of itself: Art therapy to prevent burnout. *The Arts in Psychotherapy.* 21(2) pp. 119–126.

Buday, K.M. (2013) Engage, empower, and enlighten: Art therapy and image making in hospice care. *Progress in Palliative Care.* 21(2) pp. 83–88. DOI: 10.1179/1743291X13Y.0000000050

Bull, S. & O'Farrell, K. (2012) *Art Therapy and Learning Disabilities.* London: Routledge.

Callaway, M.V., Connor, S.R. & Foley, K.M. (2018) World health organization public health model: A roadmap for palliative care development. *Journal of Pain and Symptom Management.* 55(2) pp. S13. DOI: 10.1016/j.jpainsymman.2017.03.030

Carr, S.M.D. (2014) Revisioning self-identity: The role of portraits, neuroscience and the art therapist's 'third hand'. *International Journal of Art Therapy.* 19(2) pp. 54–70. DOI: 10.1080/17454832.2014.906476

Collette, N. (2011) Arteterapia y cáncer. *Psicooncología.* 8(1). DOI: 10.5209/rev_PSIC.2011.v8.n1.7

Connell, C. (1998) *Something Understood: Art Therapy in Cancer Care.* London: Wrexham Publications.

Connor, S. & Bermedo, M.C.S. (2014) *Global Atlas of Palliative Care at the End of Life.* London: Worldwide Palliative Care Alliance.

Forzoni, S., Perez, M., Martignetti, A. & Crispino, S. (2010) Art therapy with cancer patients during chemotherapy sessions: An analysis of the patients' perception of helpfulness. *Palliative and Supportive Care.* 8(1) pp. 41–48.

Furman, L.R. (2011) Last breath: Art therapy with a lung cancer patient facing imminent death. *Art Therapy.* 28(4) pp. 177–180. DOI: 10.1080/07421656.2011.622690

Gilroy, A., Tipple, R. & Brown, C. (2012) *Assessment in Art Therapy.* London: Routledge.

Gussak, D.E. & Rosal, M.L. (2016) *The Wiley Handbook of Art Therapy.* Oxford: Wiley-Blackwell.

Hardy, D. (2001) Creating through loss: An examination of how art therapists sustain their practice in palliative care. *Inscape.* 6(1) pp. 23–31.

Hardy, D.C. (2013) Working with loss: An examination of how language can be used to address the issue of loss in art therapy. *International Journal of Art Therapy.* 18(1) pp. 29–37. DOI: 10.1080/17454832.2012.707665

Hartley, N. (2013) *End of Life Care: A Guide for Therapists, Artists and Arts Therapists.* London and Philadelphia: Jessica Kingsley Publishers.

Hartley, N. & Payne, M. (eds.) (2008) *Creative Arts in Palliative Care.* London: Jessica Kingsley Publishers.

Higginson, I.J. (2015) Palliative care delivery models. In: Cherny, N., Fallon, M., Kaasa, S., Portenoy, R.K. & Currow, D.C. (eds.) *Oxford Textbook of Palliative Medicine.* Oxford: Oxford University Press. pp. 112–116.

Hill, A. (1948) *Art Versus Illness: A Story of Art Therapy.* London: G. Allen and Unwin.

Hogan, S. (2000) *Healing Arts: The History of Art Therapy.* London: Jessica Kingsley.

Holland, C., Hocking, A., Joubert, L., McDermott, F., Niski, M., Thomson Salo, F. and Quinn, M. (2018) My kite will fly: Improving communication and understanding in young children when a mother is diagnosed with life-threatening gynecological cancer. *Journal of Palliative Medicine.* 21(1) pp. 78–84.

Holmes, J. (1993) *John Bowlby and Attachment Theory.* London and New York: Routledge.

Huet, V. (2017) Case study of an art therapy-based group for work-related stress with hospice staff. *International Journal of Art Therapy.* 22(1) pp. 22–34. DOI: 10.1080/17454832.2016.1260039

Jones, G. (2007) Complementary and psychological therapies in a rural hospital setting. *International Journal of Palliative Nursing.* 13(4) pp. 184–189.

Kubler-Ross, E. (1969) *On Death and Dying: What the Dying Have to Teach Doctors, Nurses, Clergy and Their Own Families.* New York: Scribner.

Lee, S.Y., Duck-In, J., Kyung-Joon, M., Hye-Jin, L. & Kwang-heun, L. (2016) Beneficial effect of mindfulness based art therapy in patients with breast cancer—A randomized controlled trial. *European Psychiatry.* 33 pp. S391. DOI: 10.1016/j.eurpsy.2016.01.1409

Lefèvre, C., Ledoux, M. & Filbet, M. (2016) Art therapy among palliative cancer patients: Aesthetic dimensions and impacts on symptoms. *Palliative & Supportive Care.* 14(4) pp. 376–380. DOI: 10.1017/S1478951515001017

Liebmann, M. & Weston, S. (eds.) (2015) *Art Therapy with Physical Conditions.* London: Jessica Kingsley Publishers.

Lin, M.H., Moh, S.L., Kuo, Y.C., Wu, P.Y., Lin, C.L., Tsai, M.H., Chen, T.J. & Hwang, S.J. (2012) Art therapy for terminal cancer patients in a hospice palliative care unit in Taiwan. *Palliative & Supportive Care.* 10(1) pp. 51–57. DOI: 10.1017/S1478951511000587

MacWilliam, B. (ed.) (2017) *Complicated Grief, Attachment and Art Therapy.* London and Philadelphia: Jessica Kingsley Publishers.

Magniant, R. (2004) *Art Therapy with Older Adults: A Sourcebook.* Illinois: Charles C. Thomas.

Malchiodi, C.A. (ed.) (2013) *Art Therapy and Health Care.* New York NY: The Guilford Press.

Meghani, S., Peterson, C., Kaiser, D., Rhodes, J., Rao, H., Chittams, J. and Chatterjee, A. (2018) A pilot study of a mindfulness-based art therapy intervention in outpatients with cancer. *American Journal of Hospice and Palliative Medicine®.* 35(9) pp. 1195–1200.

National Palliative and End of Life Care Partnership (2015) *Ambitions for Palliative and End of Life Care: A National Framework for Local Action 2015–2020.* Available at http://endoflifecareambitions. org.uk (Accessed 30/11/2016).

Payne, S. & Lynch, T. (2015) International progress in creating palliative medicine as a specialized discipline and the development of palliative care. In: Cherny, N., Fallon, M., Kaasa, S., Portenoy, R. & Currow, D. (eds.) *Oxford Textbook of Palliative Medicine.* Oxford: Oxford University Press. pp. 1254.

Potash, J.S., Chan, F., Ho, A.H.Y., Wang, X.L. & Cheng, C. (2015) A model for art therapy-based supervision for end-of-life care workers in Hong Kong. *Death Studies.* 39(1) pp. 44–51. DOI: 10.1080/07481187.2013.859187

Pratt, M. & Wood, M.J.M. (eds.) (1998) *Art Therapy in Palliative Care: The Creative Response.* London: Routledge.

Rubin, J. (2010) *Introduction to Art Therapy.* New York and East Sussex: Routledge.

Safrai, M.B. (2013) Art therapy in hospice: A catalyst for insight and healing. *Art Therapy.* 30(3) pp. 122–129. DOI: 10.1080/07421656.2013.819283

Saunders, C. & Baines, M. (1989) *Living with Dying*. (2nd ed.) Oxford: Oxford University Press.

Steffen, E.M. & Klass, D. (eds.) (2017) *Continuing Bonds in Bereavement*. Milton: Routledge.

Stroebe, M. & Schut, H. (2010) The dual process model of coping with bereavement: A decade on. *OMEGA—Journal of Death and Dying*. 61(4) pp. 273–289. DOI: 10.2190/OM.61.4.b

Thompson, B. & Neimeyer, R. (2014) *Grief and the Expressive Arts*. London: Routledge.

Tjasink, M. (2010) Art psychotherapy in medical oncology: A search for meaning. *International Journal of Art Therapy: Formerly Inscape*. 15(2) pp. 75–83.

Tjasink, M. & Soosaipillai, G. (2018) Art therapy to reduce burnout in oncology and palliative care doctors: A pilot study. *International Journal of Art Therapy*. pp. 1–9. DOI: 10.1080/17454832.2018.1490327

Vianna, D., Claro, L.L., Mendes, A.A., da Silva, A.N., Bucci, D.A., de Sá, P.T., Rocha, V.S., Pincer, J.S., de Barros, I.M.F. & Silva, P.R. (2013) Infusion of life: Patient perceptions of expressive therapy during chemotherapy sessions. *European Journal of Cancer Care*. 22(3) pp. 377–388. DOI: 10.1111/ecc.12041

Waller, D. & Sibbett, C. (eds.) (2005) *Art Therapy and Cancer Care*. Maidenhead, England and New York: Open University Press.

Weiskittle, R.E. & Gramling, S.E. (2018) The therapeutic effectiveness of using visual art modalities with the bereaved: A systematic review. *Psychology Research and Behavior Management*. 11 pp. 9–24. DOI: 10.2147/PRBM.S131993

WHO World Health Organisation Resource (2018a) *WHA67.19 — Strengthening of Palliative Care as a Component of Comprehensive Care Throughout the Life Course: WHA Resolution; Sixty-seventh World Health Assembly, 2014*. Available at http://apps.who.int/medicinedocs/en/m/abstract/Js21454ar (Accessed 19/12/2018).

WHO World Health Organisation (2018b) *Palliative Care: Key Facts*. Available at www.who.int/en/news-room/fact-sheets/detail/palliative-care (Accessed 16/12/2018).

Wood, M.J.M., Low, J., Molassiotis, A. & Tookman, A. (2013) Art therapy's contribution to the psychological care of adults with cancer: A survey of therapists and service users in the UK. *International Journal of Art Therapy*. 18(2) pp. 42–53. DOI: 10.1080/17454832.2013.781657

Worden, J.W. (2010) *Grief Counselling and Grief Therapy*. (4th ed.) London: Routledge.

Zhou, C., Crawford, A., Serhal, E., Kurdyak, P. & Sockalingam, S. (2016) The impact of project ECHO on participant and patient outcomes: A systematic review. *Academic Medicine*. 91(10).

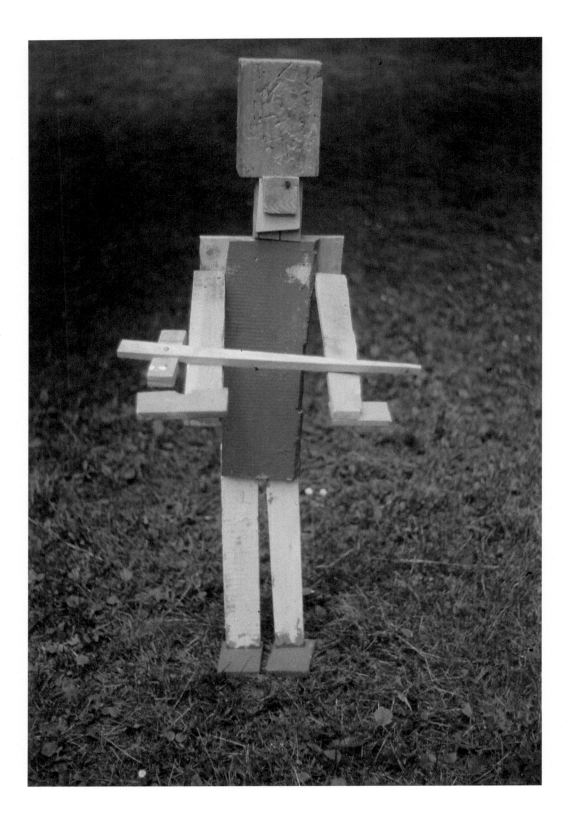

# Section One

# Art Therapy With Individuals

Individual sessions with an art therapist can be a valuable way to mobilize innate creativity and safely explore experiences of living with terminal illness, physical deterioration and grief. The chapters and snapshots of practice presented in this section are drawn from Singapore, the Russian Federation, Germany, Spain, Italy, England and the USA. They demonstrate the benefits of art therapy with individual adults and children in a variety of settings: patients' own homes, inpatient hospice and hospital wards, and community centres.

The uptake of art therapy by individuals depends on many factors, and several contributors discuss this; from the way it is introduced by the therapist (Ní Argáinin Chapter 5); the professional and cultural support of the context of care (Parker-Bell and colleagues, Chapter 7) and the tools and techniques used. In relation to the latter, Bucciarelli (Chapter 10) and Wood (Chapter 11) present the strengths and limitations of using digital technology in art therapy, highlighting the willingness of art therapists to innovate within their practice in order to increase accessibility and uptake. Throughout this section, and indeed throughout the book, there is a theme of the art therapist's research informing and changing practice. Susan Carr's (chapter 9) is one example. She shows the delicate attuning and mirroring within the therapeutic relationship of her innovative practice of portrait therapy; a collaborative process where patients co-design the art piece and the art therapist is the art-maker.

Ensuring accessibility of art therapy experiences continues to be explored in contributions from Germany and the UK. Uwe Herrmann's (chapter 4) focuses on his work with children diagnosed with a terminal neurodegenerative illness—Juvenile Batten Disease. This childhood disease leads to blindness, physical, mental and communicative deterioration and death often occurs in late adolescence or early adulthood. Despite their impaired vision, Herrmann finds that art therapy helps reduce anxiety in his young clients by providing a vehicle to explore concepts of death and dying, leading to an improved sense of self. In Snapshot 3, Lucy Pyart's work in an English hospice with an older woman losing her sight connects with Herrmann's work. With the increased potential for communication to be seriously impaired for these clients, the importance of the work that takes place within art therapy becomes even more apparent; giving form and voice to fears, painful experiences, hopes and dreams, and building a trusting therapeutic alliance.

Two moving accounts of the unspeakable grief that accompanies the death of a newborn baby are also presented here. Tripp (Chapter 8) describes using a trauma-sensitive experiential therapeutic approach with a client who moved from group to individual therapy in order to process unresolved grief for a stillborn child and the process of in vitro fertilization (IVF) treatment. The use of artwork to process her own experience of infant mortality is presented by Russian art therapist Anastasia Stipek (Chapter 7b).

Work within a multi-disciplinary context, with awareness of the intersectional concept of Total Pain, is also prevalent throughout this section. Nadia Collette (Chapter 1) writes of her work in a palliative care unit of a university hospital in Spain. She illustrates how, through the creative process, a person can make meaning of their life's story and be helped to face their own mortality. Collette argues that this increases spiritual connection and decreases suffering. Simon Bell also focuses on the concept of meaning-making and spirituality in art therapy. Using his doctoral research, Bell describes how psychotherapy and spirituality have evolved together within western cultures, highlighting the purposefulness of including spiritual exploration within psychotherapy, and art therapy in particular.

Thus, Section One gives readers a broad understanding of the conceptual underpinnings of the array of interventions used in art therapy. By examining the diverse ways in which art therapy can help individuals contemplate existential and spiritual aspects of their experiences, these chapters also provide international perspectives on grief and loss.

# 1    Deepening the Inner World

## When Art Therapy Meets Spiritual Needs

*Nadia Collette*

## Introduction

Vasili Kandinsky, in *Concerning the Spiritual in Art*, wrote, "Colour is the key. The eye the hammer. The soul is the piano with many strings. The artist is the hand that, by this or that key, makes the human soul vibrate properly" (Kandinsky, 1992). Art in its various forms is a gift of biological selection, which helps humans to better endure suffering. It is not a musician nor a painter nor a writer nor an art therapist who makes this statement but the neuroscientist Antonio Damasio, known for his experimental work and dissemination of writings on the consciousness of self (Damasio, 2010). Thus, the artistic creation's mechanisms of action and the symbolic function, complex and still poorly deciphered, are actively involved in maintaining our homeostasis, along with many other physiological functions. Damasio reminds us that they prevailed in biological evolution for their survival value (being deeply rooted in the human body), while contributing to the development of the welfare concept, "elevating humans to high peaks of thought and sensitivity," becoming something like a "biological counterpart of a spiritual dimension in human affairs" (p. 442). The neuroscientist concludes that the arts have endured thanks to their therapeutic value, as a compensation or counterweight against human calamities and suffering.

This vision invites us more than ever to consider the use of the arts in clinical interventions, particularly at the end of life. Meaning-centered group psychotherapy, designed and evaluated by Breitbart et al (2004, 2010) proposes an approach to creativity and art, between various elements such as nature, humour, or memories, as experiential sources of meaning and therefore likely to bring relief to existential or spiritual suffering.

It is important to differentiate between contact with art and accompanying someone in an art therapy process (Wood, 2015). The first one is available to anyone at anytime or accessible through directed creative arts activities. The second one allows personal insight and growth within a safe and contained setting guaranteed by the professional discipline with several requirements (Bradt & Goodill, 2013): a professionally trained art therapist who undertakes supervision of the practice; a systematic psychotherapeutic process; and a personalized treatment that involves a wide range of artistic experiences aimed at therapeutic solutions identified for each patient individually.

## Spirituality in Palliative Care

The spiritual dimension of people suffering is a pending issue for Western medicine and is even so for professionals working in palliative care. This includes questions about the meaning of one's own life, the way of being able to keep one's hope alive and of how to deal with death. The spiritual dimension also conditions us as human beings, whether we are religious or not. It expresses itself in three interrelated axes: 1) The relationship with oneself on an intrapersonal level: feeling integrity and finding meaning in existence. 2) The relationship with others on an interpersonal level: being recognized as a person and respected within dignity, loving and being loved, being in harmony with present and past relationships; and 3) the relationship with the collective unconscious or transpersonal level: the possibility of living on through the works we leave behind, being remembered and leaving a legacy, putting trust and hope in God, another higher being, the cosmos, nature, history, etc. (Mount et al, 2007; Benito et al, 2014).

"Our patients come to us complaining, not of their condition, but the subjective experience of their illness," recalls Balfour Mount (2003), the Canadian physician considered the father of Palliative Care in North America and pioneer in end of life spirituality. He explains that quality of life and feeling healthy are not necessarily interconnected with a sense of physical well-being. A person may suffer greatly in the absence of somatic symptoms; conversely severe physical impairment, including the presence of pain, can occur without anxiety or suffering. Suffering is therefore a personal and unique life experience (Cassell, 1982) and it is possible to live and die being healed.

## Art Therapy and Spiritual Care

The range of possibilities to explore in art therapy is immense, through the language of visual arts and its structures and contexts, which are alternative or complementary to words. The person is moved emotionally and physically, given the implication of perception and motor skills through the use of art materials, and this allows the patient to release an unusual type of energy. The nature of the creative experience, with gestures, colours, shapes and textures, universally fits all religious beliefs and existential convictions. Along with the essential interaction of "spirit to spirit" with the therapist, the sick person can draw parallels between what they experience during the creative process and the personal situation in which he is immersed (Wood, 1998). It requires the participation of the healthy core of the patient, which the disease is unable to reach. This enables them to face what is hurting or is making them suffer existentially.

Feelings, emotions and thoughts metaphorically represented in artworks create a bridge between body and mind (Lusebrink, 1990; Urbani Hiltebrand, 1999). It reflects a complex inner world covering the most diverse life experiences accumulated in a biography: living with joy and laughter, falling in love, feeling compassion and seeking justice, but also knowing what it is to be sick and vulnerable, what loss and hurt feelings are (Hartley, 2012). Each person can explore common and, at the same time, unique experiences through his artwork, looking for their meaning and particular value. The artwork becomes a symbolic mirror in which one can look, interpret and possibly transform oneself (Klein et al, 2008).

In his theoretical work of 1911, "Concerning the Spiritual in Art," the Russian painter Vasili Kandinsky (1992) reflects on the chromatic richness of a picture: "Colour harmony must rest only on a corresponding vibration in the human soul. This is one of the guiding principles of the inner need" (p. 59). In clinical art therapy it is striking to observe how patients, regardless of their technical skills, are the protagonists of their own artistic action and make creative decisions steered by inner guides who "tell them" to opt for a certain shape and a certain colour. It is a search for beauty, even without necessarily responding to what conventions or personal judgements consider to be beautiful. According to Kandinsky, beauty is what springs from the inner psychic need and enriches the soul in an intangible way. In painting, every colour is beautiful, as it causes a mental vibration and every vibration enriches the soul. He concludes that whatever is outwardly "ugly" may be inwardly beautiful, both in art and in life.

In the 1970s, the sculptor and performer Joseph Beuys defended the social dimension of visual arts in his "expanded concept of art" (Bodenmann-Ritter, 1995), according to which every man is an artist, starting with the fact that we are creators of our own life journey, which is potentially our best work. Art therapy is precisely based on this premise and results from current neuroscientific research seem to be gradually confirming these ideas.

The structuralist perspective of art therapy (Gontier-Asvisio, 2011) aims to strengthen the personal development of the person, in any stage of life. In her book *Matters of life and death. Key writings,* Dr Iona Heath (2008) recalls: "Dying is an integral part of living and part of the story of a life. It is the last chance to find meaning and to make coherent sense of what has gone before" (p. 46). This perspective sees the subject as a complex and unique structure to be addressed, taking in all its component parts and their reciprocal influences (the opposite of the fragmentation typical in healthcare). This encompasses the body, intellect, feelings, emotions, spirit and social dimension. All of them are mobilized, to a greater or lesser degree, by the action of creating, regardless of innate ability or acquired skill. Iona Heath considers that finding meaning in a life story is an act of creation. So art therapy complements and enhances palliative care, bringing back an ancient concept, holistic care. As medicine has become more dependent on technology, this important approach has been overshadowed. However, it is perfectly compatible with the most cutting-edge scientific advances and it is essential for the respect, harmony and integrity of the individual. When a holistic approach is absent, it can become difficult or almost impossible to find deep meaning in the story of a life.

## The Creative Process and the Inner Self Model

From the beginning of psychoanalysis, Freud (1987) expressed great interest in the inner workings of the artistic function. This interest was continued by the great psychoanalytical thinkers Carl Gustav Jung (1995), Melanie Klein (1978), Donald Winnicott (2002) and Jacques Lacan (1988). In addition, humanistic psychology, particularly phenomenology (Husserl, 1992) and gestalt (Perls, 1974), has emphasized techniques for accompanying the person or group based on somatic, emotional or artistic creative experience, which is lived as a whole experience in the here and now (Hamel & Labrèche, 2010).

Adding to these contributions, art theorists (Ehrenzweig, 1973; Fiorini, 1995) suggest that during the different phases of the creative process, the psyche of the artist goes through several states, which can be seen as related to the beneficial effect observed in art therapy (Paín & Jarreau, 1995). The first stage is the exploration phase: it begins in the world of what is already known (materials) and already established (ideas) to penetrate into an unknown world of creative chaos. The transformation phase follows (from chaos birth new forms), then the culmination phase (when the search is ending) and finally the separation phase (which is necessary to continue to another creative destiny). Once the artwork has been produced, it is self-supporting and the person who made it can move away. In this way, the creative process also involves the process of grief (López Fernández Cao & Martínez Díez, 2006), a facet that becomes particularly important at the end of life in which the experience of saying farewell, to oneself and others, is one of the main tasks of the person who understands and accepts the imminence of death (Byock, 2002).

In their model of "care of the soul" (Kearney & Weininger, 2012), grounded on Jungian psychological concepts and Buddhist philosophy, the physician Michael Kearney and the psychologist Radhule Weininger explore the relationship between fear of death and suffering. They suggest art therapy as an excellent approach for bringing awareness to the soul. Both authors create a metaphorical analogy between the soul and a wave of the sea. The crest of the wave (a very small part in relation to its whole size) represents the ego, which is conscious of but also afraid of death. The rest of the wave, down to the deepest ocean current, represents the unconscious, the part of our psyche that is not frightened of death. The wave is alone at its surface, but deeply connected at its base. For the ego "looking" from the top of the ridge, the feeling of vertigo is huge. Everything the ego sees and imagines in the depths represents a threat that causes terror: all that is unknown, different, alien, dark, associated with death. As a last, yet ephemeral refuge, it retreats in the known, rational, material, literal and controlled domain, distancing and disconnecting itself from the healing potential of the deep. The inflexibility of this anxious and terrified ego is the origin of "Total Pain," a term that expresses the maximum suffering: with the dissociation between body and soul, physical symptoms trigger feelings of alienation, isolation and meaninglessness.

If we parallel this model and the phases of the artistic creative process, we see rational understanding of the situation as the beginning of the exploration phase. This state of knowing provides temporary relief for the ego. It then passes into a deeper state where the unconscious rearranges the creative chaos into new forms (Zurbano Camino, 2007). It is during this second phase when the possibility exists for the individual artist to experience a state that resembles the "oceanic feeling." This is described as an experience where one feels a sense of belonging to a much larger whole, in a mystical union with the universe. Both the religious and non-religious may experience this. It gives a feeling of eternity and ultimate security even when faced with danger; it is the certainty that one cannot maintain himself separate from the rest of the world (Comte-Sponville, 2006). Freud (1990) also saw art as having this impact on people, and also as a powerful means of getting away from the sufferings of life.

These are complex and still little-understood homeostatic (Damasio, 2010) mental and physical mechanisms. They are informed by brain circuits that control the development of incentives (through hormones and neuromodulators) and lead us to better understand how art therapy at the end of life is able to activate the deep unconscious. It positions the participant as part of his own creation, emerging from the depths where fear seems to fade before the greater dimensions of the universe. If the patient gives of himself enough in the process of making his artwork, he will receive this "calming touch" (Kearney & Weininger, 2012) from his inner world. This can be seen as something like a harmonizing encounter with his own essence. Then he will be able to make sense of it, turning it into a meaningful experience.

However, Kearney and Weininger warn against the superficial use of this type of therapeutic approach. Its success depends on the competence of the therapist or the approach may not reach the soul. Thus, in order to direct the therapeutic work towards the depths, it is not only an ethical duty for professionals to be specifically trained in their discipline, but also to be very familiar with introspection and be aware of their quality of own presence. If not, the authors say, these approaches will be unsound, being simple ego boosting techniques, masquerading as complementary or integrative therapies.

## In Search of Something Essential: Fragments of Art Therapy Processes

The art therapy intervention in the Palliative Care Unit (PCU) of the Hospital Sant Pau in Barcelona, where I work, is based on an "intermodal" or "transdisciplinary" phenomenological model. It integrates elements of poetic writing, work with dreams and memories and the practice of conscious breathing as well as body awareness as an expressive and artistic tool. The therapeutic setting is in the patient's room, with sessions of about one hour, two or three times a week, depending on patient choice.

In our hospital, a tertiary university institution of 644 beds, the only art therapy intervention offered is that of the 10-bed PCU. It has been available since 2004, however not continuously. Until 2012, the running of the program was financed by grants. Since then, it has been externally funded by a private business (Mémora Group, a funeral services firm) and I, as the art therapist, work part-time through the hospital's research institute. Patients who accept to enter the program sign an informed consent agreement and are included in protocoled evaluation studies, authorized by the hospital Ethics Committee for Clinical Research. During the course of the study, although I am not formally part of the fixed PCU health staff, I work alongside them as another member of the interdisciplinary team.

In the following sections, we will hear the experience of art therapy for three people hospitalized in the PCU. Their process is described and analysed in the light of Balfour Mount concepts about healing connections, which can manifest in the intra-, inter- and transpersonal dimensions. Kearney and Weininger's vision about inner depth is also referred to in the analysis. All three are included in a research study (n = 83) which evaluated symptoms and the perception of help in patients and relatives after the art therapy intervention, using the Edmonton Symptom Assessment System (ESAS) and an intern questionnaire. Partial results have been communicated at a Congress of the European Association for Palliative Care (Collette et al, 2014) and the study is currently pending of publication.

## The Intrapersonal

### Victor

Victor is 57 years old and affected by a small cell lung metastatic carcinoma. At our first meeting, he sits in bed and then in the armchair. He spends a lot of time trying to find a position that will not cause too much discomfort. He intends to exercise his hands using art therapy through calligraphy, monitoring his achievements daily and hoping to regain lost feeling in his fingers. He spends the first one-hour session writing repeatedly in large letters "Hospital de Sant Pau" with a red wax crayon, then with a blue one and finally with a pen. Because of his leaning heavily on the paper, his side soon becomes more painful. He welcomes my suggestion to stop a moment, to focus attention on the breath, which gives him some relief quickly, and then he continues.

The start of the second session stretches on due to his irritation to scheduling issues in the hospital. He complains that all of us professionals visit him almost simultaneously, leaving no time to manage his phone calls about professional matters. He feels "stretched between a thousand things" and inspired in his job as a chief executive, offers a solution by asking to establish "quadrants" for visits. However, after a few minutes of being listened to and validated by me, he changes his mind and recognizes that life would actually be quite boring if we functioned in such a calculated way. I suggest to him that he make a squiggle with his eyes closed using his other hand, the one he does not write with. At first he looks worried, he asks questions about how to do it, but accepts and then draws a line quite fluidly with blue crayon. As soon as he opens his eyes, he identifies a figure: "It's me on my motorbike" and immediately highlights it with red crayon. He remembers coming and going to the hospital like this, until very recently. He states: "A whole year of chemotherapy, acting as if nothing had happened." Having defined the meaning in such a way, he finds it difficult to discern other possible forms, but amongst the elements of little interest (a lady's boot, a car, a face stuck in a shoe), he eventually "sees" a lake with a reflection of mountains. He remains absorbed when I ask him about the element that attracts his attention most and resists transforming the current image; he says: "because I would lose it." At the same time, he continues to look for more forms, while he runs his finger tracing the lake. He accepts my invitation to do this with a crayon, to record his instinctive gesture. He does so with the same blue crayon, conjuring up the lake with a more visible trace. Then he places the word "real" in the highlighted part and "reflection" on the part he identified as mountains.

When I move the drawing away to contemplate it with perspective, he notes that the motorbike is in the real and he is in the reflection. He remains very thoughtful and then says "the real is life." He questions himself about why and how these elements have come out. We decide to leave this exploration for another session. Before saying goodbye, he states that he is not interested at all in seeking magical or religious aspects, nor does he believe in "causal approaches." I ask him if what he has done so far given him such feelings or thoughts, and he says no . . . but wants to make it clear he does not want to address "the area of beliefs."

Over the weekend, his pain flares up, "wildly" in his own terms, to the extent that he claims he can locate more easily where it does not hurt than the contrary. He asks for a lot of analgesic medicines. Tuning my words to his state, I say I am sorry to see him like that, "given how well I saw you on your motorbike." He smiles, raises his arms a bit and makes a slight twisting motion with his hands, as if he was driving. Then, he is able to feel motivated to continue with some creative work. The Edmonton Symptom Assessment Scale shows a reduction of 2 points in discomfort just after the session in comparison to just before (5 to 3).

He spends all the next day resting. During my brief visit, when the pain comes, I accompany him, encouraging him to do the same exercise of conscious breathing as in previous sessions and he confirms that it gives him some relief. A day later, his general state declines. He sleeps a lot, but I use a time he is awake to visit him. He invites me to sit on

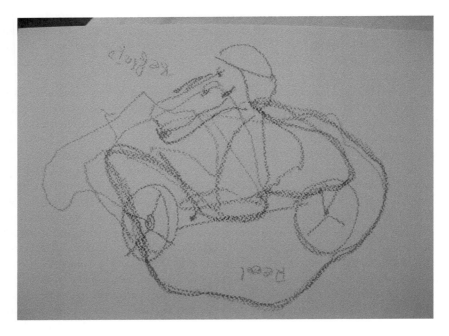

*Figure 1.1* Real and Reflection

the edge of the bed while he wants to make phone calls. In a relatively calm tone of voice, he calls his ex-wife, his sister and two close friends, asking them to come quickly because he is dying.

While waiting to greet them, he asks me if I "knew it." After inquiring into his question (did I know what?), and responding generically, he insisted on wanting a clear answer. I say yes, I knew he was dying. I ask him what allowed him to feel it and when it became clear. "It was because of many things," he answers, and the number of days that he counts corresponds to the day that he made the image of the lake. He continues, hoping I will not be angry for what he wants to say, but he sees in me the "Angel of Death," adding "Have they said it to you many times before?" I have no time to ask whether this is good or bad or how he sees it, or what it brings to him, because his relatives start arriving, and he wants privacy. He thanks me for being there.

Later, his sister tells me that, in a reconciliation gesture, Victor has asked her for forgiveness. In return, she has confirmed her commitment to be at his side. "That is all there is," she says, thanking me for the role I may have had in this. After immersing himself into progressive unconsciousness, Victor dies three days later.

What I understand as essential in this process, with regard to art therapy, is that Victor's interpretation of symbolic elements emerged from his unconscious (or maybe more specifically, his pre-conscious) and enabled him to access a more coherent identity. As in the Kearney and Weininger model, Victor's frightened ego, astride the motorbike (equivalent to being on the crest of the wave) had been dictating a disease-denial type of behaviour to him for a long time. Suddenly, this defensive, self-preserving ego had noticed its reflection in the calm waters of a lake as deep as the reflected high mountains (equivalent to the depths of the unconscious) around it. Although the symptoms took a while to reduce, they did not block the patient's reflection on his own metaphorical image. He became able to see himself in a manner more consistent with his end of life situation than with the dissociation in which he had shut himself away. From this moment, his attitude changed and he made pertinent decisions about relationship issues that were pending within his family.

## The Interpersonal

### César

César is 59 years old and affected by metastatic penile carcinoma. His general state, as observed by the medical team prior to the sessions, presents severe lability and demoralization. In the first two art therapy sessions, he experiences relaxation, excitement from memories of his childhood and reflections about his family in his native village in the Peruvian mountains. These experiences motivate him to write with a red crayon the word "Amor" (love) in one of his images that most represents his deep feeling towards his people and land.

In the third session, César is accompanied by his wife and I suggest they do some watercolour painting together, translating into shape and colour the notes and rhythms of a classical music piece I have chosen for him. While listening, César gets emotional and closes his eyes on his tears, while moving his right hand and gently following the rhythm. Then he associates the sounds with light blue and brown colours, which he draws over a paper sheet during a second listening. After completing the artwork, César interprets his mark-making. He wanted to represent another childhood memory: a hammock in blue and a piece of cord in brown, with one end in the hammock and the other in a hand that is moving it gently. He explains with powerful emotion that his mother rocked him like this, giving him peace and security. Tears come to his eyes again and he begins to hum.

Shortly thereafter, I encourage him to give his painting a title and he chooses the word "Union," to evoke the link between two sensations, one of remembering and the other of mourning. In the discussion that follows, his wife notes he "is taking it better" than herself. He expresses that, ultimately, he feels trust, no matter what happens.

In the next session, César explains in more detail how he relates to the last image he created. He begins explaining his traumatic experience from diagnosis to evidence of metastasis, going through exhausting treatments. He was not prepared for all that and found it was something unimaginable. Now, he feels he wants to move to another perception of his situation, accepting that the disease "should be in my body," he says, being unable to do anything to change this reality. He realizes that returning to his past represents for him a protective move towards his roots, doubly lost, by age and especially by emigration. He considers the drawing of the rocking hammock and the cord that connects it to the rocking hand as healing resources. They give him a sense of confidence, resurfacing from the depths of his past life experiences. From now on, he wants to remember this until his end. He wants to enjoy the time that remains for him, until his own body says he has reached the limit. He talks with a lot of emotion; he knows that there can be deep pits of sadness on the way. But he feels more prepared, looking for tranquillity in the rocking gesture that connects him with his mother's love.

After the experience of painting with his wife and finding these healing connections, he wants to do the same with his 18-year-old son, because he feels that these experiences are preparing them all to cope. I suggest an imaginary journey to a tree, their own tree as a metaphorical self-portrait, a visualization followed by the creative process. The teenager portrays himself as a central pine tree in the middle of a forest full of other pine trees. His father interprets the image as a signal that he can go quietly, because he believes that his son "will not be alone, connected with loved ones around." César has painted a walnut tree, another memory of his childhood in Peru, as well as "granadilla,"

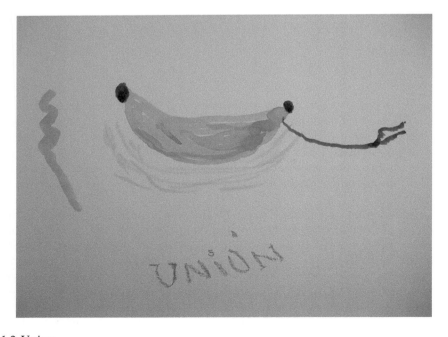

*Figure 1.2* Union

small red fruits that the tree bears. Its colour makes him think about the red bird, which was how he had represented himself in a drawing during the first session, flying nearby a ship, in search of new horizons. He explains that the horizon is now to go back to his childhood walnut tree, because just as it bears fruit, it also gives him the strength he needs to move forward.

In César's network of relationships, it is through the interpersonal ones, both past and present, that the patient is able to find more resources to address his suffering during his terminal process. He reconnects with the deep feelings of giving love and of being loved.

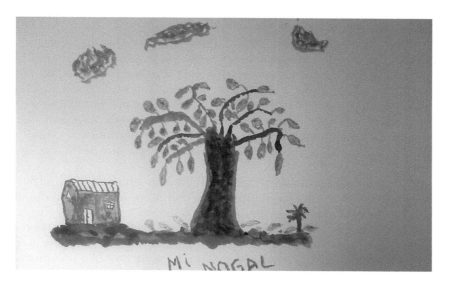

*Figure 1.3* A Walnut Tree

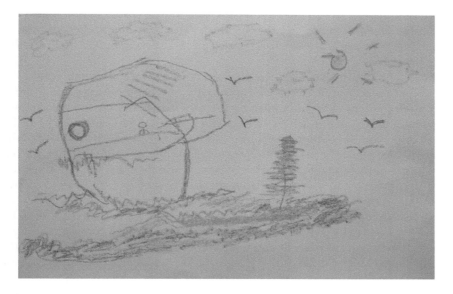

*Figure 1.4* New Horizons

## The Transpersonal

### Araceli

All her life, Araceli, the daughter of a talented painter, felt she had no right to practice art, believing she lacked the necessary technical and academic skills. Now, at 57, affected by a metastatic lung adenocarcinoma and diagnosed with depression and high anxiety, she shows me a notebook filled with minuscule figures that she had drafted in a very light pencil stroke. She mocks them, calling them "nonsense" and "clutter without importance." She picks out a drawing of a girl, who she describes as sitting on the bottom of a well, waiting. "Just like me," she says and begins to cry. Exploring what this girl awaits, she answers: "to rise again."

She is intrigued by the materials she sees in the art therapy case. She shows me a photographic article in one of her travel magazines: remarkable beings, in costumes and masks from remote villages around the world. Handmade with natural materials, all of them refer to death. The article explains that at a certain festive time of year, some chosen people carry them to bring good luck to the rest of the inhabitants of the village. Araceli insistently shows me the most disturbing elements: saw shaped teeth, long and sharp noses, claw-like fingernails and a huge ruminant skull. Then, she continues to explore the contents of the case, announcing that she will cut out images for our next meeting, but that now she needs rest.

In the next session, she shows me many small cuttings organized into three lots and stored between the pages of her notebook. I note that there is no trace of the unsettling photos from our previous meeting. She has even done some mini-collage with tiny pictures of cosy blankets ("to provide heat,") cats napping (because she adores them) and Buddha heads glued to saffron coloured paper pieces (because they give her peace.) From one of the piles of "nice things," she shows me the picture of a bouquet of flowers she thinks is very special, because its roses are already extremely wilted. "Tomorrow they will be dead," she claims. "And today?" I ask her. She pauses a moment and says: "They are full and plentiful."

When I invite her to focus on one of the many creative pathways she has been exploring during our sessions, she decides to explore the story of the costumes and masks from the travel magazine. She puts aside her work on the lovely environments because she says she can do that later by herself. She seems to prefer my company in order to go into the more disturbing images.

As she starts cutting, she has a serious expression on her face, as though she is shocked, eyes wide. Slowly, a half smile settles on her mouth. She begins a story about the characters she has selected: an Old Witch pushing the others to leave, three somewhat younger beings that have to go "no one knows where," and a Shaman, who is waiting to greet them. She identifies herself with one of the three ramblers, because with his flowery shawl he looks feminine. I suggest she take something else from her piles of clippings. She chooses a picture of a rag mouse, next to a bouquet of flowers and includes it in the previous scene, as an intruder. Ending the session, she says she is very glad with the new created image and gives voice to the mouse: "What are they doing all of them so slowly? Faster, enough dawdling!" I encourage her to summarize the session in one word, she chooses "Delight."

At the next meeting, I suggest taking a break from the collage process, and try switching to paint. When I propose brush and watercolour cardboard, she argues that the pain in her right arm will prevent her from doing what she wants and that, anyway, she is only capable of nonsense. But she trusts me and accepts my proposal of "painting music." As she listens to the music I have chosen, she relaxes and we do some conscious breathing exercises. When the notes finish, she continues humming the melody, giving it the title

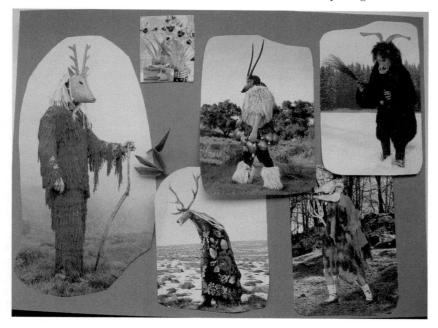

*Figure 1.5* The Witch, the Ramblers and the Shaman

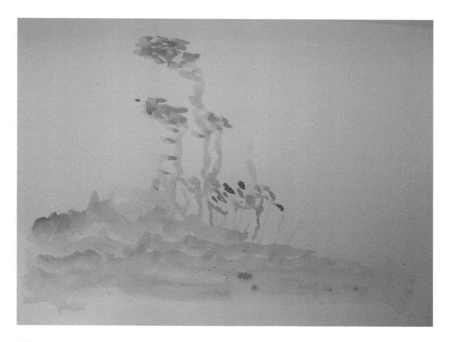

*Figure 1.6* The Dying Swan

"The Dying Swan." She associates the music with the colours "of a sunset; bluish, greenish and purple." She chooses pale turquoise and light violet watercolours. Then while listening to the music for a second time, in a very concentrated manner, she moves the brush on paper, following along with the rhythm of the musical notes.

I interrupt a moment to ask permission to take a picture with my mobile camera (one of the resources I usually use in art therapy) because I am struck by her expression. Later, when she looks at her digital portrait, the first thing she sees is her smile. While trying to explain what she felt during this moment of creation, and looking for words she cannot seem to find, I ask her to look at the gesture of her arms and hands. Only then she says "opening," "enlarged" and "expanded."

As a result of close interdisciplinary teamwork her symptoms abate and her discharge is arranged. We only have a short time to address the symbolic narrative that I invited her to write about her collage. Her story tells how much the three rambling creatures, the shaman apprentices will have to walk to respond to the claim of the Great Shaman. He is dressed in red, "magic and power in action, guardian of Far Valley" say her notes. The ramblers are urged to begin their journey by the Old Witch who calls them together in the Four Winds Wood, "when the sun sets, where the air is more transparent." They listen to the woman's appeals: "Young people, do not be lazy, do not be frightened, fear paralyzes, laziness too. Come on, come on, come on."

As she had previously identified herself with the feminine, rambling creature, can Araceli now also prepare herself to begin her long journey? Beyond the precise meaning of the metaphors present in her story, Araceli, from the depths of her creative unconscious, is appealing to essential elemental forces: to Mother Earth and to an imposing being with magical powers. These symbolize her need for confidence and her hope to belong to something very much greater, forming a whole. "Go without fear or laziness," this Old Witch advises. Is this the courage that the girl in the bottom of the well is hoping to attain in order to climb up again? Araceli, before leaving hospital, responding to our art therapy intervention assessment questionnaire, says yes, it has helped her "to widen the soul, the spirit, to feel more of the marvelous side." These are dimensions of a human being that make one feel capable of passing one's own known limits.

## Conclusions

When we advocate holistic care for a person referred to us in palliative care, we know that it cannot be achieved by drug treatments alone. Neither can it be attained only through words, nor religious rituals alone nor, of course, only with art, although it is the most beautiful and transcendent one (Hartley, 2012). However, it is important to become more aware that art and creativity are human resources with a powerful mobilizing impact on all areas that make up the person. These areas are as different as they are overlapping: body, mind, emotions, spirit (Bailey, 1997). There is a rich casuistic witness of art therapy to relate with evidence-based research into its benefits and with recent psychological theories.

The arts in therapy open up a vast world of alternative languages, accessing unsuspected treasures of inner wisdom. Individual and unique, and at the same time collective and universal, this artistic wisdom includes both ancient myths and modern ones, images, symbols, poetry, music. . . . They accompany us and sometimes, without us even noticing, provide us with the tools to help us respond to the great existential questions we humans may ask. Therefore, especially at the end of life and facing the mystery, through art therapy we can experience these profound and valuable virtues.

## Acknowledgements

The author would like to thank Marina, Gladys and Francesc, relatives of the patients Victor, César and Araceli respectively for their permission to include clinical cases and images; Grupo Mémora for funding art therapy intervention in Hospital Sant Pau; Sally Schofield, art therapist and Pamela Ferman, social worker, for their appreciated help with English translation.

## References

Bailey, S. (1997) The arts in spiritual care. *Seminars in Oncology Nursing*, 13 (4): 242–247.

Benito, E., Barbero, J., & Dones, M. (2014) *Espiritualidad en Clínica: Una propuesta de evaluación y acompañamiento spiritual en Cuidados Paliativos*. Monografías SECPAL n°6. Madrid, Sociedad Española de Cuidados Paliativos.

Bodenmann-Ritter, C. (1995) *Joseph Beuys: Cada hombre, un artista*. Madrid, La balsa de la Medusa, Visor, n° 7: 2.

Bradt, J. & Goodill, S. (2013) Creative art therapies defined: Comment on "Effects of creative arts therapies on psychological symptoms and quality of life in patients with cancer". *JAMA Internal Medicine*, 173 (11): 969–970.

Breitbart, W., Gibson, C., Poppito, S., & Berg, A. (2004) Psychotherapeutic interventions at the end of life: A focus on meaning and spirituality. *The Canadian Journal of Psychiatry*, 49: 366–372.

Breitbart, W., Rosenfeld, B., Gibson, C., Pessin, H., Poppito, S., & Nelson, C. (2010) Meaning-centered group psychotherapy for patients with advanced cancer: A pilot randomized controlled trial. *Psycho-Oncology*, 19 (1): 21–28.

Byock, I. (2002) Sens et valeur de la mort: Faits, philosophie et réflexions sur la responsabilité sociale et clinique. *Médecine Palliative*, 1: 103–112.

Cassell, E.J. (1982) The nature of suffering and the goals of medicine. *New England Journal of Medicine*, 306: 639–645.

Collette, N., Güell, E., Prada, M.L., Rufino, M., Ramos, A., & Fariñas, O. (2014) *Art therapy intervention in a palliative care unit of a tertiary hospital: Evaluation of symptoms and help perception in patients and families*. 8th World Research Congress of the European Association for Palliative Care, Lleida, Spain.

Compte-Sponville, A. (2006) *L'Esprit de l'athéisme: Introduction à une spiritualité sans Dieu*. Paris, Albin Michel, Le livre de Poche.

Damasio, A. (2010) *Y el cerebro creó al hombre: ¿Cómo pudo el cerebro generar emociones, sentimientos, ideas y el yo?* Barcelona, Destino, Imago Mundi n° 182.

Ehrenzweig, A. (1973) *El orden oculto del arte*. Barcelona, Labor.

Fiorini, H.J. (1995) *El psiquismo creador*. Buenos Aires, Barcelona, México, Paidós, Colección Psicología profunda.

Freud, S. (1987) *Psicoanálisis del arte*. Madrid, Alianza Editorial.

Freud, S. (1990) *El malestar en la cultura*. Madrid, Alianza Editorial.

Gontier-Asvisio, V. (2011) *La thérapie structuraliste: Art-thérapie et autres applications à visée structuraliste*. Paris, Editions Dangles, Groupe éditorial Piktos.

Hamel, J. & Labrèche, J. (2010) *Découvrir l'art-thérapie: Des mots sur les maux, des couleurs sur les douleurs*. Paris, Larousse.

Hartley, N. (2012) Spirituality and the arts: Discovering what really matters. In: Cobb, M., Puchalski, C., & Rumbold, B. eds. *Oxford textbook of spirituality in healthcare*. Oxford, Oxford University Press, 37: pp. 265–271.

Heath, I. (2008) *Ayudar a morir*. Madrid, Katz Editores.

Husserl, E. (1992) *Invitación a la fenomenología*. Barcelona, Paidós, Pensamiento contemporáneo 21.

Jung, C.G. (1995) *El hombre y sus símbolos*. Barcelona, Paidós.

Kandinsky, V. (1992) *De lo espiritual en el arte*. Barcelona, Labor.

Kearney, M. & Weininger, R. (2012) Care of the soul. In: Cobb, M., Puchalski, C., & Rumbold, B. eds. *Oxford textbook of spirituality in healthcare*. Oxford, Oxford University Press, 38: pp. 273–278.

Klein, J.P., Bassols, M., & Bonet, E., eds. (2008) *Arteterapia: La creación como proceso de transformación*. Barcelona, Octaedro.

Klein, M. (1978) *La importancia de la formación de símbolos en el desarrollo del yo: En: Klein M. Obras completas 2*. Buenos Aires, Paidós-Hormes.

Lacan, J. (1988) *Seminario 7 La ética del psicoanálisis 1959–1960.* Buenos Aires, Paidós.

López Fernández Cao, M. & Martínez Díez, N. (2006) *Arteterapia: Conocimiento interior a través de la expresión artística.* Madrid, Tutor.

Lusebrink, V. (1990) *Imagery and visual expression in therapy.* New York, Plenum Press.

Mount, B.M. (2003) Existential suffering and the determinants of healing. *European Journal of Palliative Care,* 10 (2) Supplement.

Mount, B.M., Boston, P.H., & Cohen, S.R. (2007) Healing connections: On moving from suffering to a sense of well-being. *Journal of Pain and Symptom Management,* 33 (4): 372–388.

Paín, S. & Jarreau, G. (1995) *Una psicoterapia por el arte.* Buenos Aires, Labor.

Perls, F. (1974) *Sueños y existencia: terapia gestáltica.* Buenos Aires, Cuatro Vientos.

Urbani Hiltebrand, E. (1999) Coping with cancer through image manipulation. In: Malchiodi, C.A. ed. *Medical art therapy with adults.* London, Jessica Kingsley Publishers, pp. 113–135.

Winnicott, D.W. (2002) *Realidad y juego.* Barcelona, Gedisa.

Wood, M.J.M. (1998) Art therapy in palliative care. In: Pratt, M. & Wood, M.J.M. eds. *Art therapy in palliative care.* London, Routledge, 3: pp. 26–37.

Wood, M.J.M. (2015) The contribution of art therapy to palliative medicine. In: Cherny, N.I. et al. eds. *Oxford textbook of palliative medicine,* 5th edition. Oxford, Oxford University Press, pp. 210–215.

Zurbano Camino, A. (2007) *El arte como mediador entre el artista y el trauma.* Tesis doctoral. Universidad del País Vasco, Facultad de Bellas Artes, Departamento de Escultura.

# 2 The Spiritual in Art Therapy at the End of Life

*Simon Bell*

There are many contemporary cultural, religious and political challenges to understanding spirituality: knowing when it appears, what it looks like, how it feels and in what ways it makes a difference to the quality of life for those engaged individually and/or collectively, and in what ways it transforms communities and society. I begin this chapter with a discussion about some significant changes in Western culture that have a bearing on how spirituality is considered in relationship to psychotherapy and its theoretical development. I then explore current definitions of spirituality and how practical theology in conjunction with qualitative research (Swinton and Mowat, 2006), with reference to the ethnographic imagination (Willis, 2000), can provide a framework and methodology to understand spirituality.

My PhD research, completed in 2008, utilised an ethnographic approach to explore the meaning-making that took place in art therapy for patients at the end of life in a palliative care setting (Bell, 2008). A retrospective analysis of nine case studies was undertaken, focusing on the art work created as part of art therapy. I make reference to practical theology and reflexivity in addition to my core methodology in order to emphasise how an ethnographic approach can elicit meaning-making and spirituality for people engaged in art therapy at the end of life. The conclusions I draw emphasise how important and significant this is for patients adjusting to the impact of a diagnosis of a terminal illness and adapting to the implications of prognosis. I make the claim that the evidence I provide as a result of the case study analysis using a qualitative ethnographic research methodology demonstrates the unique place of art therapy to facilitate the expression and exploration of spirituality.

Hospice and palliative care services, like everything else, reside within a particular cultural history and more specifically within the culture of health care represented by the National Health Service (NHS) and the charitable sector in the UK. The cultural challenges of living with a life-threatening illness and coping with the dying process and death in an increasingly technologically and economically driven system of health care throws into sharp relief many of the difficulties of meeting spiritual need at the end of life. Pressures on the funding for services have had a huge impact on the delivery of psychological therapies. Hospices in the UK have to prioritise which disciplines they employ based on their priority of need within the regime of specialist palliative care delivery. Since I contributed to a book on art therapy and palliative care in 1998 art therapy, whilst there has not been a significant decline in the prevalence of art therapy as part of hospice services in the UK, there is a continuing challenge to promote its benefits and relevance as part of contemporary palliative care provision. At the time of writing this chapter there is one part-time art therapist working in a hospice and another working for a cancer support charity in my local region, which plays host to at least five hospices.

My research demonstrated that art therapy benefits people at the end of life because it facilitates, along with other psychic needs, the opportunity to explore meaning-making and spirituality. In the sixteen years I worked for my local hospice I witnessed countless occasions when patients described and reflected on spiritual needs in the context of the art therapy I offered. Their experiences reside within a wide range of socio-economic circumstances, cultural and religious contexts and backgrounds. Capturing these experiences through a detailed case study description and analysis in my PhD enabled me to identify the meaning-making that took place as patients visualised their experiences through drawings and paintings. This creative process is intrinsic to understanding how art-making as part of a psychotherapeutic response to life-threatening illness can contribute to a deeper receptivity and responsiveness to spirituality (Bell, 2011).

## Western Culture, Psychotherapy and Spirituality

It is important to understand the cultural context within which spirituality is currently being defined in the UK and in what ways psychotherapy facilitates exploration of this area of need. The debate and growing insights with regard to the contemporary understanding of spirituality is developing apace for those who consider it to be of profound human significance. For some, however, it is quite simply irrelevant and when equated with religion is a cause of consternation in need of repudiation.

Philip Rieff (1922–2006), a sociologist and cultural critic, provides a still-relevant and imaginative discussion about the impact of psychoanalysis on the predominantly Judeo-Christian culture in the West towards the end of the 19th century onwards in his book *The Triumph of the Therapeutic: Uses of Faith after Freud*, published in 1966. He reminds us that Sigmund Freud (1856–1939) was a devout atheist and that the core tenets of Freudian psychoanalysis are culturally anti-religious. Throughout his life Freud was to regard religion as strictly outside the concern of the analytic process as it was reflective of a culture that no longer served any kind of healthy purpose for the individual. According to Rieff, ' . . . the analytic attitude is an alternative to all religious ones' (1966, p. 36). It is a 'form of re-education' and a new paradigm of 'modern pedagogies, reflecting the changing self-conception' of a far more egalitarian culture. '[I]t is the task of psychological man to develop an informed (i.e., healthy) respect for the sovereign and unresolvable basic contradictions that make him the singularly complicated human being he is' (ibid, p. 55).

Culture, according to Rieff, is about those things that bind the individual into 'communal purposes' in which the self can be realised and satisfied (ibid, p. 4). The transformation of Western culture at the time of Freud meant that the old religious symbols of salvation could no longer claim to be therapeutic. Without the opportunity for conversion and the likelihood of deconversion the individual now has to depend entirely on their autonomous, inner capacity to solve the conflicts and dilemmas of life. Rieff regards 'faith [as] an agency that mitigates suffering' and under the dying culture of 'church civilisation' therapies that were once committed to the authority of its religious representatives 'belong to the religious category of cure: that of souls'. Freud replaced faith with the 'power to choose; but, he had no intention of telling [anyone] what to choose. He wanted merely to give man more options than their raw experience of life permitted' (ibid, p. 87). In this sense it is necessary to understand that many people no longer regard themselves as living within a culture in the West that is predominantly religious. However, they may not be entirely clear about the unifying symbol system of the community they now live in. Whilst to be modern is to be entirely autonomous, individually self-actualised and self-determined, it is still virtually impossible to live apart from the spiritual and the religious in the same way that it is impossible for me not to breathe the same air as my neighbour.

Addressing spirituality therefore in the context of any psychotherapeutic endeavour means having to grapple with the current cultural context in which we live, which despite seismic shifts towards secular humanism and scientific positivism, is saturated with spiritual presentiment and religious ferment. Developments in cognitive neuroscience (Talvitie, 2009) and current influential schools of thought such as that of Mentalisation (Bateman and Fonagy, 2012) are also important when considering the concern for the spiritual in mental health and in relationship to many psychological treatment interventions that are primarily cognitive and behavioural in their orientation and that are underpinned by a burgeoning evidence base relating to the functionality of the brain. Bateman and Fonagy (2012, p. 39) advocate a 'deemphasis of deep unconscious interpretations in favour of conscious or near-conscious content'. Metaphysical consideration is again potentially regarded as a marginal concern bracketed off, along with the unconscious, as unquantifiable and not accessible to any kind of scientific scrutiny. Talvitie (2009) challenges the psychoanalytic dualism of mind versus matter and questions the original Freudian topographical and structural concept of the unconscious because of its precarious relationship to contemporary neurological understanding of the functionality of the brain. According to Talvitie, the psychoanalytic view of the unconscious is a matter of 'faith' as 'Freud was a child of romanticism . . . focused on . . . dreams, mystical experiences, mesmerism/ hypnosis, and nature' (ibid, p. 35). In this sense, despite his denial of the religious, Freud is accused of being bound to a pre-modern cultural inheritance from which his concept of the unconscious cannot escape. Talvitie suggests that there is a similarity between a dualistic view of the soul and the psychoanalytic idea of the unconscious: 'both presume a mystical sphere or entity that cannot be taken as the object of scientific study' (ibid, p. 56).

Carl Jung (1875–1961) returned to a concern for the spiritual in psychotherapy equating this with the capacity to create myths within his teleological theory of the unconscious. His departure from the psychoanalytic path towards archetypal psychology was in part due to his re-envisioning of religion as an expression of the myth-making capacity of the creative impulse inherent within all human beings and intrinsic to his view of unconscious processes.

> Jung despised the fundamental "unspirituality" implied by Freud's suspicious treatment of the dynamics of the unconscious. Just there, in the unconscious, are those superior illusions that would compensate mankind for the barren interdicts of Christianity and the almost equally barren interdicts of psychoanalysis . . . Jung thought the deeper sources of illusion were primordial and creative, unconscious though not rationalising, and mainly anti-moral, remissive rather than controlling.
>
> (Rieff, 1966, p. 121)

Jung would only entertain Christianity (along with all orthodox religion) as one amongst an infinite number of myths that human beings create in order to resolve their inner contradictions and to find some binding symbol to affirm their cohesive participation as part of the culture and community they belong to. Jung 'offered a pantheon of psychologised god-forms, from which men could choose their spiritual medicine' (ibid, p. 90). Rieff's analysis of the influence that both Freud and Jung had on the development of the modern concept of the self in Western culture is one that is divided: Freud the atheist and Jung the alchemist-cum-agnostic. Both positions cast a long shadow over psychoanalysis and the development of psychotherapy and all subsequent theory and practice when attempting to address the subject of spirituality. The changed culture in which we now live in the West means that the search for spiritual realisation is not necessarily equated with revelation or salvation. Faith is not equated with religion. Rieff's malady that 'greater freedom to choose does not cure anybody' (ibid, p. 88) reflects the loss incurred by modern culture and subsequently a 'feeling of symbolic impoverishment' (ibid, p. 242). A loss for some that is perhaps worth enduring in order to produce a third way, neither secular nor religious, not yet discovered.

In a recent episode of a BBC radio programme called *Desert Island Discs*, Kirsty Young interviews one of her many castaways, the Turkish writer Elif Shafat (BBC Radio 4, 2017). Shafat suggests that in her own journey she is seeking a new way of assimilating spiritual meaning and purpose. The following is a transcript from part of the broadcast:

**KY:** ' . . . for someone who is intellectually muscular, you are not afraid of mysticism'.

**ES:** ' . . . we live in a very polarised world especially in Turkey . . . you are either religious or you are modern and you should have no interest whatsoever in faith. I always longed for a third path. I carry no religion, however, I am someone who is interested in faith, in the possibility of God. . . . So faith for me is not necessarily a religious thing and for me what is much more interesting is this dance between faith and doubt. I like agnosticism, mysticism, people who are more confused, still searching and the journey is endless'.

**KY:** 'Would you like to be a believer?'

**ES:** 'No I don't want to be a believer'.

**KY:** 'because. . .'

**ES:** 'Just doesn't suit me that there's more certainty there when you're a believer, and also I, I don't feel close to organised religions in the sense that there is, at the end of the day, a distinction between, in all of them, between us versus them and the assumption that somehow ours is closer to the truth than them. That is not close to my heart, that dualistic way of thinking. What I like is individual spiritual journeys and those journeys are plural. Everybody's journey will be different like their fingerprints. So you might be interested in Islamic mysticism, you might end up feeling closer to Jewish mysticism, or you might start in, in one bay and swim to other shores. Everything is possible because those paths are based on that individual's own features and needs'.

Shafat seems to reflect something of the discussion I have introduced by considering the cultural context where there is a more ambiguous, pluralistic perspective with regard to spirituality and an effort to integrate 'faith' into a secular, non-religious spiritual sensibility. Responding to religious conviction, faith and spirituality in psychotherapy requires a deeper awareness of the cultural dilemmas and conflicts currently at work in society and in the world. Competing religious and political positions seem to be increasingly polarised, suppressing spiritual diversity and its means of expression, often through the arts and humanities, the consequence of which is without doubt an impoverishment of human creative meaning-making in the world. The fact that spirituality is a difficult subject to grasp and understand in a culture where religion and metaphysical considerations are being continually challenged should not therefore be proscribed within the language and practice of psychotherapy and instead given due thought and attention as an integral part of the human experience. I am certainly at the time of writing this chapter in the realm of the 'study *for* spirituality' (Watts, 2017), holding a firm conviction that spirituality is real and meaningful and an entirely legitimate and worthy focus in psychotherapy and specifically in art therapy.

## Spirituality in Mental Health and Research

What is spirituality and is there a current useful definition? In order to answer these two questions I will utilise a number of resources that provide a potentially stable and consistent framework that can facilitate the process of illuminating spirituality. Explaining spirituality and the meaning it generates for individuals and communities seems to require some understanding of the context within which it occurs, is experienced and performed. The spiritual becomes visible through ritual, the arts and religious practice and its significance and meaning can be revealed through the discipline of practical theology and qualitative research. In much the same way that the psychoanalytic concept of the unconscious is being contested by current trends in neuroscience, spirituality is being contested by the demands of a scientific evidence base in health care. Spirituality has to be considered in relationship to its cultural context in order to arrive at a more accurate understanding of its meaning and purpose. Hornborg (2011), provides an example of endeavouring to describe spirituality in two contexts, that of neo-liberal commodity capitalism within a secular Swedish society and that of native Canadian Mi'kmaq spirituality. Cultural context here is imperative to understanding the complexity of defining spirituality in relationship to numerous associated variations, variables and influences. Equally, it is important to consider how the theory and practice of psychotherapy is approached in multiple cultural and national contexts in order to get a sense of what level of sensitivity and responsiveness there is towards spirituality by its practitioners.

Swinton (2001) provides some clarity and a way forward when facing the challenge of meeting spiritual needs within the UK. His approach is considered with regard to mental health but is equally relevant and transferable to that of other health and social care needs including palliative and end of life care. Swinton believes that in order 'to develop a therapeutic understanding of spirituality it will be necessary to learn to be comfortable with uncertainty and mystery' (p. 13). This emphasis is entirely right and is important as a counter to the scientific hegemony in Western culture which is always important to acknowledge but, as many accept, it is not the only significant way of interpreting human experience and building an evidence base for particular facts and realities. Swinton defines spirituality as:

> . . . an intra, inter and transpersonal experience that is shaped and directed by the experiences of individuals and of the communities within which they live their lives. It is *intrapersonal* in that it refers to the quest for inner connectivity. . . . It is *interpersonal* in that it relates to the relationships between people and within communities. It is *transpersonal* in so far as it reaches beyond self and others into the transcendent realms of experience that move beyond that which is available at a mundane level.
>
> (p. 20)

He goes on to expand on five central features of spirituality: meaning, value, transcendence, connecting and becoming. However, there are notable variables and changes of emphasis when considering non-religious spiritual needs and spirituality as a religious concept (pp. 25–28).

Cook (2016) provides another useful definition of spirituality used by the Royal College of Psychiatrists and a discussion relating to the use of narrative in psychiatry to develop a better understanding and response to spirituality in mental health.

> [Spirituality is] a distinctive, potentially creative and universal dimension of human experience arising both within the inner subjective awareness of individuals and within communities, social groups and traditions. It may be experienced as a relationship with that which is intimately 'inner' immanent and personal, within the self and others, and/or as relationship with that which is wholly 'other', transcendent and beyond the self. It is experienced as being of fundamental or ultimate importance and is thus concerned with matters of meaning and purpose in life, truth, and values.
>
> (Cook, 2004, pp. 548–549 quoted in Cook, 2016, p. 5)

Cook et al (2016) provide a comprehensive reflection of how the narratives people share about their experience of mental health provide a rich imaginative and creative terrain for understanding and making sense of spirituality. Powell (2016, p. 48) addresses the two predominant positions of the physicalist perspective of classical science and the metaphysical view and appeals for tolerance between the two as both recognise that human experience is more than the sum of its parts. In support of encouraging a 'soulful narrative' Powell (p. 49) suggests that '[s]pirituality has two dimensions: the quest for answers to the ultimate meaning and purpose of life, and the experience of wholeness of being that can bring inner strength and peace'.

Swinton acknowledges the challenges of remaining attuned to spirituality and religion given the historical evidence since Freud of prejudicial and hostile attitudes within medicine, psychiatry, psychology, psychoanalysis and quantitative research paradigms.

> Statistics, averages and universal norms may be useful for certain purposes, but they cannot capture the intricacies and richness of the experience of being human. Reflections on what it means to live as a human being draws us beyond the confines of empiricism and a mechanical view of persons, towards an understanding of human existence that is multifaceted, mysterious and frequently deeply spiritual. People live their lives in a constant process of exploration, mystery and wonder within which issues of love, hope, meaning and transcendence are of fundamental importance.
>
> (p. 53)

Swinton goes on to apply a research methodology that is sympathetic to these general principles. He focuses on understanding 'the ways in which meaning is constructed in and through human experience' as all lived experience is regarded as intrinsically meaningful and requires interpretation (pp. 99–104). Swinton and Mowat (2006) further develop the ground and foundations for a rigorous research methodology with regard to understanding spirituality, incorporating practical theology which they define as ' . . . theological reflection on the practices of the Church, as they interact with the practices of the world, with a view to ensuring and enabling faithful participation in God's redemptive practices in, to and for the world'(p. 6). They advocate an interdisciplinary approach. This approach offers anyone interested in spirituality a context and framework that has the integrity of scholarly theology and a potentially robust research methodology. My argument here is that to understand spirituality in different contexts there needs to be an explicit position from which this is being explored, not in the service of ascendancy but to contribute to a creatively engaged, mutually receptive and responsive conversation.

A further dimension to this approach would be the work of Paul Willis (2000) and the ethnographic imagination. Meaning-making is a form of cultural production which occurs in daily life and is in itself a form of mediation between 'individuals and structures'. This is a creative process between human beings and their material surroundings in order to express individual and shared beliefs, values and purpose. Willis celebrates the human practice of creating meaning through cultural objects and artefacts embedded in an exquisite range of sensibilities and sensuality (ibid, p. 29).

A robust qualitative research methodology conjoined with practical theology as a scholarly framework is capable of providing further insight and knowledge from across a diverse spectrum of spirituality from the avowedly secular to religious faith; an approach that unashamedly resides at the deep end of subjectivity, creativity and the imagination where human beings engage in *socio-symbolic* meaning-making in everyday life which has the potential to transcend conventional social structures (Willis, 2000). The implication here is that spirituality may also be a dimension of cultural production that enables individuals to overcome social divisions and mediate between the individual and social structures to transform relationships and communities into a more harmonious culture where difference is tolerated and diversity is embraced.

## Saad's Story

When working with Saad, I visited him in his home on an urban estate. He was in his late forties and lived alone in a small terraced property that had been adapted to accommodate his wheelchair and other aids and adaptations due to the advanced stages of his diagnosis of motor neurone disease. His bedroom was adjacent to a small living room and there was a galley kitchen to the right of the front door. Often, when I arrived to meet with him a relative would be about to leave having cooked some samosas and prepared some daal, filling the house with the fragrance of spices. Saad would be waiting and ready to meet, always enthusiastic and welcoming. There were many occasions during these visits when I met family members leaving or arriving shortly after our session, some of whom had journeyed from Pakistan to see him.

With great concentration, Saad could mobilise himself around the cramped space of his home in his wheelchair. He could still communicate but with great effort. He was unable to use his left arm and had limited use of his right arm and hand. He often regarded the art-making as a physical challenge and as a means to overcome the impact of his condition on his mobility. He would usually use a pencil or felt tipped pen and sometimes ventured to use a small brush to dab water colour paint onto a sheet of paper on the tray attached to his wheelchair. Saad was a Moslem and had regular visits from his imam and other more devout relatives who would sit and read the Koran to him. He worked on abstract patterns and shapes, sharing the meaningful interaction of engagement and relationship through the images he created and the sense of reaching beyond his difficult circumstances. He was supported by a cultural and religious context of faith and family devotion and in the art therapy there was a deep concern for the validation and worth that he experienced by handling art materials and making images in the context of the non-verbal purposeful dynamics of the therapeutic relationship. My acknowledgement of the religious orthodoxy and cultural heritage of Saad's life and circumstances and the attention to meaning-making in art therapy affirmed his inherent human value and enabled him to transcend his physical limitations by connecting and becoming more of himself. Spirituality in this context is identified as both relating to religious faith and the therapeutic process that he engaged with in art therapy that enabled Saad to experience a deeper sense of his self-worth and purpose in addition to a greater integration of his physical and mental wellbeing despite his deteriorating condition.

This vignette is reflective of the case studies in my PhD research which describe the many ways in which spirituality emerges as part of the process of art-making in art therapy. The proximity of dying and death when living with a life-threatening illness intensifies the likelihood of a search for meaning and purpose. This can initiate a process of preparation in response to the level of 'mortality salience' that is experienced. This is the human capacity to be aware of one's own mortality (Kearney, 2000, p. 17). According to Becker this awareness can evoke profound fear and anxiety. In the face

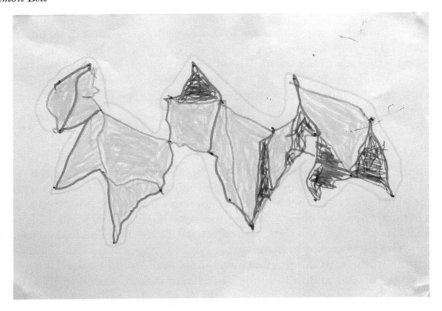

*Figure 2.1* Abstract

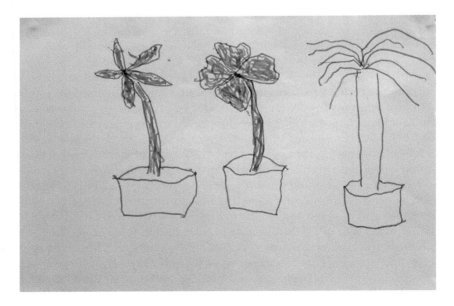

*Figure 2.2* Plants

of the enormity of a poor prognosis and all the implications, spirituality often becomes significant as a means of validating and affirming personhood and identity when coping with progressive physical deterioration, the dying process and the anticipation of death.

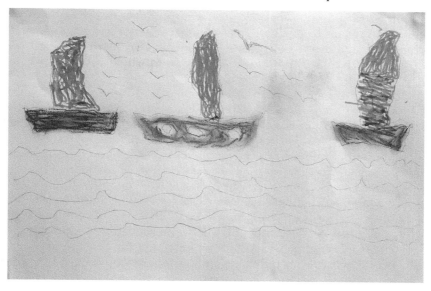

*Figure 2.3* Boats

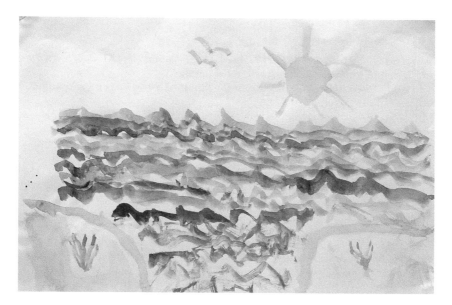

*Figure 2.4* The Coast

## Conclusion

Spirituality in art therapy at the end of life is a key aspect to the attention given to human suffering as part of a holistic approach. For art therapists to be able to address meaning-making and spirituality it is helpful to consider the historical and cultural place of metaphysical considerations as part of a psychotherapeutic intervention and in view of such developments as transpersonal psychology (Powell and MacKenna,

2009). The theoretical development of diverse approaches to psychotherapy and current practice with regard to psychological therapies cannot easily ignore the continuing relevance and significance of spirituality, reflected by modalities such as psychosynthesis psychotherapy and the tradition of psychospiritual psychology (Simpson et al, 2013).

I have emphasised the importance of developing a strong theoretical and research framework to support the evidence for spirituality. My references to practical theology, an ethnographic research methodology and the cultural debate relevant to all efforts to define and respond to spirituality in psychotherapy are an attempt to bring together a combination of interdisciplinary interests to shed further light on this significant aspect of human experience. Art therapy is well placed to facilitate this, along with many other end-of-life concerns, as it offers a creative, imaginative context within which the person living with a life-threatening illness can explore meaning and purpose. Spirituality is a fragile and elusive term referring to a diverse understanding of the cultural and psychological significance of creating and discovering meaning within the confines of physical existence and the mystery of all those aspects of life that are beyond full comprehension. In this sense I am reflecting my personal commitment to spirituality as real and true and wish to join with those who, like me, whether persuaded by religious orthodoxy, agnosticism or secular mysticism, are curious about why it is that human beings continue to be preoccupied with spiritual matters in art, in life and in our dying and death.

# References

Bateman, A.W. and Fonagy, P. (eds) (2012) *Handbook of Mentalization in Mental Health Practice*, Washington and London: American Psychiatric Publishing, Inc.

BBC Radio 4 (2017) *Desert Island Discs*, Broadcast on 28th June 2017, Presenter: Young, K. Producer: Taylor, S. London: BBC.

Bell, S. (2008) *Drawing on the End of Life: Art Therapy, Spirituality and Palliative Care*, Unpublished Ph.D. thesis, Sheffield: University of Sheffield.

Bell, S. (2011) 'Art Therapy and Spirituality', *Journal for the Study of Spirituality*, 1 (2), pp. 215–230.

Cook, C.C.H. (2004) 'Addiction and Spirituality', *Addiction*, 99, pp. 539–551.

Cook, C.C.H. (2016) 'Narrative in Psychiatry, Theology and Spirituality' in Cook, C.C.H., Powell, A. and Sims, A. (eds) *Spirituality and Narrative in Psychiatric Practice: Stories of Mind and Soul*, London: The Royal College of Psychiatrists.

Cook, C.C.H., Powell, A. and Sims, A. (eds) (2016) *Spirituality and Narrative in Psychiatric Practice: Stories of Mind and Soul*, London: The Royal College of Psychiatry.

Hornborg, A. (2011) 'Are We All Spiritual? A Comparative Perspective on the Appropriation of a New Concept of Spirituality', *Journal for the Study of Spirituality*, 1 (2), pp. 249–268.

Kearney, M. (2000) *A Place of Healing: Working with Suffering in Living and Dying*, Oxford: Oxford University Press.

Powell, A. (2016) 'Helping Patients Tell Their Story: Narratives of Body, Mind and Soul' in Cook, C.C.H., Powell, A. and Sims, A. (eds) *Spirituality and Narrative in Psychiatric Practice: Stories of Mind and Soul*, London: The Royal College of Psychiatrists.

Powell, A. and MacKenna, C. (2009) 'Psychotherapy' in Cook, C.C.H., Powell, A. and Sims, A. (eds) *Spirituality in Psychiatry*, London: The Royal College of Psychiatry.

Rieff, P. (1966) *The Triumph of the Therapeutic: Uses of Faith After Freud*, London: Chatto and Windus.

Simpson, S., Evans, J. and Evans, R. (eds) (2013) *Essays on the Theory and Practice of a Psychospiritual Psychology: Volume 1*, London: The Institute of Psychosynthesis.

Swinton, J. (2001) *Spirituality and Mental Health Care: Rediscovering a 'Forgotten' Dimension*, London and Philadelphia: Jessica Kingsley Publishers.

Swinton, J. and Mowat, H. (2006) *Practical Theology and Qualitative Research*, London: SCM Press.

Talvitie, V. (2009) *Freudian Unconscious and Cognitive Neuroscience*, London: Karnac Books Ltd.

Watts, G. (2017) 'Of' and 'For': Studying Spirituality and the Problems Therein', *Journal for the Study of Spirituality*, 7 (1), pp. 64–71.

Willis, P. (2000) *The Ethnographic Imagination*, Oxford and MA: Polity in association with Blackwell Publishers Ltd.

# 3  Snapshot of Practice
## Art Therapy and Acquired Visual Loss

*Lucy Pyart*

## About Me

I have a background in physiotherapy and recently completed the MA Art Psychotherapy, at the University of Roehampton. I'm currently employed as an art psychotherapist within a primary school setting and additionally have an interest in art psychotherapy in medical contexts. As a student I completed a placement in a hospice setting and wished to write about this, as the work I completed with one client still informs my practice, serving as a reminder of the power of the symbolic image as a mediator for change.

## About the Context in Which I Work

This vignette presents a client who was referred to art therapy whilst receiving respite care in a hospice. The client was initially an inpatient at the hospice but was subsequently discharged home and attended art therapy on an outpatient basis. The hospice provides care for adults in an urban setting on the south coast of England.

## Case Example

The client: Ella Craze, who wished for her real name to be used, was registered blind, having lost her sight shortly before starting art therapy. Her primary diagnosis was; "orbital (relates to the eye) and abdominal malignancy, with metastatic spread". She was 60 years old.

For her initial session, Ella chose air drying clay to work with and moulded it whilst we spoke. Ella had required multiple medical procedures as a baby, due to a tumour in her eye, which had caused prolonged periods of separation from her mother. She spoke about two adult romantic relationships that had ended; she did not have any children. She also discussed anxieties about trusting someone new in relation to a new carer and I felt it highly likely this would also relate to me as a new person.

Figure 3.1 shows Ella's initial sculpture. Looking at the pieces she made, I wondered about the separateness of her experience and her potential need for holding herself together within relational contexts (Bick, 1968, pp. 484–486).

In the session that followed Ella explored her cancer via dream imagery of a "gnarled tree which changes shape" (Figure 3.2). She also discussed another dream where a friend left her alone in town. Whilst she discussed this, Ella made a coil pot which then broke

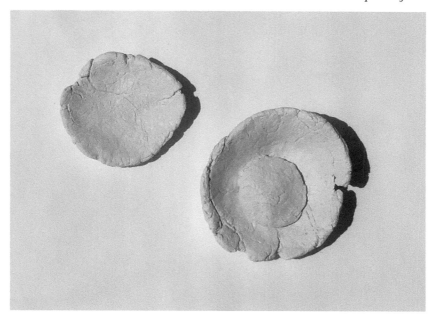

*Figure 3.1* Initial Session With Ella (Air Drying Clay, 4 cm and 3 cm Diameter)

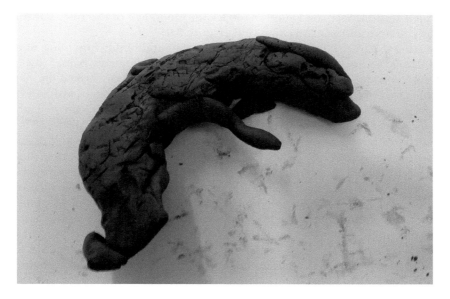

*Figure 3.2* Sculpture of a Tree From a Dream (Session 2 Clay, 10 cm)

(Figure 3.3) as she discussed her frustrations with relationships. My countertransference was of a great sadness and I wondered out loud about her longing for a deeper connection with people and a close romantic relationship.

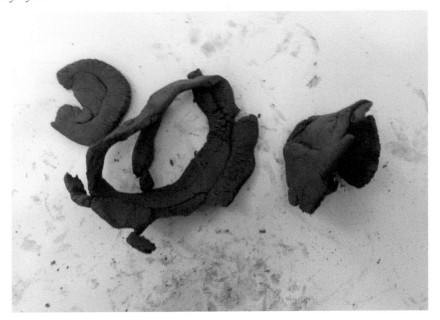

*Figure 3.3* Coil Pot (Clay, 5 cm Diameter)

In the next session, Ella continued to work with the image of the tree, but this time it had changed shape, and was 'reaching out' (Figure 3.4).

After making the tree, Ella began talking about pain and bodily functions. She asked if she could lie on the floor, as this is how she would normally manage pain. I invited her to try some guided imagery in this new position of lying on the floor. I asked her to hold the image of the tree in mind and to see if she could feel the 'reaching out' with her body. She then began to reach her hands away from her body; she lay like this for several minutes until the end of the session.

In the sessions that followed, Ella reported that she was taking risks and reaching out; like the tree she embodied in the session. This felt significant; she reported that she was offering hugs to friends and family, which is not something she would normally do. She also reached out to me, stating that she wished we could both have riser recliner chairs, like the one I provided for her "so we could both be together and comfy". She had also had success in finding a volunteer befriender with whom she has a 'mind to mind' connection.

Towards the end of our work together Ella began to talk about poetry and that she had been thinking of words, to which I acted as a scribe. She decided she would like these words published, which they were after her death, in the hospice newsletter. I am now also continuing this wish by publishing them here:

*You Never Know by Ella Craze*

*You never know when it's the last time you will see your own reflection or see the sea,*
*Feel moved to pick up a paintbrush,*
*You never know when the end is going to be.*

*Walking on warm sand, small waves lapping at my toes . . .*
*For the very last time?*

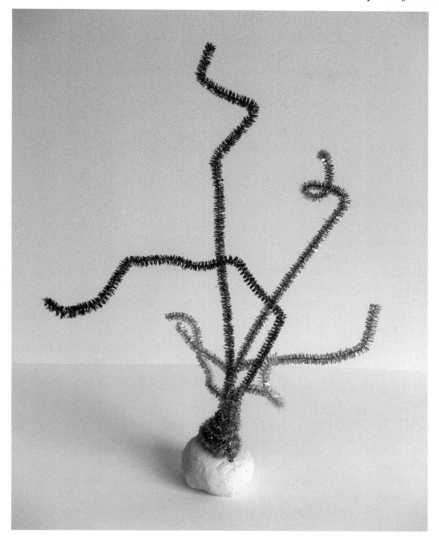

*Figure 3.4* Tree Reaching Out (Session 3 Plasticine and Pipe Cleaners, 18 cm in Height)

*A pen laid down where it was last used,*
*A tissue scrumpled in the corner of a pocket,*
*Inadvertently thrown away.*

*Dancing to Billy Ocean's red light,*
*Spells danger . . .*
*Can't hold on much longer.*

*Your voice, my voice;*
*Bird Song . . .*

*Ahhh yes . . .*
*But I don't half like toast.*

## Advantages of Art Therapy in My Context

This vignette demonstrates that art therapy was a potent psychological medium for a 60-year-old visually impaired women, who faced her individuation process with courage in the context of life-limiting illness. Ella was keen to engage with art therapy and described herself as an artist prior to her loss of sight. I was struck when I first met her, that she had continued to sculpt at home, even after her loss of vision. Herrmann (1995, p. 230) highlights that for those who have lost their vision, a "reservoir of visual memories" will persist. It seemed Ella had been searching for ways to stay connected to her old self prior to her loss of sight, to the arts and to find satisfying relationships. I believe art therapy enabled her to achieve some of these goals.

## One Idea That Shapes My Work

Jung's concept of individuation shapes my work. Jung saw life as a developmental process towards 'individuation', which links with the "resolution of . . . opposites" and the experience of the wholeness of self which lies 'beyond the ego' (Storr, 1995, pp. 98, 88). In short, 'individuation' could be described as; "becoming who one really is" and symbolic images are seen to have a central function, acting as a mediator between the ego and self (Schmidt, 2005). For Ella, there seemed to be a continual yearning for a close relationship and the symbol of the tree reaching out felt significant. It is argued here that by externalising this symbolic imagery within the context of the therapeutic relationship, Ella was brought into contact with deeper parts of herself. These parts appeared to relate to her need to reach out to others, right up to the point of her death and beyond via her poetry.

## References

Bick, E. (1968). 'The experience of skin in early object—relations'. *International Journal of Psychoanalysis*, 49 (2), pp. 484–486.

Herrmann, U. (1995). 'A Trojan horse of clay: Art therapy in a residential school for the blind'. *The Arts in Psychotherapy*, 22 (3), pp. 229–234.

Schmidt, M. (2005). 'Individuation: Finding oneself in analysis—taking risks and making sacrifices'. *Journal of Analytical Psychology*, 50, pp. 595–616.

Storr, A. (1995). *Jung*. London: Fontana Press.

# 4 Art Therapy and Juvenile NCL

*Uwe Herrmann*

## Introduction

Juvenile Batten Disease is a progressive and terminal neurodegenerative illness that gradually deprives children and adolescents of mental and physical faculties, until they die by the end of their adolescence. Drawing on 25 years of art therapy practice with this population at a large state school for the blind in Germany, the chapter highlights issues for long-term art psychotherapy accompanying young clients through the stages of their illness. It describes how making art facilitates clients unable to speak to express and work through their illness-related fears and complete vital 'life tasks' in their remaining years. Addressing the need for an adaptive and active therapist in response to the clients' physical and mental decline, the chapter also speaks to the specific countertransference that the illness evokes and how the clients' art objects constitute lasting mementos of their existence.

## Juvenile Batten Disease: Medical, Psychological and Educational Positions

The term Batten Disease describes a group of hereditary, progressive and terminal neurodegenerative illnesses caused by genetic mutations, also known as NCLs (*neuronal ceroid lipofuscinoses*). The juvenile type of Batten Disease, JNCL, affects children from around the age of six. The first symptom is sight deterioration around age six, eventually leading to complete blindness. In their teens, children progressively lose all physical, mental and communicative abilities. Epileptic seizures and dementia set in and active speech deteriorates, while the understanding of language remains for several more years. Parkinson-like symptoms affect posture and movement, and fine and gross motor skills are gradually erased. Clients with JNCL are confined to a wheelchair in mid-adolescence, eventually become bedridden and have to be fully nursed. Death sets in by late adolescence into early adulthood (Hofman, 1990; Kohlschütter, 2001; Hobert & Dawson, 2006; Jain & Aggarwal, 2016; Ostergaard, 2016).

Much of the literature on JNCL seems concerned with the medical and educational implications of this rare condition. In schools for the blind, where many children with JNCL spend the major portion of their life, the illness poses a challenge to educational paradigms and practices. Von Tetzchner et al. (2013) outline that educationalists must be adaptive and closely observe the children's changing needs to help them build up skills and abilities in spite of an overall tendency of decline.

Earlier educational papers have drawn attention to the condition's psychological implications. Gombault and Vermehren (1989) describe the disintegration of language as a continuous source of frustration for the child, while Koehler and Loftin (1994) observed that children with JNCL tended not to disclose their anxieties in interviews, but non-verbally in everyday situations. Gayton (1987) advocates searching for alternative, non-verbal means of communication, to be established as early as possible.

The literature on JNCL seldom addresses whether children are aware that their condition is terminal; as the fatal diagnosis remains undisclosed to many of them, this is a critical concern. In 25 years of practice I have encountered only one family deciding to share this knowledge with their child; in all other 14 children I worked with parents instructed staff not to disclose any details of the illness to their children, and not to address the subject of death. This stance can also be found in the literature: Koehler and Loftin (1994) observe that rather than death and dying, anger is the central concern of children with JNCL. They caution not to ascribe all of the children's emotions to being ill and thus "paint an overly pessimistic portrait of the child" (p. 320). However, Gombault (1992: 17) sees the process of physical and mental deterioration as "a source of repeated new distresses and worries" and suggests that children grapple with feelings of guilt and with anticipating their early death.

The children's deterioration over more than a decade towards an early death is a heavy psychological burden for them, their families and carers. From early on children show emotional problems, including aggressive outbursts and phases of depression, and sleep disturbances, hallucinations and paranoia in later stages. Hofman (1990) connects many of these problems with losing environmental control and the ability to express oneself, causing anxiety and confusion in the child, while the erosion of language hampers psychological assessment. Though some of the medical and educational literature acknowledges the psychological strains in children with JNCL, few mention their need for psychotherapy. While the slow progression of the illness would allow for many years of psychotherapy, psychotropic drugs seem the main treatment for the psychological symptoms connected to JNCL (Kohlschütter, 2001; Bäckman et al., 2001; Ostergaard, 2016).

The reasons for this gap in the literature can only be speculated: hospitals and schools, as the institutions mainly concerned with JNCL, may respond to the illness with their respective medical and educational means; while psychotherapy may be practised with JNCL clients but not described in the literature, it is equally likely that the prospective loss of speech discourages carers from seeking verbal psychotherapy for these children. It is here that Gayton's (1987) call for alternative, non-verbal means of communication makes the arts therapies a particularly worthwhile option.

## Art Psychotherapy Positions on JNCL

The few papers I have written seem to be the only art therapy publications on JNCL to date (Herrmann, 1995a, 1995b, 2001). This coincides with a scarceness of art therapy literature on blindness, with the exception of some case vignettes in Edith Kramer's and Judy Rubin's work and my own publications (Kramer, 1971, 1979, 2000; Rubin, 1976, 1978; Herrmann, 1995a, 1995b, 2006, 2009, 2010, 2011a, 2011b, 2016a, 2016b). It seems that along other blind children those with JNCL have received especially little attention from art therapy. On the other hand, art therapy has shown its efficacy for people with life threatening illnesses and in palliative settings (Dreifuss-Kattan, 1995; Wood & Pratt, 1998; Waller, 2002; Waller & Sibbett, 2005; Liebman & Weston, 2015).

In my earlier papers on JNCL I made several observations: while children experienced the persistent loss of physical and mental functions as disruptive and traumatic, the art process served as a 'filter' helping to repress their anxieties and concerns. As they could examine, mourn and integrate preliminary or permanent losses of physical abilities into a changed sense of self, the art object had an anchoring and reassuring effect in therapy. However grave any progressive shift of the illness had been, the art object displayed a noticeable capacity to keep the children's sense of self intact into the late stages of the illness.

Further, many of the children, though shielded from their diagnosis, showed a high concern with death and dying in their artwork, pointing to their latent knowledge of their illness as terminal; in the symbolism of their art objects, their apprehensions could be expressed and worked with discretely even when verbal discourse on these subjects was eschewed by their carers or had become physically impossible.

I described how the clients' physical and mental deterioration makes giving them assistance increasingly crucial and makes massive demands on the art therapist's adjustability, alongside adapting the understanding of the art object and process to the clients' dwindling verbal, mental and physical abilities.

I also addressed the specific countertransference that working with a slowly deteriorating client evokes in the therapist. This may surface in the concern and care that a practitioner may develop for the artwork; i.e. whether a client would remain physically capable and/or live long enough to complete a particular art project and whether it was crafted well enough way to have an 'enduring life' (Herrmann, 2001).

I will revisit some of these points and add further reflections from the perspective of continued practice.

## Art Therapy Within a School for the Blind: The Service in Context

Clients with JNCL have traditionally attended schools for the blind. Though special school practitioners have extensive experience in working with physical conditions, the child's slow decline towards death goes against the grain of educational practice, dedicated to enhancing children's intellectual and physical progression. Having a therapist among one's ranks to cater to the psychological needs of *dying* blind children was therefore one of several reasons for establishing art therapy at the Hanover State School for the Blind some 25 years ago, and in later years counselling, verbal psychotherapy and music therapy were introduced to the school's therapy department.

Since the beginning of my practice, children with JNCL have used art therapy along other blind clients in weekly individual sessions. Most of the 15 JNCL clients I have worked with began therapy a year or two after their transferral to the school for the blind, typically at age seven to nine, when their emotional instability gave cause to their referral. Clients with JNCL normally stay in art psychotherapy for eight to twelve years until their condition necessitates their transferral to home nursing or a hospice; in a single case I could maintain itinerary art therapy in-home sessions for a girl into the last months of her life until she died at age 22.

The multitude of stimuli and social demands of the bustling classroom often stresses and overwhelms children with JNCL, who are already grappling with losses of physical and mental faculties, and with not achieving curricular goals. In contrast, art therapy provides a calm and non-demanding environment. Falk (2002: 117), working with Alzheimer patients, similarly describes artmaking as "a place of refuge". It is therefore a common phenomenon that the disruptive behaviour of JNCL clients rarely occurs in art therapy and tends to peter out in the classroom a few months after their referral. A considerable portion of this phenomenon is to do with the dynamics of artmaking and the therapeutic relationship, and with allowing a client to retreat to an adaptive therapy setting and to work on his or her internal conflicts, as described by Dalley (1990) for art therapy in mainstream education. Art therapy as an in-school service for JNCL clients has an added effect on educational staff: the child's temporary withdrawal from the classroom for the therapeutic session relaxes the classroom situation, and simply knowing that the art therapist is a 'specialist' ally in working with a dying child relieves teachers from having to take on a therapeutic role that outstretches their professional role and training. Further, art therapy's psychodynamic frame of reference contributes to the reflections of the educational team: it adds the dimension of the unconscious, symbolic communication and the transference relationship to how a child with JNCL is perceived and understood.

Though art therapists experience the same difficulties as other professionals working with JNCL, art therapy's aesthetic and symbolic traits may be particularly suited for responding to the losses and psychological problems associated with JNCL, beginning with the role that art can play when the illness begins to erase speech.

## Lost Speech and the Symbol

Blindness creates a sensory divide between the visually impaired child and the sighted therapist, and I have addressed the psychodynamic implications of this blind–sighted encounter elsewhere (Herrmann, 2011b, 2016b). When working with JNCL the deterioration of speech is another building block in the isolation increasingly affecting the therapeutic relationship.

In the early stage of JNCL art is a means of expression that eases the child's frustration with many losses, including speech. Similarly, Magee (2002), Falk (2002) and Tyler (2002), working with other progressive conditions like Huntington's and Alzheimer's disease, have remarked how music and art provide an alternative means of communication when speech is compromised. In the advanced stage of JNCL talking is reduced to stammering, then to mere sounds and finally to silence. To keep the art process afloat the art therapist must learn to read the minimal communicative clues and to anticipate the wishes and thoughts of a blind and increasingly apraxic, muted and demented client. Though we may possess these skills in essence, they are seldom part of our training and we must develop and hone them as we practice.

When 13-year old Miriam, my first JNCL client, was wheeled into the art therapy room for her first session, I felt very uneasy. She was in the advanced stage of JNCL, completely blind, could hardly use her hands and spoke very little. Trying to connect with her I had to slow down, use simple language, and break down the range and exploration of tactile art materials into digestible units. Miriam's condition required my learning to be a very *active* therapist, able to adjust and structure our encounter, and to bridge the sensory gap between her and the studio's contents. To me, this was a yet unfamiliar experience and I will later address it in terms of therapeutic interventions and countertransference.

Initially Miriam used two-word sentences to indicate which project and materials she wanted. It was unsettling when after a few months her language was reduced to 'yes' and 'no', until I discovered that Miriam could steer her art process with these two words quite effectively as long as I provided a systematic verbal rundown of options from which she could choose. Though this procedure complicated our work and made me worry about future sessions, it was reassuring that Miriam and I could access her ideas, wishes and predilections.

Then a series of severe epileptic seizures kept Miriam away for several weeks; when she returned with no speech at all, a sense of hopelessness hung over the session. Miriam seemed completely locked in and I seemed locked out. However, I eventually realized that she responded to my words with almost unnoticeable head movements indicating confirmation or refusal of what I offered to her. Painstakingly slow, Miriam expressed what she wanted to make, from which material and how precisely it should be fashioned. Over two sessions, she modelled a barren clay tree, growing on a rocky outcrop, some of its branches scattered on the ground, others still attached on the tree's trunk (Figure 4.1).

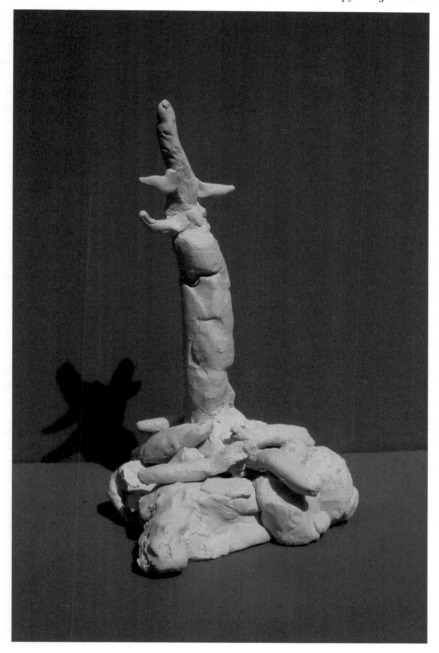

*Figure 4.1* Miriam: The Tree After a Storm (White Stoneware)

When the work was finished, we could unpack what Miriam thought; I voiced what I saw and thought, and gave her alternative options to confirm or disclaim by slightly moving her head. As we explored the sculpture, I put its story of loss and resilience into words for both of us. I described how the tree seemed to have suffered, how maybe some storm brought down boughs and branches while others still seemed in place. When I said that the tree, though seemingly having suffered great damage, was still standing, Miriam gave the slightest nod and breathed a deep sigh.

Before Miriam was transferred to nursing care and died the year after, she made a final clay tree. With its branches unscathed and covered in an abundance of leaves and blossoms, it is a most improbable and defiant image of resilience in adverse conditions. It is through such imagery, related to a client's story and yet detached enough to be a consolation, that art can relate, transform and transcend suffering in the complete absence of speech.

Having addressed the physical inability to speak in the late stage of the illness, it is important to acknowledge that language loss connected to JNCL is twofold: in the condition's early stage the fatal prognosis constitutes a taboo, keeping children, parents and practitioners from addressing illness-related worries. It is here that art can help articulate things that cannot or must not be spoken.

## The Symbol and the Unspeakable

Having lost speech, Miriam's art expressed her concerns and experiences, which I could clad into words. However, even when speech is still functioning, the spectre of the illness often forfeits words. Being ill at ease with discussing illness and dying unites most parents and practitioners working with JNCL. Adults may want to protect children from knowing about their illness and likewise children may want to protect adults from knowing that they know, which has been described for JNCL (Gombault, 1985, 1992) and other terminal conditions (Wass, 1995; Vernick & Karon, 1965; Spinetta & Maloney, 1974; Bluebond-Langer, 1978, 1995; Chaflin & Barbarin, 1991). We may think about this verbal deadlock as a pre-emptive, selective 'loss' of speech. Here, art therapy can address the unspeakable in a moderated, yet effective way for the aesthetic and symbolic elements of its practice, as the following case vignette illustrates.

Shortly after his 10th birthday he started making a boat from scrap wood and other materials, equipping the vessel with a mast and sail, an anchor, a lifebelt, a German flag, lights and paper decorations (Figure 4.2).

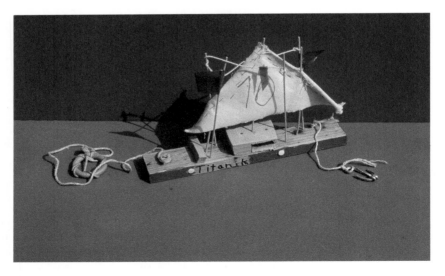

*Figure 4.2* Slavik: Titanik (Wood and Mixed Media)

As a final touch, he wrote 'Titanik' on the boat and a big 10 on its sail. I understood the idiosyncratic spelling of 'Titanik' as a double entendre of his name Slavik, his Slavic origin and the *Titanic* disaster. As our conversation flowed, Slavik started talking about the *Titanic* and her fate; how all seemed great as the ship headed for America; how it hit the iceberg, and how lights could still be seen and music could still be heard until it went down to the bottom of the sea with its passengers. With his artwork, Slavik linked the doomed ship's story to his own and mastered the impossible task of discussing death without compromising the taboo of addressing it as a personal subject. It seemed that he anticipated the seriousness of his condition as much as its certainty. This may be understood in the light of findings that children with another undisclosed diagnosis of terminal illness similarly develop an increasing awareness of their illness and its implications based on an array of internal and external perceptions (Bluebond-Langer, 1978, 1995).

In following months Slavik did not dwell in the state of doom that making his 'Titanik' might have suggested, but began squaring matters between death and him. He often enquired about death as a philosophical conundrum and I responded with reading him myths and fairy tales that addressed and illuminated the subject. Alongside we made art, often to a point that stretched my willingness to comply with his wishes, as in the case of making a life-sized wooden coffin. He had conceived this idea from a popular children's book on a little vampire befriending a mortal boy, and the book's use of the term 'underground furniture' for the little vampire's casket made Slavik chuckle. As he crafted the coffin, made shelves for books and CDs, and finally transformed it into a boat, it became clear that he greatly relied on me as an ally of a particular sort: an adult who was willing and able to help him navigate difficult waters through the use of art as a symbolic, discrete and most importantly, transformative activity.

Slavik often returned to the question why the artists aboard the *Titanic* had persisted with their music even though they knew they were going to die. We arrived at the conclusion that making their art might have been a consolation and an act of defiance through creating beauty. Indeed, much of the strength associated to art seems to lie in its reparative potential, capable of redressing suffered or imminent losses and to complete vital life tasks.

## Symbolic Reconstruction and Completion

As Erikson (1959) describes, the tasks of adolescence are geared towards independence and autonomy. Adolescence is a very vulnerable period of human development, and as the most rapid and fundamental loss of abilities in clients with JNCL happens in that time, this creates a painful dichotomy between ideal and reality. Each new physical or mental loss threatens the evolving personality of the JNCL adolescent and must be integrated towards a changed idea of his or her self.

As one of the tasks of adolescence is to physically and emotionally detach from one's parents, JNCL clients often perceive the art object and the therapist as more suitable and 'neutral' containers into which they can evacuate aspects of their former healthy self to be safely and permanently 'stored', as in the case of Claas, a 17-year-old boy in the advanced stage of JNCL. The illness had taken most physical abilities from this previously active, football-loving teenager. In his second art therapy session, he modelled a clay football player and in the ensuing sessions made an almost life-sized superhero with a sword from scrap wood (Figure 4.3).

Reflecting on his creations, I wondered if they had names. Claas promptly and proudly responded that his sculptures represented 'tough guys' named after both of us:

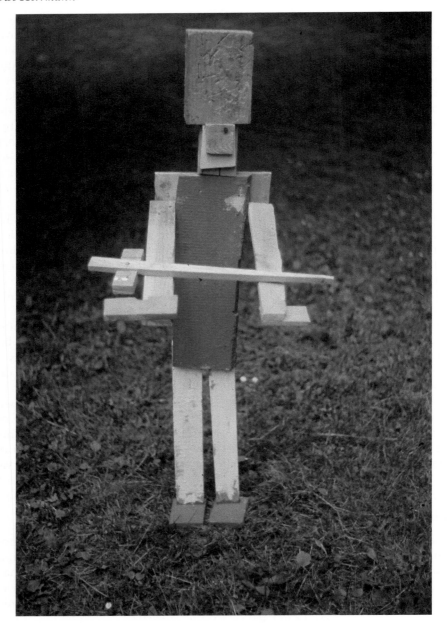

*Figure 4.3* Claas: Superhero (Acrylic on Wood)

'Claas-Uwe'. As Claas, clients may temporarily merge themselves, their artwork and the therapist as 'one'. Such a merger can serve them as a reassurance that physical abilities, though irretrievably lost to them, are still safe and accessible within the 'other', the therapist and the artwork, as an imaginary extension of their self. This does not change the raw facts of loss, but makes them more bearable until the client's ego is sufficiently restored to face them. This capacity is not only inherent to art in therapy but to art as such: Dreifuss-Kattan (2016) has recently emphasized the helpful role that art plays for loss and mourning by researching the biographies of renowned artists.

Making art also facilitates completing other tasks of adolescence and adulthood that are far beyond the scope of what clients can reach within their short life span, in an imaginary and yet concrete way. Slavik and Miriam spent much time building houses with everything but the kitchen sink, and so have most of the 15 clients I have worked with. Making model houses, with miniature human inhabitants, gardens and animals, trees and wells, or sculpting landscapes of countries never to be travelled in reality, belong to the repertoire of art projects that most of my JNCL clients at some point or other choose in therapy. Such work is of utmost importance to them and provides an immense sense of contentment. I suggest that the cause of this satisfaction lies in the feeling to have completed some crucial part of the human experience. Even if only in a bonsai fashion, art thus creates a sense of completion in spite of the artist's world falling to pieces, or as the American poet Kenneth Rexroth (1987: 43) put it, "against the ruin of the world, there is only one defense—the creative act".

For a progressively ill client the creative act comes with increasing difficulty, and this makes demands on the art therapist's ability to assist.

## Decline and Intervention

Working with deteriorating clients stirs uncertainties how to respond to their decreasing ability to handle materials, to think or to remember and to make choices about material, form and content. This concerns the crucial question of how to intervene in therapy, what to say, how to react and how to assist the patient to be of good use to her or him. Art therapy pioneer Edith Kramer (1986, 2000) terms this ability the 'Third Hand' that the art therapist must lend to the client, which is, other than the auxiliary ego, of a mental *and* physical nature. Such an intervention can take many forms, from a verbal comment to suggesting a material, a technique or physically assisting the client's mastery of a difficult task.

A patient's decline calls for an increasingly active therapist providing such interventions; this role may not always sit easy with the paradigms and practices of nondirective art psychotherapy but is a vital issue to resolve. A passive therapist may remain separate from the client and assume that this keeps therapy 'pure' of external influences. In the case of JNCL and similar debilitating conditions however, a non-participating therapist can be experienced as unhelpful, rejecting or persecutory. Unless a therapist becomes a 'co-creator' in the late stages of the illness, he or she will merely be an extension of the client's suffering.

When working with Miriam, developing our part verbal, part gestural exchange was key to her pursuing her artwork. Alongside, I increasingly had to assist her modelling with my own hands. In the very late stage of JNCL this may extend to modelling on clients' behalf and according to their instructions, or catering for a very minimalistic working procedure, as in the case of Maik, who arrived to art therapy distressed and angry. Seventeen years of age, Maik had no fine motor abilities, and his violent, insistent pounding on his wheelchair had become his only communication and only functioning movement. When I handed him clay, Maik's distress soon disappeared as he shaped the material, grabbing and repeatedly slamming it onto the working surface, and finally let go of it. Over a year, Maik produced thirty odd abstract sculptures all bearing the imprint of his fingers (Figure 4.4).

Touching the finished and fired objects, his fingers would automatically slide into the indentations that they had left in them, and when this happened, his face lit up with pleasure, if not recognition. When Maik successively dropped his sculptures into the glaze, he giggled each time when opening his hand was rewarded with a splash. This meditative and ritualistic work made Maik happy and in retrospect seems a manifestation of two basic

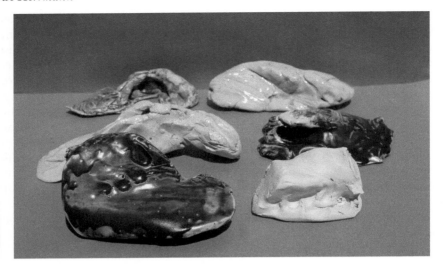

*Figure 4.4* Maik: Clay Sculptures With Fingerprints (White Stoneware, Partly Glazed)

functions making up an important, yet difficult part of our inner lives: holding on and letting go.

Though the art therapist's increasingly active involvement is paramount to maintain the therapeutic process with JNCL clients, it also opens the doors to strong countertransference feelings.

## Decline and Countertransference: The Prism of Death

The slow decline intrinsic to JNCL frustrates and debilitates client and therapist. It threatens their relationship, as feelings of isolation and desperation increasingly enwrap the session. In the advanced stage of the illness, working with a client who has neither functioning speech nor vision and only minimal dexterity may make the art therapist feel unskilled, ineffective and hopeless, and such countertransference feelings may sometimes come close to a parental response of despair and anxiety. With each new project that Miriam and many other clients began, I found myself worrying that they might not have time to complete them, or ensure that they were crafted well enough not to disintegrate. Such worries on the therapist's side must ultimately be understood as related to his or her knowledge that therapy will not be ended by the clients' improvement, but by their death.

'Mors ultima linea rerum est'—Death is the ultimate boundary of things, Horace writes (*Epistulae*, c. 21BC/1888: 32). Though death seems to end all our strivings, as time undoes all our doings, repression shields us from this becoming a permanently conscious insult to our ego. Horace's quote can be flanked with another Latin quote from the Middle Ages: *Mors certa, hora incerta*—Death is certain, its hour uncertain. This dichotomy of uncertain certainty underlies consciously or unconsciously what we do with our lives and why. Working with a terminally ill client the therapist's awareness of death can serve as a prism, focussing therapy on what the present moment has to give. Making art rather than orbiting around fears and worries, ego functions may be strengthened. While a patient seemingly looks away from fears, anxieties and losses and concentrates on mastering the art process, frightening affects or thoughts can be contained, reworked and reformulated towards the temporary formal and psychological solution that the artistic symbol can provide. Art might thus be understood as the epitome of the present moment used well.

However, knowing about clients' terminal condition can sometimes cause distortions in the way we look at their artwork or behaviour, as we may lose using the present moment over being too focussed on death and dying. This may then indeed lead to the projective reading of the one's own death anxieties into the client's every move and sentence, which Koehler and Loftin (1994) cautioned against. Artwork is especially prone to such projections, as its ambiguity invites interpretation. If the art therapist views the client's artwork exclusively through the prism of death, this may foreshorten its rich and stratified meanings that may not only express reflections on dying but simultaneously a love for life and the present moment.

One of the particular countertransference responses I frequently observe when working with JNCL clients is connected to the further fate of their artwork, i.e. where it will be placed and cared for after the termination of therapy and/or the client's death. Such concerns tint the transference relationship from both ends and amplify the 'caring', curatorial element in art therapy working with a terminally ill client.

## The Making of a Legacy: Artwork, Afterlife and Countertransference

When we die most things we leave behind will eventually be discarded. Other than most human belongings, art is often preserved for posterity and leaves an account of its subject and its maker. Shakespeare summarizes this in Sonnet No 18 when he talks about how this poem immortalizes his beloved: "So long as man can breathe and eyes can see/So long lives this and this gives life to thee".

If a visit to a museum does not evoke the same ambivalent feelings as a stroll on a graveyard, it is probably because artwork, though its makers are long dead, can still speak to the living in a sustaining way. Artwork not only immortalizes the artist, but conveys how he or she looked at things and offers the spectator an invigorating dialogue across time: in a painting, Jacques Lacan (1977) observes, the painter's gaze is left behind, preserved and transmitted across centuries, and meets the gaze of the contemporary spectator. The aesthetic surge that art offers to the viewer as a 'bait', titillating his or her sensory and intellectual response, may be the strongest reason to collect, preserve, research and display art for prosperity. In my experience, this also applies to clients' artwork after they have died.

As the ceramic artist and writer Edmund de Waal wrote, "some things seem to retain the pulse of their making" (2011: 16). I find this pulse is alive in the physical traces that the clients' hands have left in their sculptures, and as I helped them create, my involvement has also become part of it. After children with JNCL have died they leave behind a large legacy of artwork that speaks of them. As I am aware of this, so are the children. Differing from other blind clients those with JNCL repeatedly ask about the material longevity of artwork in general, and their work in particular. Hearing that clay objects can survive for millennia is a great reassurance for them. Often clients are very outspoken that their sculptures be on permanent display for others. While some families ensure that all their children's artwork is transferred to their home after terminating art therapy, others prefer not to. Then the department offers a home to this work, to be documented, stored and displayed.

Over the years I thus gradually became a curator of sorts for a collection that seems insignificant compared to a museum's holdings. The feelings of care that such artwork still evokes in me long after therapy terminated can be understood in terms of countertransference. It is based on my being witness to its creation and my sometimes 'as-if' parental response, but also by my being a fellow artist who helped bring a sculpture into existence.

In her essay *Dead Stock: The Researcher as Collector of Failed Goods,* Celeste Olalquiaga (2008: 39) illuminates that particularly collections of the non-sellable kind represent a surplus, leftover or residue which she characterizes thus: "Bereft of primary cultural value and/or circulation, the items (. . .) are no longer in use, and the pleasure they offer is derived in part from their inherent anachronism and/or marginalization, which renders them witness, or traces, of a different time". For me the artwork that JNCL clients have left in the department contains the residue of our relationship, speaks of their stories, of our time together and how we spent it. For other clients with or without JNCL this legacy transcends being a memento: it offers them objects of beauty to view, touch and be encouraged and inspired by as they attempt their own creative act.

## References

Bäckman, M.L., Aberg, L., Aronen, E. & Santavuori, P.R. (2001) New antidepressive and antipsychotic drugs in juvenile neuronal ceroid lipofuscinoses—a pilot study. *European Journal of Pediatric Neurology,* 5, February, Supplement A, 163–166. DOI: 10.1053/ejpn.2000.0455

Bluebond-Langer, M. (1978) *The Private World of Dying Children.* Princeton, NJ: Princeton University Press

Bluebond-Langer, M. (1995) Worlds of dying children and their well siblings. In: Doka, K. (ed.) *Children Mourning—Mourning Children.* Bristol, PA: Hospice Foundation of America/Taylor & Francis.

Chaflin, C.J. & Barbarin, O.A. (1991) Does telling less protect more? Relationship among age, information disclosure, and what children with cancer see and feel. *Journal of Pediatric Psychology,* 16, 169–191.

Dalley, T. (1990) Images and integration: Art therapy in a multi-cultural school. In: Dalley, T. and Case, C. (eds.) *Working with Children in Art Therapy.* London: Routledge.

de Waal, E. (2011) *The Hare with Amber Eyes: A Hidden Inheritance.* London: Random House.

Dreifuss-Kattan, E. (1995) *Cancer Stories: Creativity and Self-Repair.* Hillsdale, NJ: Analytic Press.

Dreifuss-Kattan, E. (2016) *Art and Mourning: The Role of Creativity in Healing Trauma and Loss.* Abingdon, Oxon: Routledge.

Erikson, E.H. (1959) *Identity and the Life Cycle: Psychological Issues, I, Monograph I.* New York: International Universities Press.

Falk, B. (2002) A narrowed sense of space: An art therapy group working with young Alzheimer's sufferers. In: Waller, D. (ed.) *Arts Therapies with Progessive Illnesses.* Hove: Brunner-Routledge.

Gayton, R. (1987) Juvenile Battens disease. *The British Journal of Visual Impairment,* Summer (V: 2), 55–57.

Gombault, E. (1985) Sehgeschädigte mit Vogt-Spielmeyer-Stock-Syndrom. In: Rath, W. and Hudelmayer, D. (eds.) *Pädagogik der Blinden und Sehbehinderten* (Handbuch der Sonderpädagogik, Bd. 2), 444–453. Berlin: Carl Marhold Verlagsbuchhandlung.

Gombault, E. (1992) *Hilfen für das Kind bei seiner Auseinandersetzung mit der eigenen Situation.* In: Landesbildungszentrum für Blinde, Hannover: Bericht zur Tagung zu Fragen der pädagogischen Betreuung von Kindern, die von juveniler NCL betroffen sind. Tagung am LBZB Hannover vom 22. und 23.05.1992. Conference report.

Gombault, E. & Vermehren, B. (1989) *Der Alltag mit den Spielmeyer-Vogt- Kindern.* In: Auf dem Weg in die Hilflosigkeit? Leben Lernen mit der Spielmeyer-Vogt- Krankheit. Tagungsbericht der Tagung für Angehörige und Betreuer der betroffenen Kinder, 13. — 15. Oktober 1989, Bad Segeberg, Tagungsstätte der Ev. Akademie Nordelbien. Conference report.

Herrmann, U. (1995a) Kunsttherapie mit einem mehrfachbehinderten blinden Mädchen. *Lernen Konkret,* 1 (2), 28–29.

Herrmann, U. (1995b) A Trojan horse of clay: Art therapy in a residential school for the blind. *The Arts in Psychotherapy,* 22 (3), 229–234.

Herrmann, U. (2001) Mein eigenes Haus. Kunsttherapie als Psychotherapie für Kinder und Jugendliche mit NCL. In: *NCL: Zur Lebenssituation von blinden Kindern und Heranwachsenden mit einer unheilbaren Abbauerkrankung: Beiträge aus Pädagogik, Therapie und Medizin.* Compiled by Hartmut

Schlegel. Schriftenreihe zur Theorie und Praxis der Blindenbildung. Hannover: Landesbildung-szentrum für Blinde/VZFB.

Herrmann, U. (2006) Blick und Blindheit in der Kunsttherapie. *Kunst & Therapie*, 1, pp. 42–54.

Herrmann, U. (2009) Der Blick der tastenden Hand. Kunsttherapie mit Geburtsblinden. In: VBS (Hg.) *Teilhabe gestalten*. Würzburg: Edition Bentheim.

Herrmann, U. (2010) Braucht das Selbst ein Bild? In: Wendlandt-Baumeister, M., Bolle, R. & Sinapius, P. (ed.) *Wissenschaftliche Grundlagen Der Kunsttherapie*. Bern: Peter Lang.

Herrmann, U. (2011a) The tangible reflection: A single case study investigating body image development in art psychotherapy with a congenitally blind client. In: Gilroy, A. (Hg.) *Art Therapy Research in Practice*. Bern: Peter Lang.

Herrmann, U. (2011b) *Art Psychotherapy and Congenital Blindness: Investigating the Gaze*. Unpublished Ph.D. Thesis, Goldsmiths University of London.

Herrmann, U. (2016a) Der Blick des blinden Schöpfers: Kunsttherapie mit Geburtsblinden. In: Dannecker, K. & Herrmann, U. (Hg.) *Warum Kunst? Über das Bedürfnis des Menschen, Kunst zu schaffen*. Berlin: Medizinisch-Wissenschaftlicher Verlag.

Herrmann, U. (2016b) Touching insights: Visual and tactile cultures in researching art psychotherapy with congenitally blind children. In: Docter, D. & Zárate, M. (Hg.) *Intercultural Arts Therapies Research*. ICRA/ECArTE arts therapies research series. London: Routledge.

Hobert, J.A. & Dawson, G. (2006) Reviewneuronal ceroid lipofuscinoses therapeutic strategies: Past, present and future. *Biochimica et Biophysica Acta*, 1762, 945–953.

Hofman, I. (1990) *The Batten-Spielmeyer-Vogt Disease, Bartiméushage*. Doorn, NL: Bartiméus Foundation.

Horace (Quintus Horatius Flaccus) (c. 21 BC) Epilstulae, edited by A.E. Wilkins, London: Macmillan & Co, 1888

Jain, D. & Aggarwal, H. (2016) Batten disease: A rare case report and review of Literature. *Archive of Clinical Cases*, 3 (4), 126–132. DOI: 10.22551/2016.13.0304., D.10081

Koehler, W. & Loftin, M. (1994) Visually impaired children with progressive, terminal neurodegenerative disorders. *American Journal of Visual Impairment & Blindness*, July-August, 317–328.

Kohlschütter, A. (2001) Juvenile neuronale Ceroidlipofuzinose (juvenile NCL): Medizinische Gesichtspunkte. In: *NCL: Zur Lebenssituation von blinden Kindern und Heranwachsenden mit einer unheilbaren Abbauerkrankung: Beiträge aus Pädagogik, Therapie und Medizin*. Compiled by Hartmut Schlegel. Schriftenreihe zur Theorie und Praxis der Blindenbildung. Hannover: Landesbildung-szentrum für Blinde/VZFB.

Kramer, E. (1971) *Art as Therapy with Children*. New York: Schocken Books.

Kramer, E. (1979) *Childhood and Art Therapy*. New York: Schocken Books.

Kramer, E. (1986) The art therapist's third hand: Reflections on art, art therapy and society at large. *The American Journal of Art Therapy*, 24 (2), 71–86.

Kramer, E. (2000) *Art as Therapy: Collected Papers*, edited by L.A. Gerity. London: Jessica Kingsley Publishers.

Lacan, J. (1977) *The Seminar of Jacques Lacan, Book XI: The Four Fundamental Concepts of Psychoanalysis 1964–1965*, edited by J.-A. Miller. London: The Hogarth Press and the Institute of Psycho-Analysis.

Liebman, M. & Weston, S. (2015) *Art Therapy with Physical Conditions*. London: Jessica Kingsley Publishers.

Magee, W. (2001) Case studies in Huntington's disease: music therapy assessment in the early to advanced stages. In: Waller. D. (ed.) *Arts Therapies and Progressive Illness: Nameless dread*. Hove: Brunner-Routledge.

Olalquiaga, C. (2008) Dead stock: The researcher as collector of failed goods. In: Holly, M.A. and Smith, M. (eds.) *What Is Research in the Visual Arts?* New Haven and London: Sterling and Francine Clark Art Institute/Yale University Press.

Ostergaard, J.R. (2016) Juvenile neuronal ceroid lipofuscinosis (Batten disease): Current insights. *Degenerative Neurological and Neuromuscular Disease*, 6, 73–83.

Rexroth, K. (1987) *World Outside the Window: The Selected Essays of Kenneth Rexroth*, edited by B. Morrow. New York: New Directions Publishing.

Rubin, J. (1976) The exploration of a 'tactile aesthetic'. *New Outlook for the Blind*, 70, 369–375.

Rubin, J. (1978) *Child Art Therapy*, New York: Van Nostrand Reinhold.

Spinetta, J. & Maloney, L.J. (1974) Death anxiety in the outpatient leucemia child. *Paediatrics*, 65, 1034–1037.

Tyler, J. (2002) Art Therapy with older adults clinically diagnosed as having Alzheimer's disease and dementia. In: Waller. D. (ed.) *Arts Therapies and Progressive Illness: Nameless dread.* Hove: Brunner-Routledge.

Vernick, J. & Karon, M. (1965) Who is afraid of death on a leucemia ward? *American Journal of Diseases of Children*, 109, 393–397.

von Tetzchner, S. et al. (2013) Juvenile neuronal ceroid lipofuscinosis and education. *Biochimica et Biophysica Acta*, http:// dx.doi.org/10.1016/j.bbadis.2013.02.017

Wass, H. (1995) Death in the lives of children and adolescents. In: Wass, H. & Neimeyer, R. (eds.) *Death: Facing the Facts.* Washington/Bristol/London: Taylor & Francis.

Waller, D. (ed.) (2002) *Arts Therapies with Progessive Illnesses.* Hove: Brunner-Routledge.

Waller, D. & Sibbett, C. (2005) *Art Therapy and Cancer Care: Facing Death.* Maidenhead: Open University Press.

Wood, M. & Pratt, M. (1998) *Art Therapy in Palliative Care: The Creative Response.* London: Routledge.

# 5  Blurry Vision

## Introducing Art Therapy to Palliative Care Patients

*Deirdre Ní Argáin*

Palliative care is a well-established and valued part of the Irish health services. Largely funded by public donations, it has been an area of innovation where professionals work together holistically and think outside the box, to support and empower patients to play an active role in their health journey. As such it has been open to the idea that creative arts can contribute to healthcare and has supported art therapy, which is a relatively new profession in Ireland.

When I returned from training in London in 1988, I was one of a handful of art therapists in the Republic of Ireland. When we met with music therapists, drama therapists and dance movements therapists we could all fit easily in a sitting room. Together we formed a professional body, the Irish Association of Creative Arts Therapists (IACAT) and formed links with the Northern Ireland Group for Art as Therapy (NIGAT). Today there are 150 art therapists registered with IACAT and professional trainings in Cork and Belfast. There has been a similar growth in the other creative arts disciplines and we continue have a joint professional body and to lobby together for statutory recognition as allied health professionals.

Much of my art therapy journey has been under the auspices of palliative care. Over the past 20 years I have worked in three different hospices in Ireland, firstly as a sessional art therapist one day a week, secondly as the first art therapist in a setting that already had art facilitation and currently as a sole practitioner in a setting that has had experience of art therapy.

Each setting has brought its own challenges to the process of establishing my role in a multi-disciplinary team and introducing art therapy to clients. As more palliative care providers in Ireland employed art therapists I was able to compare my experience with that of others through qualitative research. (Ní Argáin 2008). I am particularly interested in patient's perceptions of art therapy and recent quantitative research in psycho-oncology has proved to be a valuable lens through which to view my work in palliative care (Nainis *et al* 2006, Forzoni *et al* 2010). This chapter describes how experience and research has helped me to clarify my role.

### Sessional Work—Depending on the Team to Mediate

Nonverbal expression and communication is one of the great strengths of art therapy and is often a reason that an art therapist is seen as a valuable addition to a team. However, it is in the nitty gritty of verbal interaction that introductions are forged and the benefits of art therapy explained to prospective clients. As a sessional art therapist, I often depended on others to make the initial approach to patients. This wasn't ideal as most members of the multidisciplinary team struggled to 'explain' art therapy (personal communication). Staff education sessions and patient information leaflets all brought home to me the need to find simple accessible language to outline what art therapy could offer palliative patients. But as someone very new to palliative care myself I was on a learning curve and so the language I used relied heavily on theoretical definitions of art therapy and aspirations to be a psychotherapeutic magic bullet.

Very few patients come into palliative care settings looking for art therapy and this creates a dynamic where the therapist is entering their space and suggesting something that may be quite unfamiliar. This can add to the anxiety of both the patient and the therapist. This is best described for me by Bocking (2005) in her wonderfully honest 'don't know' story.

> Bald heads, tubes and dangling bags of urine, body fluids in recycled cardboard kidney dishes, drips and monitors. Coughs, smells lumps and bandages, cards, flowers, fruit bowls. Vulnerability and suffering. I walk into people's personal spaces with my box of paper and art materials and our eyes meet. Is what I am offering appropriate just now? Is it a yes or no moment?
>
> (Bocking 2005, p. 212)

And what is the art therapist offering? Some colleagues seemed to feel that I was there to distract the patients whilst others felt that art would be the key to unlock the most withdrawn and non-communicative of people.

Paola Luzzatto (1998) succinctly describes her dilemma on moving from psychiatry to oncology:

> I felt pulled in two directions: either keeping my emphasis on the mind of the patient as I used to do in working with psychiatric patients, or turning towards the body with my full attention, and accepting the physical need for relief, for relaxation, for soothing experiences that the patients were presenting.
>
> (Luzzatto 1998, p. 170)

When I did get the opportunity to be the one introducing art therapy I needed to prepare for the fact this could turn into an impromptu session. This need to be able to move from introduction to first and perhaps only session depending on the patient's time and energy is reflected in the literature (Coote 1998, Wood 1998, Balloqui 2005).

As I finished that sessional post and prepared to move to a new part of Ireland I reflected that the work that stood out was that where the patients had a clear idea of why they wanted to do art therapy.

## Working With Others—Roles and Definitions

Hyland Moon (2002, p. 17) wrote, 'What I want is one riveting story. I want it to introduce succinctly . . . instead multiple stories surface bobbing up like buoys on the water'. Art therapists working in palliative care are familiar with these multiple identities—enlightened teacher, recreational therapist, hospital artist and psychotherapist.

In my second post I was fully integrated into the team. I was the first art therapist to work in this setting but not the first artist. There was already a dedicated art room and regular recreational art groups. My challenge in introducing art therapy here was to distinguish it from art facilitation or teaching. Art therapy has its roots in arts practice in healthcare (Hogan 2001). It is not just that patients don't understand the distinction; they often don't experience it. Listening to the general discourse in the day room it was common for me to be called teacher and for clients to say how therapeutic they found the art facilitation sessions. Both myself and the art facilitator aspired to create a system whereby selection of patients for art therapy or art group was based on their expressed needs and preferences. To explore the dynamic between our two roles we devised a kind of Maslow's pyramid of art-based aims in care settings (Maslow 1943).

This helped us to define a theoretical transition point where in order to proceed the skills and training of an art therapist were needed. In practice we found that for clients the process of art therapy often began in the earlier stages. To use a model from the integral philosophy of Ken Wilbur (2000), art therapy transcended and included art facilitation, as opposed to being parallel processes. The difficulty in defining art therapy with its diverse aetiology and eclectic practice was reflected in an on-the-ground struggle to clarify what we were offering to patients. Colleagues working in settings without art facilitation still experienced ambiguity about their role and emphasised the range of ways that clients might use sessions. Offering choices and alternatives and making the introduction as broad based as possible was the strongest shared theme to emerge from my research (Ní Argáin 2008).

Taking this eclecticism as my starting point I began to look for information about patient's perceptions of art therapy. Quantitative studies of art therapy in oncology are establishing an evidence base for its efficacy in treating psychological symptoms of cancer patients (Nainis *et al* 2006, Monti *et al* 2006, Thyme *et al* 2009). Some of these studies also give us insight into patients' perceptions of art therapy, insights that I believe are transferable to the palliative context. An empirical study in Chicago (Nainis *et al* 2006) was one of the first attempts to quantify the anecdotal evidence that art therapy could help patients. It found that one session of art therapy can have beneficial effects on relieving both physical and psychological symptoms. Over 110 patients were approached to take part in this study, which used pre- and post-test measures to assess the effect of one session of art therapy on nine common symptoms. Of the patients approached, 50 accepted and 63 refused. The effects on the people who engaged in the session were very positive, with significant reductions in all symptoms except nausea, in a very diverse patient population. However, the authors note that despite these benefits a significant number of patients are 'reluctant' to try art therapy and that additional research is needed to understand the reasons why people refuse art therapy. I wonder if patients who benefit from art therapy are self-selecting and could more people benefit if the effects of art therapy were more widely understood and communicable?

As part of the experimental protocol this paper does tell us that subjects were asked 'what goals he or she had for the exercise'. Although there is no information on what the patients' stated goals were there is a breakdown of how they felt that the session had affected their well-being:

> When asked how they perceived art therapy changed their overall well being, 45 (90%) stated that the session distracted them and focused their attention onto something positive. Eighteen subjects (36%) responded that the therapy was calming and relaxing, 6 (12%) felt productive and worthwhile, and 12 (24%) felt that it was a pleasant activity. Three subjects (6%) commented that the art therapy had no effect.
>
> (Nainis et al 2006, p. 166)

It is worth noting the gap between what was being measured (symptoms), the stated objective of art therapy (to allow awareness and expression of an individual's deepest feelings), the protocol (which sounds more like a tuition session) and the patients' feedback. The latter tells us that patient experience when engaging in art therapy may be as much an escape from their deeper feelings as an engagement with them. This is not so very far from the 'relief from morbid introspection' described by Adrian Hill (1951) in the early literature on art therapy.

Is there any quantitative evidence of the more profound effects of art therapy that most art therapists witness and that have been documented in numerous case studies? An Italian research project is a better model for this type of research (Forzoni *et al* 2010). The methodology here involved interviewing a randomised group of 54 patients who had attended art therapy sessions during their chemotherapy treatment. Unlike the previous study, the patients had seen the art therapist for an average of four to five sessions. The semi-structured interviews were conducted after treatment by a psychologist who first asked whether art therapy had been helpful or not. The answer was remarkably similar to the earlier single session study as participants overwhelmingly experienced the sessions as helpful; only three patients felt art therapy was not helpful (5.5%) and 51 patients (94.5%) described art therapy as helpful. The psychologist then went on to explore what the patients perceived as being most helpful.

> It became quite clear that there was a continuum, from a more light, often physical experience (e.g., 'I was able to relax') to more profound experiences (e.g., 'I got in touch with my unconscious') triggered by the art therapy process.
>
> (Forzoni 2010, p. 43)

From content analysis of these interviews three main groups emerged:

Patients who described their experience as relaxing, creative and pleasurable. The researchers called this generally helpful (37.3%).

Those who perceived art therapy as helpful because art making encouraged them to talk about themselves and be listened to by the therapist. The researchers called this helpful because of the dyadic relationship with the therapist, (33.3%).

A third subsection saw art therapy as being helpful because of the dynamic between themselves, their artwork and the art therapist. These patients talked about 'expressing emotions and searching for meanings'. They felt that the images 'spoke to them'. This the researchers termed the triadic relationship (29.4 %).

These results are giving structure to our observations that art therapy can operate at different levels. One of the most important things I got from reading this paper was the simplicity of the language used. Was art therapy helpful? And if so, how?

I used this language to devise a tool/prop that I felt would clarify the introduction process and also act as a sort road map for the patient allowing us to have a conversation about where they wanted to go and most importantly how we might start. This consists of a laminated A4 sheet headed *How Could Art Help?* I deliberately wanted the sheet to visually communicate something about art therapy so it uses imagery and looks handmade—writing not typing. The text outlines some of the ways that patients may find art therapy helpful in ordinary everyday language.

## Sole Practitioner—What Kind of Art Therapist Are You?

I brought this tool to my next post with the Galway Hospice Foundation. Here I found myself as a sole practitioner in an institution that had a commitment to providing art therapy for its clients for the previous decade. I had two predecessors and each had made a significant contribution to the development of the post in different ways. As I introduced myself to colleagues I was struck by their curiosity to find out 'which kind of art therapist' I would be.

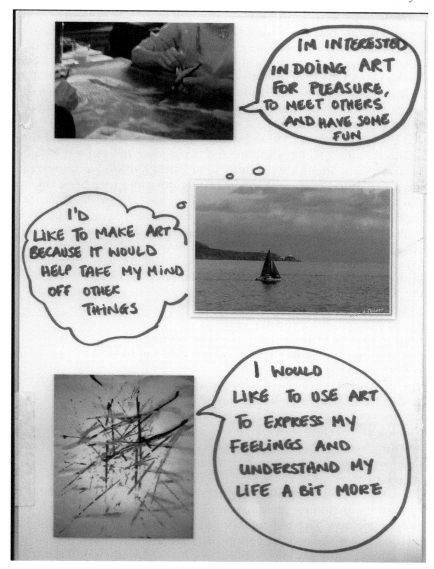

*Figure 5.1* How Could Art Help?

I explained that I saw myself as someone with expertise in how art can be 'good for you'. This firmly shifts the emphasis from art being a skill that you need to 'be good at'. Working out how art can be helpful involves getting to know the person and listening to their problems and what they are comfortable with. I realised at this stage that the eclectic practise art therapists described in my research involved knowledge and expertise in art media and methods, good communication and listening skills, understanding therapeutic dynamics and the dynamics of the creative process. What 'kind of art therapist' we are surely depends on the needs of the patient.

In a recent audit of introductions to 21 new referrals for art therapy I used my standard introduction tool with 14 patients. The referrals came from both daycare (8) and IPU (13). Of the seven patients where I didn't use the standard introduction, six were inpatients. Three of these patients were too tired/ill to engage even in an introduction. Of the three others, one had dementia and a more hands-on introduction in the art room was appropriate; the other two were very open to art therapy and didn't need any introduction. The one daycare patient who I didn't use the tool with had profound fatigue and sight problems. All the patients who engaged informally used art recreationally. The 14 patients who received a formal introduction were evenly divided between daycare and the IPU. After careful consideration, two inpatients and one daycare patient declined art therapy. Of the 11 patients who engaged in art therapy five wanted to have some pleasure and enjoy creative activity, three wanted to take their minds off things and three wanted to use art to express their feelings and try and make sense of what was happening. This small audit was my first attempt to quantify what I believed was an improvement in the quality of my initial engagement with clients. Using this tool I have been able to see each encounter as a small piece of research leading to greater practice wisdom (Scott 1990). From my experience people respond well to the laminate and often end up discussing the images as well as the text. For some the images have even been a starting point for their own artwork. As reflected in the sample audited most people are drawn to the idea of using art to relax and have some focus outside their illness. But many people comment on all of the options and this leads to a discussion about how art can help in different ways:

Being a source of pleasure and fun
Being a way to focus outside the illness
Being a way to express feelings and explore meanings
This leads to conversations about art making in relation to:
Quality of life issues
Management of anxiety associated with illness
Expression of feelings and development of insight

The third option has elicited different responses including people putting their hands over it and saying *'not that'*, but more often a puzzled *'I'd be interested in that but I wouldn't know how to use art that way'*. Does this latter comment indicate a space for a more directive approach to art therapy?

Included in the semi-structured introductory session are questions about the person's artistic history, including dressmaking, DIY, and gardening. I also ask about any previous experience they have of counselling or therapy. Having a standard beginning has allowed me to be more receptive to individual differences and preferences. While the patient art therapy journey may begin in one place they often find the sessions helping in ways they had not planned. In the language of the Italian study, they may begin using art in quite a light way and move through the sessions to the formation of a dyadic relationship and even on to insights generated through the creative process (triadic relationship). When reviewing work we may often return to the original laminate and discuss how different pieces of art making have helped in different ways. So as well as influencing the language used when introducing art therapy assessing client's needs and wishes, this study has also provided a framework for evaluating the art therapy journey.

The following case examples are illustrations of diverse beginnings and journeys where life meets art.

## The Importance of a Creative Space

June's independent and active life was changed hugely by her illness. No longer able to help her children and grandchildren she herself now needed their care and support.

With great strength of character she adapted to this challenge and continued to enjoy her family life and inspire those around her. When June came to the art room she explained how she was even limited in going to an art class as she had to avoid infection. Looking at the laminate she felt that art would help to bring some pleasure and fun into her life. She had always been a creative person and had even considered going to art college as a young woman but her activity now was limited to reading. This is just one of the images that June has made in the art therapy room.

It was inspired by a photograph and she loved the deep rich colours and its vibrancy. This piece required huge levels of engagement with mixing colour and close active looking. June got great pleasure from the process, which also reconnected her with a sense of 'being able' when so much of the past three years had involved 'not being able'. She continued to develop her creative practise, exploring a wide variety of media and making work full of meaning that reflects her engagement with life.

## Putting a Story Down on Paper

Michelle was one of the people that I didn't use the laminate with; she had recently been diagnosed and she went straight into telling her story. Her anxiety levels were very high; however, Michelle had an innate faith in the creative process and almost needed no introduction. Michelle's first image was painted over several weeks and encapsulated her illness and her hopes of recovery on one side of a path, on the other side she painted significant parts of her life to date.

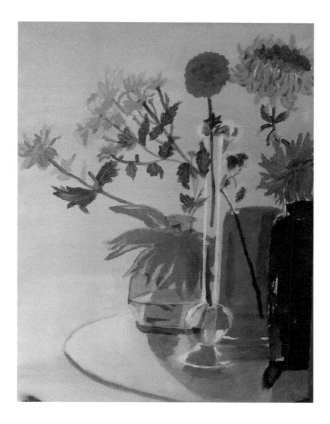

*Figure 5.2* June

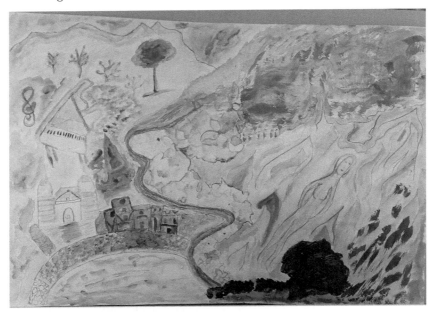

*Figure 5.3* Michelle (See Plate 6)

It is an example of art helping in a dyadic relationship. Having put her story down on paper Michelle described a sense of relief and a desire to continue painting for pleasure and as a way of *'not getting bogged down in the illness'*. Michelle has discovered a real passion for painting and continues to develop as an artist outside the art therapy sessions.

Both the preceding examples show how a sense of pleasure and creative involvement can contribute to a healthy sense of self even when dealing with illness.

## The Power of Symbolism

Darren was a young man who had defied the odds and was living with inoperable metastatic cancer way beyond medical expectations. He was not sure about art therapy but agreed to come to the art room to find out more. When Darren read the laminate he said that he wanted to express feelings and gain insight but doubted that he could do that using art material. I asked him a little about his experience of art. He was very good at mechanical drawing and had also built electronic devices. I suggested bringing in some objects from this part of his life to make a relief sculpture.

The following week Darren brought in two pieces of a computer component—he explained to me that each side of the component were different and this represented the different sides of his personality—the technical scientific side and the creative side. He was looking for some way to combine them in the clay and settled on superimposing one over the other so forming a cross. When Darren stepped back from this he was really surprised at what the resulting image conveyed to him. The image of the cross revealed a third aspect of his sense of self and one that was deeper and most important to him—his spiritual self. Once this became apparent the rest of the image flowed—the foot and hand and speech bubble with heart are symbols of his spiritual journey and the importance of love. A further stage of revelation happened when we made the reverse plaster image from the clay mould.

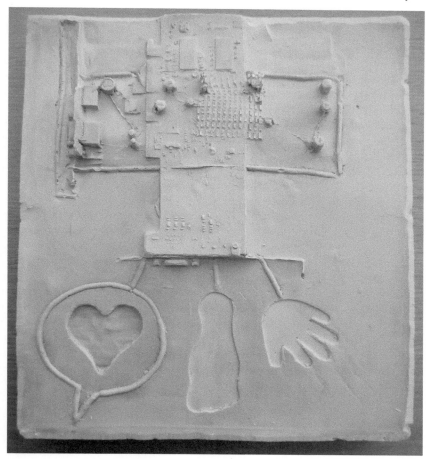

*Figure 5.4* Darren

Darren saw the cross as also resembling an aerial view of a fortress and /or safe place where the individual could gather the strength and nourishment needed for life's struggles and challenges. Darren felt that the power of visual art was in combining so many layers of meaning in one piece. He was excited by the possibilities for expression that this opened up but aware of the therapeutic boundaries needed to navigate this safely. This was an example of art helping through the triadic relationship.

## The Art of Living

Walter was an elderly man who had developed motor neuron disease (MND). He had been a particularly active man, a soldier, a fire chief and involved in his local community. He was now confined to a wheelchair, with limited movement in his hands and difficulty speaking. I asked Walter if he would like to explore art as a form of communication. Walter seemed to really like the laminate as he could point at words and images; it was a good start. He chose the third option, but he wasn't sure how he could physically use the art materials. My rule of thumb is that if someone can feed themselves they can draw. I presented Walter with a range of drawing implements from crayon to paint and asked him to try making a journey from one side of the paper to the other and then to rate the drawing implement. This placed the emphasis on what was good for Walter—what served him best as opposed to 'being good at art'.

Two things emerged from this simple beginning. Firstly Walter really enjoyed the independence of being left with some art material and an empty page. Secondly when we looked at the different marks he could relate them to imagery seeing clouds gathering over a mountain. This associative imagining does not come readily to everyone.

From then on Walter chose to work with the paint and brush, producing a series of paintings based on his long and active life. This image combined paint and pastel to make a portrait of a fellow firefighter.

At this stage it felt like Walter was benefitting from the dyadic possibilities of art therapy. Images generate rich data and discursive communication which is exactly what is missing when speech is a struggle and everything has to be spelt out. Between the image and my increasing ability to tune into Walter in the relaxed atmosphere of the art therapy room we rarely needed to use the alphabet sheet and our conversations became longer and deeper.

Despite enjoying the independent activity Walter was frustrated by his inability to make the marks he wanted. We had occasionally looked at the work of other artists when exploring a theme or colour and he began to ask to do this more and more and so a few weeks passed without any making. As part of a review session I used the laminate again reminding him of his original reason for engaging in art therapy and asking him how he felt that art therapy could continue to help. Walter again pointed to the section about expression but also explained that the image on this section had meant as much to him as the text. The colours reminded him of fire and the shape was like the grid of a city. We talked about Walter's frustration with painting and drawing and I suggested that he might like to try collage.

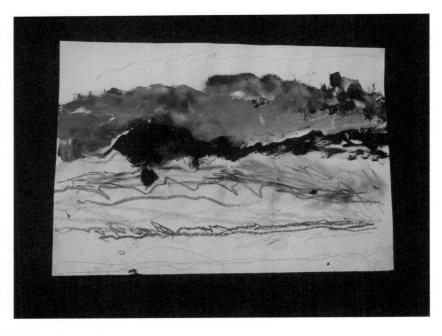

*Figure 5.5* Walter (Image 1)

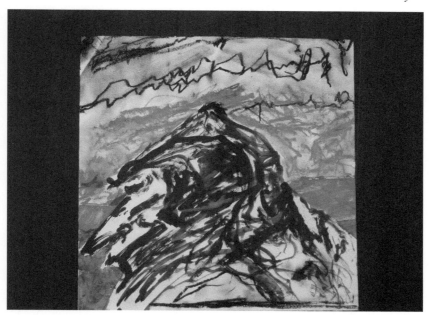

*Figure 5.6* Walter (Image 2)

Over the next few sessions Walter sifted through images and selected those he wanted, putting them together to make an image that expressed his experience of living with such a difficult illness.

Called 'Cause and Effect', it began with the light coming from the sky and representing power or God, and the rest of the piece seemed to be a conversation with this initial image. The next layer down represents the creation, nature, the world. Underneath this is the human layer which started off with the image of the man with the frying pan and the woman with the fire extinguisher. Walter described them as a poor man and a rich woman; despite their different circumstances they are the same to God. They will also both age as represented by the older figures. Walter was quite frustrated by the lack of images of older people in magazines and particularly asked me to get images of people who were old but not healthy. Parts of the collage have his characteristic humour.

In this piece Walter was putting his own experience, so difficult to rationalise on an individual level, into the bigger existential picture which can't be fully understood. In this piece he seemed to move from the dyadic to the triadic experience of art therapy, as the collage had its own dynamic in which Walter discovered meaning. This was the last image that Walter made.

## Concluding Comments

I began my work in palliative care with a very blurry vision of what art therapy could offer in this context. I found it challenging to enter into people's space and encourage them to try something new and different when their energy was low and their time precious. Research, both my own and that of others, has helped me to clarify my role and improve my practice. Maintaining choice but improving clarity has led to better therapeutic work, assessment and evaluation and included the patient in all these processes.

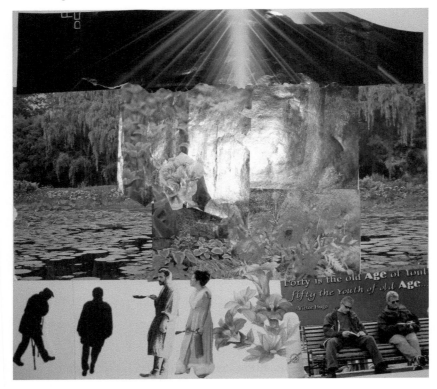

*Figure 5.7* Walter (Image 3)

Art therapists may see the relationship between these three ways of helping as hierarchical, with the holy grail of the triadic relationship being at the centre. But the truth is that we don't know if that is how it is experienced by patients who may view it as more interlinked. I certainly have experienced patients moving between expression and pleasure and distraction. There is room for further research in this area. Our knowledge of human psychology has moved on hugely since the foundation of the profession and the establishment of training. Both art and therapy are broad churches—contributing to resilience building, mindful awareness and cognitive change as well as cathartic expression, recognition of unconscious processes and increased self-awareness.

## References

Balloqui, J. (2005) The efficacy of a single session. In: *Art Therapy and Cancer Care*, ed. D. Waller and C. Sibbett. Maidenhead, England and New York: Open University Press.

Bocking, M. (2005) A 'don't know' story: Art Therapy in an NHS medical oncology department. In: *Art Therapy and Cancer Care*, ed. D. Waller and C. Sibbett. Maidenhead, England and New York: Open University Press.

Coote, J. (1998) Getting started: Introducing the Art Therapy service and the individuals' first experiences. In: *Art Therapy in Palliative Care*, ed. M. Pratt and M. Wood (London and New York: Routledge).

Forzoni, S., Perez, M., Martignetti, A., and Crispino, S. (2010) Art therapy with cancer patients during chemotherapy sessions: An analysis of the patients' perception of helpfulness. *Palliative and Supportive Care* 8: 41–48.

Hill, A. (1951) *Painting out Illness* (London: William and Norgate Ltd).

Hogan, S. (2001) *Healing Arts: The History of Art Therapy* (London and Philadelphia: Jessica Kingsley).

Hyland Moon, C. (2002) *Studio Art Therapy* (London and Philadelphia: Jessica Kingsley).

Luzzatto, P. (1998) From psychiatry to psycho-oncology. In: *Art Therapy in Palliative Care*, ed. M. Pratt and M. Wood (London and New York: Routledge).

Maslow, A. (1943) A theory of human motivation. *Psychological Review* 50 (4): 370–396.

Monti, D.A., Peterson, C., and Kunkel, E.J. (2006) A randomised control trial of mindfulness- Based Art Therapy (MBAT) for women with cancer. *Psycho-Oncology* 15: 363–373.

Nainis, N., Paice, J., Ratner, J., Wirth, J., Lai, J., and Shott, S. (2006) Relieving symptoms in cancer: Innovative use of Art Therapy. *Journal of Pain and Symptom Management* 31 (2).

Ní Argáin, D. (2008) Peeping in the door. *JIACAT: Journal of the Irish Association of Creative Arts Therapists*: 13–21.

Scott, D. (1990) Practice wisdom: The neglected source of practice research. *Social Work* 35 (6).

Thyme, K.E., Sundin, E.C., Wiberg, B., Oster, I., Astrom, S., and Lindh, J. (2009) Individual brief art therapy can be helpful for women with breast cancer: A randomised controlled clinical study. *Palliative and Supportive Care* 7: 87–95.

Wilbur, K. (2000) *A Theory of Everything* (Boston and London: Shambala).

Wood, M. (1998) The body as art: Individual session with a man with aids. In: *Art Therapy in Palliative Care*, ed. M. Pratt and M. Wood (London and New York: Routledge).

# 6 Snapshot of Practice

## A Case of Individual Art Therapy

*Grace Ong*

## About Me

I am a 34-year-old Chinese female residing in Singapore. Graduating from LASALLE College of Arts in 2012 with a master's in art therapy, I spent the first four years post graduation working as a full-time art therapist at Assisi Hospice. Founded by the Franciscan Missionaries of the Divine Motherhood in 1969, Assisi Hospice provides inpatient, day care and home care services. There are currently two full-time art therapists and both group and individual art therapy are available for inpatient and day care residents. Only individual therapy is available for those in home settings. I also have previous internship experience at a children's home while doing my MA Art Therapy training at LASALLE. This experience with children has helped me to provide child bereavement support through art therapy at Assisi Hospice. Currently, I am pursuing a diploma in Montessori to deepen my understanding of child development.

## About Singapore Palliative Care Services

Singapore has been making efforts in improving its quality of palliative care services over the past seven years since it was assessed on the first release of the quality death index in 2010. At that point in time, Singapore ranked 18 out of 40 countries and a national strategy for palliative care emerged in 2011 to move hospice and palliative care forward (Duke NUS & Lien Centre for Palliative Care, 2011). In 2014, the national guidelines for palliative care were adopted by the Ministry of Health and implemented. With this guideline, improvements have been made to care for terminally ill patients and to improve manpower skills. As of 2015, Singapore is now ranked 12th on the quality death index. However, room for improvements include re-looking at the financial model for palliative care. In terms of psychosocial care, more could be done to help de-stigmatize death and death taboos within the Singaporean society (Law, 2015). The Ministry of Health and the Singapore Hospice Council are currently working towards generating more discussions about end-of-life care at an earlier stage. These include conversations and information kits on advanced care planning or making advanced medical directives. The aim is to integrate social support with medical care as an entire care package (Lai, 2017).

## Case Example

Sally (pseudonym) was referred via the home care service for emotional support during her disease progression. She had been admitted to the hospital and during her stay had verbalized suicidal ideation. She had requested the art therapy service because she had previous experience in a group setting at another medical institution. I visited Sally at home, and this is where we conducted art therapy sessions.

### Accessing Personal Resources and Gaining Control

During the first visit, she said that she wanted to use the art for self-expression. She said that she felt very drowsy and that the level of sleepiness was not in line with her expectations of disease progression. I invited her to create an image of herself on the paper. Sally had prepared her own painting materials which were a gift from her colleagues. She was eager to use the paints but was unsure about how well she could use them. Taking tentative steps, she painted her first strokes but gained confidence with each step.

In the first few sessions we explored her disease progression, her feelings towards her disease and the sense of helplessness she felt when she experienced physical pain. These would often lead her to want to commit suicide. This was not because she wanted her life to end, but for the pain to end. It was also overwhelming to feel as if her body was unable to do what it used to do and that her mind was feeling physically different. Therefore, art making was a way for her to process these feelings. As seen through the artwork, the first one started out with only the use of paints, with more abstract form. However, as the sessions progressed, she was able to develop more coherence in the images. At the same time, her medications were being adjusted and she was more able to gain the clarity she needed in her mind.

### Tying in the Past With the Present

As trust and rapport developed in the therapeutic relationship, Sally began to share about some of the relationships she had been through in her images. This process raised some

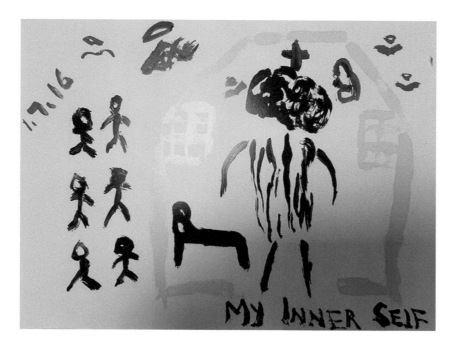

*Figure 6.1* My Inner Self

insights for Sally as she realized that there were patterns to relationships she had with the male figures in her life. Her father was someone close to her and she was more comfortable with him than with her mother. However, there was a yearning from him that was not fulfilled and she missed him after his death. Similarly, in the two male relationships she had, they were both long distance, separated both by geography and culture. She admitted that these relationships had caused hurt and never fulfilled her completely. Eventually, through spiritual discernment she believed that it was her "call" from God to become the "spouse of Jesus Christ". Similarly, both art therapist and Sally reflected on the distance between her spouse and herself. She was always yearning to be with him and could only do so in death. She explained that because of this, there was a frustration of waiting for the final moment to come.

Exploring these relationships also led her to realize a need to reconcile herself with her family, especially her mother who now had dementia. Through facilitation by the medical social worker, they had the chance of a family session where Sally was able to express her feelings and desire with regards to end-of-life care.

### Coping With Expectations

As her condition deteriorated, the pain was more difficult to manage and the home care nursing team found it difficult to manage her accompanying anxiety. In one session, we used a pack of cards to create a story. In the first three images, she shared about a holiday she wanted to have but was no longer important to her at that point. In the fourth card, she spoke about her eyes being drawn to the steeple in the background and how that was a symbol of God for her. When asked about the foreground she did not put much thought into it. However, when she was invited to make art in response to these images, she chose to replicate the foreground. She said that it was the suffering and the "cross" she had to carry to show her obedience to God. Her art did not take away the pain or the anguish of her illness, but it gave her a space to speak about her fears and to express what she wanted.

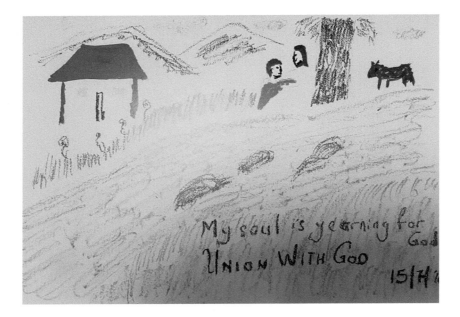

*Figure 6.2* My Soul Is Yearning for God

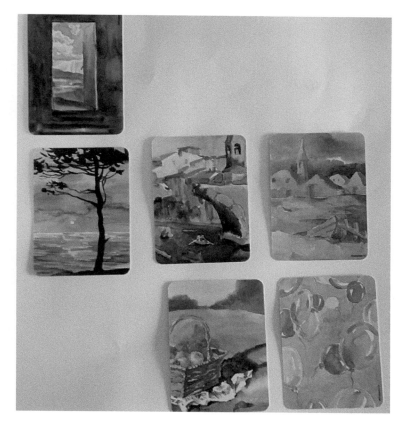

*Figure 6.3* Narrative of Her Current Situation

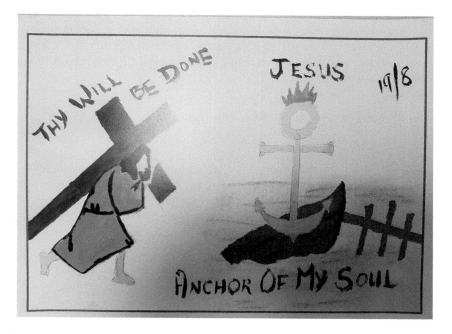

*Figure 6.4* Anchor of My Soul

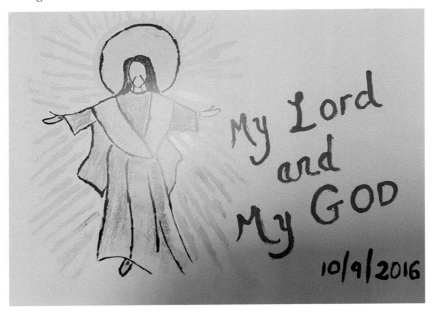

*Figure 6.5* My Lord and My God

*Closure*

Towards the end of the journey, she struggled greatly with wanting to pass away and yet not being able to as the disease was progressing slowly. During this time, she was admitted to the inpatient unit so that her family could focus on being with her while the hospice team took care of her medical and nursing needs.

In the last month before her passing, she did her final image where she looked towards meeting her "spouse" and God. In this time, she journaled and prayed in preparation for the final moments of the journey. Her image almost seemed like a resurrection, a moving on to a new life, as per her beliefs as a Catholic. She died comfortably, with the pain managed and her family with her.

## Advantages of Art Therapy in My Context

### 1. Legacy Work

Creating gifts and objects of significance for patients' loved ones. These may be done in the presence of the loved one or separately with the art therapist. If items are to be passed on only after the death of the patient, the art therapist has the responsibility of contacting the family member(s) involved. This process may form part of bereavement care, helping family members speak about the loss, relive good memories or to process the final moments of the patient.

### 2. Facilitate Conversations Between Family Members and Patient

Art images can become powerful tools of communication between family members and the patient. The symbolic meaning behind the artwork can open up conversations which may sometimes be awkward to initiate, such as expressing love, forgiveness and appreciation to each other.

### 3. Children of Patients—To Express and Process Death

Art therapy in a palliative care setting is a valuable tool in helping children explore their thoughts and feelings before the death of a loved one. The provision of art materials creates an environment that shifts the focus away from the patient to the child. Having a space where they can focus on their experience gives them a chance to express what they sometimes would not be able to if they were in the company of the patient and other family members. At other times, open studio sessions can help both children and adults change their perception of what a hospice is. The non-threatening space to enjoy art making in the company of others who might be in the same position can be comforting. Some feedback has been that the open studio offers respite for the child and allows them to do something for themselves or the patient if they choose to do so.

### 4. A Space to Be Together

At times, art therapy is simply a place to be. After the artwork is done and completed, the presence of the art therapist as a containing function is very important. Sitting with the loss, simply experiencing what the patient is experiencing is at times more powerful than the art making. It is in this being together that the authentic relationship is formed between the patient and art therapist, allowing the patient to feel less lonely.

## One Idea That Shapes My Work

The needs of the patient always come first. The first few questions to answer are "Who is Mr/Mrs/Ms xxx in front of me? What are his/her needs? What are the struggles they have been facing and are facing?" Once these questions have been answered, art materials are then offered and art therapy can begin. Many patients have never had an experience of doing art; in fact, it may sometimes seem like a luxury and a waste to do art at the end of life. However, developing a trusting relationship with the art therapist who understands their needs and concerns can help them to overcome their vulnerabilities and use art to create a space of deeper sharing.

## References

Duke NUS & Lien Centre for Palliative Care (2011, October 4). Report on the national strategy for palliative care (Rep.). Retrieved September 6, 2017, from www.duke-nus.edu.sg/sites/default/files/Report_on_National_Strategy_for_Palliative_Care%205Jan2012.pdf

Lai, L. (2017, July 27). MOH to embark on three-year project with Singapore Hospice Council to plug gaps in end-of-life care. *The Straits Times*. Retrieved September 6, 2017, from www.straitstimes.com/singapore/health/moh-to-embark-on-three-year-project-with-singapore-hospice-council-to-plug-gaps-in

Law, F. (2015, October 7). Singapore makes strides in palliative care. *Today Online*. Retrieved September 5, 2017, from www.todayonline.com/singapore/singapore-moves-quality-death-index

# 7a Religious Practice in Russia, Medical Settings, and End of Life Rituals

*Barbara Parker-Bell*

To provide a cultural context for the next chapter, this section is offered to assist the reader's understanding. During the communist times of the Soviet Union (1922–1991), Russians experienced a state-imposed atheism and a deconstruction of religious institutions (Evans & Northmore-Ball, 2012). Accordingly, religious practice of all denominations was severely restricted and people could not openly practice their faiths.

It is only after the dissolution of communism in the early 1990s that restrictions relaxed, and new and even collaborative relationships between state and church were forged, specifically with the Russian Orthodox Church (Benovska-Sabkova et al., 2010). According to Benovska-Sabkova et al., separation between church and government is still officially declared, but in actuality, the Russian Orthodox Church "receives substantial symbolic and material support from the state" (p. 17). Over half of religious institutions now registered in Russia (over 5000) are Russian Orthodox Churches (Embassy of the Russian Federation, 2017). The second greatest number of religious institutions registered are for practice of the Muslim faith (over 3000 institutions). Other religious groups that are recognized and registered with significantly smaller numbers include, but are not limited to, Baptist, Seventh Day Adventist, Evangelical, Roman Catholicism, Judaism, and Buddhist faiths. The greatest number of Russians who recognize an affiliation with a religious group identify their affiliation as belonging to the Russian Orthodox Church.

Evans and Northmore-Ball (2012) studied religious affiliation and practice trends in the Russian Federation by examining cross-sectional surveys conducted from 1993–2007. Data analysis uncovered significant resurgence of Russian Orthodoxy and a steady increase of religious identification and practice in the Russian population. In 1993 half of Russians identified as Russian Orthodox. This number grew to 80% in 2007. Data also showed that younger Russians rather than older adult Russians have been more likely to report religious affiliation as well as practice, represented by active churchgoing. Evans and Northmore-Ball (2012) posited that younger Russians have embraced the role of the Russian Orthodox Church to represent and uphold traditional values of moral conservatism. Younger adults who stated that they practiced Russian Orthodoxy attended church occasionally, which was more often than declared by older Russian adults.

As a part of this cultural transformation, a dialogue between the Russian Orthodox Church and the State regarding health and social services provided to Russian citizens has also been established (Diocese of the Russian Orthodox Church, 2017). For example, church collaboration with the Russian Ministry of Health has resulted in many hospitals having a room available for prayer. Alternatively, notices of services and contact information for the church may be available in a hospital. Patients may call the number to request an Orthodox priest to perform religious rites or to request religious items such as icons, educational materials, and prayer sheets, which may be distributed by church volunteers.

At the hospital in which Anastasia experienced the loss of her son, such a prayer room existed, but the room was consistently closed and unavailable for use. Clergy was not present at the hospital, but a phone number for the local church was available on the prayer room door for those who wished to reach out for religious and/or spiritual support. Based on anecdotal information, other religious group resource information is not generally displayed or available in Russian hospital settings.

Overall, when considering religion and spirituality in Russia, one must be mindful that that individuals will vary in terms of how they may embrace religion, spirituality, or secular values in their daily lives and life cycle events. However, given the predominance in Russian culture of the Russian Orthodox faith, some information will be provided about Russian Orthodox traditions regarding end of life rituals. In the context of Eastern Orthodox Faith, the broader umbrella under which Russian Orthodox faith falls, and in Russia in particular, deaths may be seen as good or bad deaths with each type of death having positive or negative repercussions for living family members or horrible illnesses.

After the loved one's death, careful preparations of the deceased's body for burial are followed to ready the person for the afterlife. (World Funeral Customs: Eastern Europe, 2017). Special items may also be left in the casket to provide comfort or afterlife use. Traditional practice calls for 40 days of mourning including ceremonies that are conducted at different stages throughout the 40 days, related to the soul leaving the body on the third day, the spirit leaving the body on the ninth day, and the body no longer existing, on the fortieth day. The body is laid in an open casket for viewing for a few days prior to the funeral service, which is typically held on the third day, after the soul has left the body. Burial is required in the Russian Orthodox faith as it is believed that the soul will reunite with the body at the time of the Last Judgment. After the funeral, any handkerchiefs used by mourners should be thrown away to "signify that everyone's sorrows should start to diminish once the funeral has passed, and not be carried much farther into the future" (World Funeral Customs: Eastern Europe, 2017, Russia, para. 6).

## References

Benovska-Sabkova, M., Kollner, T., Komaromi, T., Ladykowka, A., Tocheva, D., & Zigon, J. (2010). "Spreading grace," in post-Soviet Russia. *Anthropology Today*, 26(1), 16–21.

Diocese of the Russian Orthodox Church. (2017). *Church and medicine: Do not leave the hospital without pastoral care.* Retrieved April 16, 2017 from: www.mepar.ru/library/vedomosti/75/1618

Embassy of the Russian Federation. (2017). *Religion in Russia.* Retrieved April 7, 2017 from: www.rusemb.org.uk/religion

Evans, G., & Northmore-Ball, K. (2012). The limits of secularization? The resurgence of orthodoxy in post-Soviet Russia. *Journal for the Scientific Study of Religion, 51*(4), 795–808.

World Funeral Customs: Eastern Europe. (2017). *Russia.* Retrieved April 4, 2017 from: https://imsorrytohear.com/blog/tag/russian-funeral-traditions/

# 7b Addressing End of Life Care, Loss, and Bereavement in the Russian Federation

*Barbara Parker-Bell, Tatiana Vaulina, and Anastasia Stipek*

## Introduction

The creation story of this chapter is a rich one. I have been tremendously blessed to have the opportunity to visit and collaborate with many wonderful professionals and advocates of art therapy in the Russian Federation during the autumn and early winter of 2016 as a part of a Fulbright Scholar Grant. Without my Russian colleagues' assistance in terms of research, translation, questionnaire responses, and willingness to share cultural, professional, and personal stories related to end-of-life care, loss, and bereavement, this chapter would not have come together. I extend my thanks to art therapy practitioners who helped me find professionals working in this specialty throughout the Russian Federation. I particularly want to thank my coauthors who wrote from the heart and helped me gain a fuller understanding of Russian perspectives.

My own personal experience with end-of-life care, loss, and bereavement stem from my private practice art therapy work in Northeastern Pennsylvania, USA. End-of-life issues, loss, and bereavement are natural themes that enter into all people's lives and I have had the privilege of supporting many people through these life passages in creative ways. No matter one's country of origin, end-of life is experienced. Yet, how one may reflect on, prepare, or seek support for end-of-life or loss of loved ones is influenced by one's social and cultural lens. In addition, historical, geographic, and institutional conditions impact the resources one may have for personal or family medical or psychological care. In this chapter, I hope to illuminate some of the aforementioned dynamics in the Russian Federation. Availability of end-of life care, service providers' roles, as well as prevalent attitudes towards seeking psychological help will be addressed. Additionally, perspectives and experiences of art therapy service providers will be offered, followed by a story of healing from loss achieved through the artistic process and reflection written by my Russian coauthor Anastasia Stipek.

## End-of-Life and Hospice Care in the Russian Federation

"The palliative care movement in eastern Europe started during the communist era, when the needs of the dying were much neglected" (Luczak, 2000, p. S.23). For example, in Poland, the movement originated with volunteers who wished to ease the suffering of cancer patients in medical wards. Additionally, visiting hospice advocates from Britain provided information to Polish medical professionals about hospice concepts and the use of oral morphine to help ease pain. In the 1990s, the palliative care movement spread slowly across Eastern Europe and eventually into Russia after the dissolution of the Soviet Union. Luczak noted that international organizations were significant catalysts in the development of hospice care in the Russian Federation.

Accordingly, much of the literature available in English about the development of hospice in the Russian Federation has focused on international exchanges of information and training of medical professionals in the Russian Federation by international guests (Becker, 1999; Matzo et al, 2007; Paice et al, 2008). Nurses were often the benefactors of this training because, according to Paice et al., nurses had great potential to impact end-of-life care due to the greater amount of contact time they had with patients and families. Matzo et al. described the End-of-Life Nursing Education Consortium (ELNEC) efforts in Russia that occurred between 2005–7. Matzo et al noted that at that time in the Russian Federation, only a limited number of nurses had received any formal education in palliative care during their professional studies. They further stated that Russia was considered a "palliative care poor country" (Matzo et al, 2007, p. 247) due to the small number of healthcare centers that had incorporated palliative care into treatment, particularly in relationship to the large population and expanse of national geography. Conferences were held and curricula included material related to sharing terminal diagnoses with patients and family, pain management, comfort care, burnout prevention (for nurses), and home-care. ELNEC trainings in Russia were conducted with nurses that worked in neonatal units as well, and with members of faith-based communities or lay caregivers who were frequent providers of "care, social services or spiritual support to hospice patients and people living with or affected by HIV or AIDS" (Matzo et al, 2007, p. 249). ELNEC continues to provide training to medical professionals around the world. Educational topics such as involving families as part of the care team and attending to psychosocial and spiritual needs in addition to the care recipients' physical needs, are a part of the curriculum.

Importantly, ELNEC emphasizes the ethics of cultural competency for its trainers, and the necessity of addressing and respecting cultural values and traditions regarding healthcare and the death and dying process (Ferrell et al, 2015). For example, in Russia, it is the role of the physician to discuss prognosis, comfort care, or matters related to death or dying with those affected. Consequently, nurses have often been restricted from communicating with patients and family members regarding these topics reducing the potential for nurse provision of support and psychological care at the end of life. In this context, trainers who were nurse educators did not impose their systems or values on the trainees to promote a different system. Yet, as a result of trainings further dialogues about roles of professionals in palliative care have occurred among doctors and nurses.

In contemporary Russia, the availability of palliative care for adult patients is now approved and mandated to be a part of healthcare systems by the Russian Ministry of Health (Krom et al, 2016). Three types of palliative care services have been identified as important to cultivate and provide: a palliative approach to those in emergency care, general palliative care that is provided to patients with chronic diseases at non-terminal stages of treatment, and specialized palliative care that is provided for patients in a terminal state. However, the development of systems that assure educational training for care professionals and institutional provision of palliative treatment is still in progress. For example, professional end-of-life care within hospital or inpatient clinics is more apt to be found in larger cities and is often not available in vast regions of rural Russia. Krom et al (op.cit) suggested that an emphasis on building a network of outpatient clinics and home-based services needs to occur to fill the gap of care that exists outside large city centers. The authors assert that the promotion of palliative care outpatient clinics throughout Russia will improve the medical and psychological care of patients with chronic noninfectious diseases. Some of the primary challenges to the achievement of these developmental goals relate to the complexity of facilitating collaboration among interdisciplinary organizations. Interdisciplinary professionals participating in end of life care may include physicians, nurses, social workers, and psychologists.

## Psychological Help in the Russian Federation

The role of mental health professionals in the context of end-of-life care in Russia is less available in the literature. Only one source (Matzo et al, 2007) mentioned the presence of a psychologist at end-of-life care trainings. Part of this omission relates to Russian cultural history and educational traditions and practices related to the provision of psychological help. Currie et al, (2012) explain some of the history of professions such as psychology, social work, and counseling. While interest and practice of Freudian psychology existed in Russia before the Communist era, after the Russian revolution in 1917, psychological practices were restricted to those that supported Marxist and Leninist ideology and its enforcement. It was not uncommon during that time that psychiatric diagnosis and treatment was assigned based on the perceived threat the person may present to society based on ideological non-conformity versus psychiatric or psychological conditions (Currie et al, 2012). A history of any psychological treatment or hospitalization also became a part of a person's work documentation and negatively influenced potential for subsequent employment. Consequently, Russians took great care to avoid mandated or voluntary usage of psychological services. Conversations about personal or emotional concerns were generally reserved for very close family and friends. Even after Russia experienced transformational changes in governmental structure and societal philosophies providing citizens with more life freedoms at the end of the century, feelings of distrust of mental health professionals continued to linger (Currie et al, 2012). Alternatively, people could turn to the Russian Orthodox Church for direction or comfort concerning life problems. Historically, the church has been seen as a suitable place for care of the Russian soul and may often be a preferred resource for psychological help.

Still, mental health professions, beginning with social work, re-emerged and grew after the fall of Communism in the 1990s to address the population's new social needs (Currie et al, 2012). Following years of detachment from Western psychology, interest in studying and practicing psychological concepts increased and educational institutions teaching such concepts began to appear. In the Russian Federation, psychological care professionals include medically trained psychiatrists, psychologists, social workers, and counselors, a subset of the social work field.

Art therapy is not yet considered a separate mental health profession (Karkou et al, 2011; Russian Art Therapy Association, 2017). Generally, art therapy practitioners are psychiatrists or psychologists or artists with additional training or experience with art-based psychotherapeutic interventions. Therefore, it is difficult to enumerate how many mental health professionals consider themselves art therapy practitioners. Formal art therapy educational programs for helping professionals have only recently come into existence on a post-graduate basis (Russian Art Therapy Association 2015; ECARTE, 2017). Other exposure to art therapy may occur in elective classes in a psychology degree program, or a special topic or master class (Parker-Bell & Vaulina, 2015). Educational conferences hosted by creative arts therapy organizations and associations are regularly held in Moscow and St. Petersburg and provide additional avenues for art therapy learning. Unfortunately, such conferences are not commonly available in Asian regions of the Russian Federation.

## Art Therapy in the Russian Federation

Yet, much has been accomplished. In 2017, the Russian Art Therapy Association will celebrate its 20th anniversary. For 20 years, many passionate individuals have worked vigorously to support the continued growth and recognition of the field through communicating the benefits of art therapy via research, writing, professional presentations, and public information. Other groups, such as the International Art-Therapeutic Club and the Expressive Therapies Association in Moscow, also bring professionals together to provide opportunities for trainings. Russian art therapy journals, the *International Journal of Art Therapy: "Healing Art,"* and *"Art & Therapy"* (English translation of Russian journal titles Международный журнал арт-терапии "Исцеляющее Искусство" and "Арт & Терапия") sponsored by the Russian Art Therapy Association and the International Art-Therapeutic Club respectively, are written in the Russian language. In addition, organizations and universities host international guests to provide lectures and workshops to expand the scope of information available to Russian clinicians. As a result of these developments, practitioners of art-based interventions work in a variety of places. These environments include schools, psychiatric institutions, drug and alcohol treatment centers, and more recently, medical and rehabilitation settings. Innovative art therapy services have expanded to museums (The Russian Museum, 2017) and family therapy clinics (Shestakova & Kerr, 2015) as well as private practices.

## Art Therapy in Hospice Settings

To obtain more particular information about art therapy contributions to end-of-life psychological care, Russian professionals were consulted. Coauthor Tatiana Vaulina, psychology professor at Tomsk State University, made calls to hospice care centers in the Tomsk region to inquire about available services. While hospice centers did exist in this city of over 500,000 people, none of the hospice centers had psychologists or others specifically on staff to address psychological care. The search was expanded and the authors connected with psychology and art therapy practitioners in Moscow and St. Petersburg, the largest cities in the Russian Federation. Key contacts responded quickly with names and e-mail addresses of those who had some experience in this area. Questions were crafted in English and then in Russian by Dr. Vaulina. Professionals were asked to address where they were located, how their work was involved in hospice or bereavement care, the amount of time they have worked in this area, philosophies that guided them, and how they incorporated creative arts into treatment. Additionally, respondents were asked to share a case example if they wished and if permission had been received from the client and/or clients' family.

In total, four individuals from different areas in Russia; Moscow, Ulyanovska Region (south and east of Moscow), and Tomsk (in Western Siberia) completed the questionnaire. Their experience in psychology and art therapy with end-of-life care and bereavement spanned from 3–5 years to more than 15 years and they practiced in hospitals, a woman's health center, private practice, and family homes. When they provided art therapy services, a variety of structures were utilized such as individual, group, and family formats. In terms of guiding philosophies, the humanistic philosophy was unanimously endorsed. In addition, respondents identified existentialism, family systems, cognitive behavioral approaches, and Ericsonian hypnotherapy. Three of the practitioners worked with those undergoing cancer care, and the private practitioner worked with clients experiencing bereavement when that was germane to clients' cases.

When asked why and how they used art therapy processes in treatment, the respondents cited the capacity of the creative arts to transform clients' negative emotions and feelings, thereby providing the client with some relief, as a primary motivation for art therapy use in treatment. They noted that art engagement contributed to psychological and emotional adaptation and distraction from thoughts of the illness, negative predictions, pain, and fear. Through the tangible and pleasurable process of working with materials, defenses surrounding exploration of psychological concerns were decreased. Art methods helped clients verbally express their fears and helped them find new meanings. One respondent asserted, in a particular case of child who experienced life-threatening cancer and a series of challenging cancer treatments, that the creative and supportive experiences of art therapy helped the child garner his strengths so that the end result was a shift from a hypothesized terminal diagnosis to a sustained remission diagnosis. The practitioner cited that the art therapy work provided joy, strength, and solace to the child and his family during the very difficult times.

## Methods and Examples

Based on respondents' case descriptions, two main art therapy strategies emerged, one focused on spontaneous artmaking with individuals (adults and children) and thematic work conducted in group treatment processes with cancer patients in hospital or outpatient settings. Practitioners were sensitive to media qualities and how these qualities related to client comfort and need for control or expression. A range of art materials such as pencils, collage, paints, or clay were offered. When artmaking themes were provided, they were often broadly cast allowing for symbols and metaphors to emerge.

During individual art therapy conducted with the young child mentioned above, the practitioner described the child's spontaneous artwork as relating to protective figures doing battle with monster figures that represented his cancer. Symbols of death also entered into his artwork and his characters worked to avoid those symbols. His prolific and absorbed creativity using diverse media was supported by the practitioner, his family, and the staff of the oncology setting, as it helped him cope with the physical and emotional effects of the cancer journey and the possibility of death (E. Usanova, personal communication, December 3, 2016).

In the context of group art therapy, another Russian practitioner noted offering a group of clients the direction to make a whole world out of clay. As the group worked to build their world and observed each other's creations, the participants recognized that they were grappling with symbols of death, and were challenged to consider how these symbols fit into the world they created. While symbols of death were initially seen as unwelcome guests within their collaborative art piece, discussions among the group, facilitated by the professional, allowed the participants to transform their hostility regarding death's presence into a greater sense of acceptance.

## Strengthening Support for Work With Life-Threatening Illness, End-of-Life Care, and Bereavement

In all the reports from the professionals working in the hospital setting, a strong message related to the need for institutional, educational, and community support for art therapy use in life threatening illness and end-of-life care was asserted. Respondents expressed concern that many people facing issues of potentially terminal illness and end-of-life care are not being provided psychological care in any form. As mentioned previously, hospice and end-of-life care practices are relatively new to Russia. Therefore, governmental regulations to set standards for hospice and end-of life care are better developed in reference to medical aspects of care and less developed and implemented in regard to psychological care. If provision of psychological care in such medical settings is considered rare, art-based psychological care is even more rare, as there is no officially recognized or sanctioned art therapy profession. Practitioners that do provide art-based services in medical settings often contribute to client care as volunteers, which makes this type of career focus unsustainable over the long-term. One survey respondent proposed a three-step remediation process. The first step would be to establish the consistent presence of psychologists in hospital units that address life-threatening and terminal illness. The next step would be to unite the psychologists and other practitioners who utilized art-based interventions in this clinical specialty. After this was achieved, this group of professionals could advocate for art-based psychological care in hospice and end-of-life care settings.

## Barbara's Introduction to Anastasia's Story

When gathering information for this chapter in Tomsk, I was fortunate to meet the third author, professional psychologist, researcher, and art therapy practitioner, Anastasia Stipek. Over coffee, Anastasia and I discussed her interest in using art therapy to support healthy bereavement processes. It was at that time, she began to tell her own story of loss and grief, and the pivotal role that art had played in helping her heal and return to living following the death of her newborn child. Anastasia was fortunate in that she had access to inner resources and skill sets in art and psychology to help her make sense of her experiences. Others experiencing such loss may not have possessed the same level of resources and resiliency. In the hospital and neonatal settings Anastasia found herself in, no professional came forward to address her or her husband's emotional well-being regarding their child's life and death struggle and eventual loss to that struggle. No referrals to psychological help or support groups were made, and the topic of loss seemed to be avoided, making the family feel more alone in their grief. As previously explained, there are systemic and cultural factors that contribute to this omission. As a survivor of this traumatic loss, Anastasia has committed herself to finding ways to offer art therapy services to neonatal units and parents who experience this sadness. She is well on her way in this journey; please read her story, the final section of this chapter.

## Anastasia's Introduction to Her Story

I am Anastasia A. Stipek, wife, artist, practicing psychologist and art therapist, senior researcher of the Department of Psychology at Tomsk State University in Tomsk, a Russian city in western Siberia. It will be my role in this chapter to provide some understanding of cultural tendencies regarding grief and loss in the Russian Federation as well as to report on my own grief and healing experiences. In Russia, people tend to grieve silently so that no one can see you or even notice that you are in grief. Many times, people in Russia do not grieve at all. They try to forget their tragedy as soon as possible and never go back to it. Only later do they notice that the pain is still there; it was hidden inside and prevented them from living a fuller and happier life. Historically, Russians were this way. They were too busy working on the fields of crops that fed them; the summer is short and the winter long. Their spiritual experiences were limited to some religious holidays which were carefully followed. Later, they experienced dreadful revolution and war experiences, perestroika—a political movement for reformation within the Communist Party of the Soviet Union during the 1980s which consisted of the restructuring of the Soviet political and economic system to capitalism—and prior to that, the Soviet Union, which required working as much as one could for the sake of the country. People had to survive; they did not have time to grieve about all their losses. There were too many losses in every family during those times. And people did not know how to grieve. Currently, this situation is changing, but slowly. The saying "be strong and go on" still remains in cultural memory.

For many Russian people, the tragic experiences they face in life evoke and initiate a search for spiritual fundamentals, with the goal of receiving some explanation or assistance with accepting the unchangeable. My search for spiritual fundamentals began a long time ago with Russian classic writers and thinkers like Tolstoy, Dostoevsky, Nikolai Berdyaev, Ivan Ilyin, and some others. Later, I understood that they were the founding fathers of Russian existential philosophy. I also am guided by Burno's (2005, 2011) fundamentals and principles of therapy by means of creative self-expression, and by Alekseichik (1993, 1998, 2007), who is the creator of Russian existential psychotherapy originating from Russian Orthodox culture. Dr. Alekseichik created a psychotherapeutic approach which is called Intensive Therapeutic Life (ITL). This approach refers to the Orthodox psychotherapy principle of spiritual growth and development. ITL includes a large range of carefully worked out levels of organization of the therapeutic process and is an opportunity for clients to consider their lives in the physical, social, psychological, and spiritual dimensions, with an emphasis on the spiritual dimension. ITL helps clients move from problems to resolving problems and towards dealing with core existential issues.

Additionally, I grasp, with all my heart, the words and ideas I read in sermons by Orthodox Metropolitan Anthony of Sourozh (2003) and texts by Optina Elders (Rozhneva, 2014). These sermons address and reveal new meaning for me in regard to concepts of life, death, health, truth, freedom, soul, spirit, eternity, hope, faith, love, disease, renewal, and many others. An example prayer of the Optina Elders (Optina Elders, 2017, bullet 21) is provided below:

> Grant unto me, O Lord, that with peace of mind I may face all that this new day is to bring.
> Grant unto me to dedicate myself completely to Thy Holy Will.
> For every hour of this day, instruct and support me in all things.
> Whatsoever tidings I may receive during the day, do Thou teach me to accept tranquilly, in the firm conviction that all eventualities fulfill Thy Holy Will.
> Govern Thou my thoughts and feelings in all I do and say.
> When things unforeseen occur, let me not forget that all cometh down from Thee.
> Teach me to behave sincerely and rationally towards every member of my family, that I may
> bring confusion and sorrow to none.
> Bestow upon me, my Lord, strength to endure the fatigue of the day, and to bear my part in all
> its passing events.
> Guide Thou my will and teach me to pray, to believe, to hope, to suffer, and to love.
> Amen

All these great people and their messages helped me to keep my bearings and grow spiritually. In their books, they revealed Orthodox meanings of grief, pain, creativity, purpose of life, and much more. With their help, I understood that my grief was not larger than anyone else's. I read that my favorite writers and thinkers also lost their children, newborn, infant, or later in life. Their stories consoled me and gave me strength. Tolstoy and his wife lost five of their thirteen children (Porter, 2010; Tolstoy, 2015). Fyodor Dostoevsky and his wife (Dostoevsky A., 1977; Dostoevsky F., 1979) lost two of their four children. They grieved but did not fall into dark despair. Tolstoy (2015) wrote in his diaries that he saw mysterious and higher meaning in the deaths of his children. He achieved a greater connection to his spiritual center through the processes of loss, grief, and reflection.

## An Art-Therapist Who Lost Her Newborn Baby: To Our Beloved Son Illiam

We lost our newborn son. My pregnancy proceeded without complications and the delivery was to term but it was not easy for our baby to be born. He was born with excessive cord encirclement, he did not cry out and his lungs did not open. After birth, he spent seven days in intensive care and he developed aspiration pneumonia and his little heart gave up. Our baby died. Now three months after the tragedy, I am writing this text with hopes that my story and my experience will help my many sisters in grief. Since 2010, I have been a practicing psychologist and have specialized as an art therapist the last five years. I learned that creativity through art could easily be applied as psychotherapy to adults, children, and me.

At my son's birth, it was unbearably difficult for me to be with people who wanted to help me. I even asked my parents and close relatives to keep their distance as I was not ready to deal with their pain, expectations, and questions. I was sinking. The physical and spiritual pain was beginning to drown me. While this was happening, the clinic seemed to ignore my experience. Only my husband's encouraging words, expressed through his own pain and tears, his strong and bright soul which could accept what was happening and overcome it, saved me and brought me to life. He was by my side when the ground crumbled under my feet; he was there for me and his presence lifted me back up. Everything happened so fast, I did not have time to realize what was happening and how we were going to live life. But, when my husband and I would talk, my spirit revived and I began to see a future life.

The first few days after labor I needed to physically feel that my life would continue as usual, as if this confirmed that I was still alive. Simple things confirmed reality such as eating, drinking, showering, and flossing my teeth. Really, I did not care about those things, but these everyday activities gave me a strong connection to life, allowing me to "land" on my two feet. Again, a few days after the funeral, it was important for me to fill our life with normal things like cooking, cleaning, etc. I felt a great need to understand and see what my life was going to look like because the life I prepared for was not destined to come. The feeling of emptiness and depletion felt like it would never heal. I knew creativity was always healing for me, but I was afraid to start creating again as if I wanted to stay in my grief. I lacked courage and strength to overcome my despair and to make that first step.

With the death of our son, my ability to love and to create did not end, it was just hard to open it. But with help, I pulled my oil paints out of the drawer, prepared several canvases and began to paint simple things: branches and leaves. It was slow at first, but I began to paint one painting after another. I did not think about sophisticated images, I simply painted what I saw. It was October, and fall was beautiful and bright. I remembered how two years ago, I painted a picture of fall (Figure 7.1). That painting is one of our favorites as it reminds us of our favorite song "Autumn Leaves," the one my husband and I sang to our baby boy in intensive care, changing some words in it, but keeping the melody. Many romantic events in our family life were connected with this song: how we missed each other during some business trips, lazy weekends after a working week, birthdays, etc. Autumn and leaves were something from the past that connected me to the future. Here's a portion of what I wrote about that painting two years ago:

> After my evening walk in the park. I was so inspired by all those leaves on the ground with their harsh scent and beauty . . . I could see so clearly and irresistibly that I must

paint immediately all this life of the evening park. Procrastination would be death and you would not believe it but the next morning all those leaves were covered with the first snow. I was amazed. The mystery of what had happened was revealed to me. The snow covered everything so thoroughly I could not see that colorful carpet of leaves I admired last evening. That life not only ended but had become quite different in one night. While I was painting, the world was changing and by the morning my work had been completed and the world was reborn.

I consumed this text and felt that I was going in the right direction. I was painting autumn which connected me with the essentials of life: hope, faith, and love. With each new painting, I became stronger, and my pain opened new meanings for me, made me look into my inner depths, and gave me the inspiration to turn around and live. Another helpful activity for me was keeping a diary. Putting my thoughts and feelings into words helped me feel alive and real, to think clearly and understand what had happened, to comprehend reality and reveal new meanings. I tried to write down everything I had gained in our tragic experience.

My first painting after Illiam's death (Figure 7.2) allowed me to look back at the memories of fall when my son was born and died, and I wanted to keep all the memories, to never lose them. My September was filled with the expectations of "That Great Day" of excitement when I would meet our baby and this experience will not be forgotten.

More painting came, and the smallest painting among them was that bright, sunny, sad, and joyful autumn. I wanted to see bright colors and a turquoise river on that painting. I named that tiny painting "Reading the Forest in Autumn." I named it so because I was inspired by an illustration from a children's book, "Springlet," the book I read to my son when he was in intensive care. A little story from that book was called "Forest in Autumn."

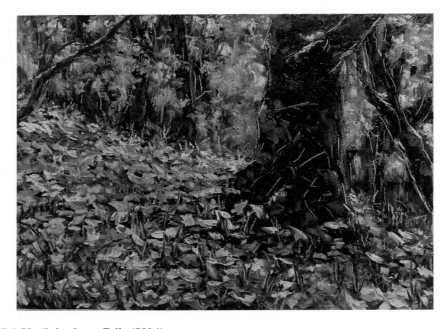

*Figure 7.1* Until the Snow Falls (2014)

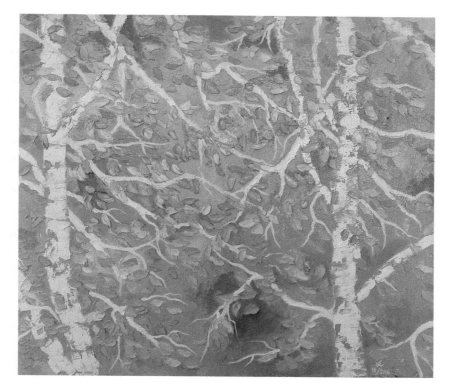

*Figure 7.2* My September-Like October (2016) (See Plate 1)

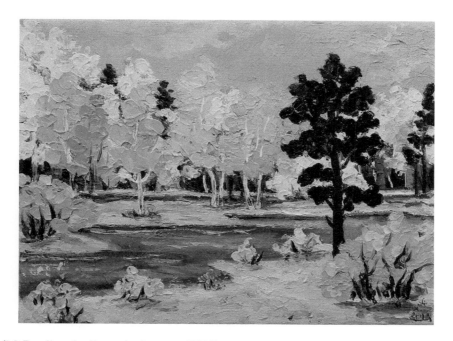

*Figure 7.3* Reading the Forest in Autumn (2016)

For me, it is very important not to forget everything I gained in my loss. I know that people can easily devalue what is so important for them; I often face such situations when working with clients. Taking notes in my diary and painting were the ways for me to remember my son and to keep my spiritual gains. Many times, I blamed myself for all that had happened. It is difficult and really not possible to find the ones at fault, or to understand the point of this loss and suffering. What saved me from the pain and agony of tearing my heart apart was looking ahead, not justifying myself, not blaming anyone, but simply continuing to live life.

My son's death showed me how much I am afraid of my own death. With this fear ringing loud in my heart, everything lost value and became meaningless for my existence or someone else's. I could feel that it was not right and it was impossible to live with this fear since it had a paralyzing effect. It was not the first time that I looked at death and felt this fear. But never before did I see that abyss so vast, overwhelming, and dreadful. I said to my husband "I feel like I'm going to fall into this, what shall I do?" He knew that the phrases like "do not be afraid" would not help me. He replied with a question: "What can you create right now?" I remembered that I wanted to paint a winter tree that I had seen, and with his push of encouragement, I took a canvas and start painting the tree.

It was very difficult for me to get started, making the way through my fears, but at the same time, I felt how I was looking straight into my fears through my unstoppable tears. Soon something happened while I was painting and struggling with my fear, something flashed before me and my fear disappeared, as if my fears began to burn out—I stared death in the face. From that moment to now, that experience is with me and simply recalling it relieves my anxiety and fears.

The words of one of my friends gave me consolation when she said, "Your baby came into this world not to learn something, but to give you love and humbleness." I believe this is so. Our son brought us his gift and this I will never forget. This solace helped me remember my pregnancy. I recollected and wrote down everything we did with my son in my belly. Our life was wonderful! I found great comfort and strength in my memories. I was a mother then, and in some sense, I continue to be a mother.

Still, at this time, it is not easy to continue life after it changed so suddenly. It is not easy to meet people and talk to them about what happened. Questions about the baby are unavoidable because people saw me pregnant, a happy expectant mother. I am ashamed to look at them and meet their eyes. Here, Figure 7.4 represents my question: Why am I ashamed?

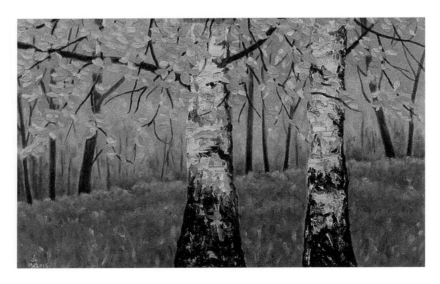

*Figure 7.4* Clarity (2016)

In conclusion, I would like to provide points that may help my fellow professionals be more effective with mothers who have lost a baby:

- **Healing presence.** It is important to ensure that a "genuine spiritual presence" is available to the woman in grief. Spirituality in this context transcends specific religious expressions and its attachments to religious values and rituals. It refers to a subjective experience of one's own inner dimension and includes belief in personal growth, universal human morals, values, and traditions. Therefore, the aim is to help loved ones be next to her, not as a formal presence but a presence of being in which emotional and spiritual energy may resonate. This healing presence may take place in silence, or in a conversation. Avoid phrases like, "Everything will be alright," "Do not worry," "Do not cry," etc.
- **Daily routine.** It is important to help a woman to continue living life and working on routine things, especially those that have always been a part of her everyday life, those that are regular, repetitive or even ritualistic in nature. It is important to help a woman to find "her activities," to identify them, and in some sense, to "make sure" that she implements them.
- **Hope of life.** It is very important in the first weeks to half a year, to help a woman keep focused and see that new plans can be made, life goes on. However, she should face her grief at her own pace without rushing, and then turn towards her new life content. After the loss of a baby, life content changes radically. Filling life with new content is accomplished gradually as healing from the wounds of loss takes place.

A woman creates new life and it is important to show her that any loss does not cease her creativity. Love extends beyond Death.

## Final Notes

In the Russian Federation, art based end-of-life and bereavement care, deeply rooted in Russian philosophy and cultural knowledge, currently occurs in small pockets of places throughout the expansive nation. Like Anastasia, people may heal themselves through art and reflection processes after loss, but many more could benefit from the support of a therapeutic presence skilled at helping people move through emotional and spiritual processes to achieve healing resolution. As Russia continues to develop its network of end-of-life care systems, and as attitudes towards acceptance of psychological help softens, perhaps practitioners of art-based care will experience the institutional conditions and acknowledgment they need to reach more people. We, as chapter authors, appreciate the opportunity to communicate this wish.

## References

Alekseichik, A. Ye. (1993). 'Voskhozhdeniye na vershinu'. [Climbing to the top]. *Moskovskiy Psikhoterapevticheskiy Zhurnal, 4*, 112–122. (in Russian)

Alekseichik, A. Ye. (1998). 'Intensivnaya Terapevticheskaya Zhizn'. [Intensive therapeutic life]. Retrieved from: http://valery-159.narod.ru/psykhologi/psy/psy_010.htm (in Russian)

Alekseichik, A. Ye. (2007). 'Intensivnaya, terapevticheskaya, tselebnaya vera'. [Intensive, therapeutic, healing faith]. *Lithuanian Association for Humanistic Psychology*. Retrieved from: www.lhpa.net/ru/index.phpoption=com_content&view=article&id=281:2014-01-16-02-13-59&catid=6:2009-06-05-08-10-02&Itemid=13 (in Russian)

Becker, R. (1999). Adult/elderly care nursing: Teaching communication with dying across cultural boundaries *British Journal of Nursing, 8*(14), 938–942.

Burno, M. Ye. (2005). Native psychotherapy in Russia. *Archives of Psychiatry and Psychotherapy, 7*(1), 71–76.

Burno, M. Ye. (2011). Therapy by means of creative self-expression by M. Burno—TCSEB as the Russian native method-school of therapy by means of Spiritual Culture. *World Journal Psychotherapy, 1*(4), 45–49.

Currie, C.L., Kuzmina, M.V., & Nadyuk, R.I. (2012). The counseling profession in Russia: Historical roots, current trends, and future perspectives. *Journal of Counseling and Development, 90*(4), 488–493.

Dostoevsky, A. (1977). *Dostoevsky: Reminiscences.* New York, NY: Liveright Publishing Co.

Dostoevsky, F. (1979). *The Diary of a Writer.* Lewiston, NY: Olympic Marketing Corp.

European Consortium for Arts Therapies Education (ECARTE). (2017). *Membership Directory: State Academy of Post-Graduate Pedagogical Training St. Petersburg.* Retrieved February 1, 2017 from: www. ecarte.info/membership/directory/state-academy-st-petersburg.htm

Ferrell, B., Malloy, P., & Virani, R. (2015). The end of life nursing education consortium project. *Annals of Palliative Medicine, 4*(2), 61–69, DOI: 10.3978/j.issn.2224–5820.2015.04.05

Karkou, V., Martinsome, K., Nazarova, N., & Vaverniece, I. (2011). Art therapy in the postmodern world: Findings from a comparative study across the UK, Russia, and Latvia. *The Arts in Psychotherapy, 38,* 86–95.

Krom, I.L., Yerugina, M.V., Dorogoykin, D.L, & Shmerkevich, A.B. (2016). Tendencies of institutionalization of palliative care in modern Russia: Interdisciplinary analysis. *Saratov Journal of Medical Scientific Research, 12*(2), 196–199. (in Russian)

Luczak, J. (2000). Hospice care in Eastern Europe. *Lancet,* December Supplement, *356,* S23.

Matzo, M., Kenner, C., Boykova, M., & Jurkevich, I. (2007). End-of-life nursing education in the Russian Federation. *Journal of Hospice & Palliative Nurses Association, 9*(5), 246–253, DOI: 10.1097/01. NJH.0000289659.93666.39

Metropolitan Anthony of Sourozh. (2003). *Sermons and Talks.* Retrieved from: www.mitras.ru/eng/ eng_archive.htm

Optina Elders. (2017). Prayer of the Optina Elders. *The Orthodox Page in America: Orthodox Prayers.* Retrieved April 16, 2017 from: www.ocf.org

Paice, J.A., Ferrell, B.R., Coyle, N.oyne, P., & Callaway, M. (2008). Global efforts to improve palliative care: The international end-of-life nursing education consortium training programme. *Journal of Advanced Nursing, 61*(2), 173–180.

Parker-Bell, B., & Vaulina, T. (2015). Russian-American collaboration in art therapy and psychology: Methods and outcomes. *Global Partners in Education Journal, 5*(1), 4–14.

Porter, C. (2010). *The Diaries of Sofia Tolstoy.* New York, NY: Harper Perennial.

Rozhneva, O. (2014). *The Optima Elders and Their Sayings.* Retrieved from: www.pravoslavie.ru/ english/74512.htm

Russian Art Therapy Association. (2015). *Art Therapy and Art Therapists: The Status, Performance Standards and Training.* Retrieved from: http://rusata.ru/d/263056/d/15387459.pdf (English Translation)

Russian Art Therapy Association. (2017). *What Is Art Therapy?* Retrieved from: http://rusata.ru/ cho_takoe_art_terapiya (English Translation)

Russian Museum. (2017). *Educational Projects: Art Therapy.* Retrieved from: http://en.rusmuseum.ru

Shestakova, A., & Kerr, C. (2015). Russian family art therapy: New perspectives. In: C. Kerr (Ed.), *Multicultural Family Art Therapy* (pp. 123–137). New York, NY: Routledge.

R. F. Christian, Leo Tolstoy (2015) Tolstoy's Diaries Volume 1: 1847-1894. London: Faber & Faber Ltd.

# 8 Stillbirth

## Mourning Unspeakable Loss With Art Therapy and EMDR

*Tally Tripp*

## Introduction

According to the Center for Disease Control and Prevention, the loss of a baby after 20 weeks of pregnancy is termed a "stillbirth" and is a sad but undeniable reality for about 1% of all pregnancies in the United States (Center for Disease Control and Prevention 2017). Stillbirth, a type of perinatal loss, connects two of the most fundamental human experiences, birth and death, in a single moment. This cruel juxtaposition of the promise and joy of new life and the sudden loss of that life and its associated hopes and dreams, is a complicated matter. For grieving parents, the aftermath of a stillbirth can result in a sense of isolation and disenfranchisement. The "invisible loss" of a pregnancy or an un-realized life may not be viewed in the same way as more traditional losses such as the death of a parent or an older child (Barr & Cacciatore, 2008; Lang et al, 2011; Seftel, 2006). Society's lack of acceptance of the family's right or need to mourn the stillbirth can interfere with grieving and healing, leaving parents feeling vulnerable, helpless and alone (Harr & Thistlethwaite, 1990; Lang et al, 2011). Often well-meaning friends, relatives and even medical providers pull back from the family, not knowing how to respond or simply overlooking the psychological needs that may be present (Lang et al, 2011; Speert, 1992). The bereaved may experience a whirlwind of negative, contradictory emotions including shame, guilt and even envy (Barr & Cacciatore, 2008). Related thoughts and feelings associated with ambiguous loss can intensify, interrupt or perturb the healing process and contribute to further depression and relationship problems (Boss, 2006). The trauma of stillbirth can result in fundamental shifts in the mothers' basic assumptions about herself and her view of the world, which is "forever changed" (Cacciatore & Bushfield, 2007).

Trauma-sensitive, experiential therapeutic approaches are needed to address the range of intense, complex emotions resulting from stillbirth. The creative process can access emotions and facilitate expression of feeling states that often are, essentially, wordless. Experiential, art, and body-based therapies that do not rely on words to "tell the story" can provide strengths based, focused and creative outlets for mourning unspeakable loss. According to Seftel (2006):

> No matter what the expressive medium, when we give form to this invisible grief, even if it is difficult to gaze upon, these images invite us beyond the state of overwhelming or frozen emotions. And if we put forth our images and tell our true stories, we break the isolation that too often surrounds us when we need connections the most.
>
> (pp. 173–4)

This chapter will describe the case of a 36-year-old woman who suffered the consequences of the stillbirth of her full-term baby. In individual and group therapies, the author introduced trauma-informed tools to help the bereaved mother focus productively on the perinatal loss. A blended approach utilizing art therapy, sensorimotor psychotherapy and a modified EMDR protocol using bilateral stimulation facilitated working through the aftereffects of the stillbirth and paved the way for a successful pregnancy and birth experience in the future.

## Case of Joanne

"Joanne" (a pseudonym) began seeing me for therapy approximately one year after the heartbreaking event of the stillbirth of her first-born child. Joanne is a well-educated, professional woman with a strong spiritual practice anchored in Buddhist tradition. In our initial session, it was noted that she was depressed, avoidant and highly anxious. Many of Joanne's troubling symptoms lined up with a diagnosis of post-traumatic stress disorder (PTSD). She complained that her worldview had "totally changed" in the aftermath of losing her infant son; she could no longer feel safe or expect positive outcomes in life; she had lost trust in the community of caregivers and doctors; she felt different from others and even detached from her self. Self-blame and blaming the body for a stillbirth is not an unusual occurrence and Joanne repeatedly questioned her own role in the traumatic event: How could *she* have let this happen? What could *she* have done differently? Why had *she* "failed?" Joanne's memories of her labor and delivery were vivid and disturbing and she experienced frequent nightmares and flashbacks that interfered in daily life. She struggled with basic activities such as getting up and going to work. She experienced difficulty with trust and intimacy in her marriage. She had begun to isolate from her previously important social networks, avoiding events where there might be pregnant women or babies present, as she believed this would add to her overwhelming sadness and pain.

## Family History

The youngest daughter from a large Catholic family, Joanne had been raised to be stoic and self-sufficient. Hard work was praised, and feelings were largely ignored in her household. Joanne's father, a well-known and respected businessman in the community, was an alcoholic who kept his public and private persona separate. He suffered from serious bouts of depression and very likely had an undiagnosed bi-polar disorder that he may have managed through substance use. Mother was anxious, unhappy in her marriage, and emotionally distant from the family. Joanne was in the middle of her first semester of college when her father, without warning, committed suicide by a gunshot wound to the head. This horrific event took place in the family's garage and it was her mother who discovered his lifeless body. The aftereffects of this event were quite challenging. Joanne's mother was resentful of her husband's suicide and retreated into her own depressive state, dismissing her grief and refusing to talk about the experience with her children. For Joanne, and likely for the entire family, this traumatic loss was never fully resolved. This would be an important piece of the overall tapestry of unprocessed memories we would address in our grief focused trauma work.

## Overview of Treatment

Prior to beginning treatment with me, Joanne had been engaged in psychoanalytic psychotherapy for about 10 years. While she had made progress and felt a good connection with her analyst, she reported feeling increasingly frustrated by an approach that relied primarily on words. Joanne's therapist had heard about my Women's Art Therapy Trauma Group and recommended she join, believing it would be a good addition to their individual verbal therapy. Joanne was indeed a good fit for the group and found its experiential and creative orientation provided her a unique opportunity for exploring grief and loss.

## Group Art Therapy

Joanne was a member of the Art Therapy Trauma Group for approximately 9 months. In many of our group sessions, I directed the women to create artworks in response to common themes of loss, grief and trauma. Joanne found setting aside a weekly time and space for personal art making in this group to be extremely beneficial. She focused mindfully on creative expression that dealt with her perinatal loss. One striking piece was made using a glass jar that she filled with sand and small objects representing the life that, had he lived, her son might have had. She often spoke of wanting to remember and "honor" his short life, and she often found sharing these feelings in our intimate group setting provided comfort and support.

While the group was composed of female survivors with many types of abuse and interpersonal trauma, Joanne maintained that the experience of the stillbirth made her unique. There was a hint of defensiveness in the way she approached other members, possibly related to unresolved feelings about her ambiguous loss. Several of the women in the group had children in their lives, and it was often uncomfortable for Joanne to participate when this became a topic of conversation. In some sessions, Joanne would become so disturbed that she would have to excuse herself to get up and walk around the room. Because trauma groups can be "triggering" by the very nature of the topics discussed, our group had already set ground rules that included ways to manage potentially difficult situations. Getting up, briefly excusing oneself, etc. were considered understandable if not expected ways for members to cope with the overwhelming feelings that could arise in any session.

As time went on, Joanne had to travel more for work and this resulted in missing a number of meetings. Once she began her in vitro fertilization (IVF) treatments, she experienced some uncomfortable side effects that also interfered in her regular attendance. Some of her absences may have been compounded by the emotional difficulty of being in a trauma-focused group setting, but there was also the reality of her fragile and somewhat unstable physical state. Ultimately Joanne decided to leave the group and begin working more intensely with me in individual sessions. Our focus was on processing the unresolved grief surrounding the stillbirth of her first born.

## Individual Therapy

Joanne and I worked together individually for another year, dealing with several subsequent pregnancies and miscarriages. We began by developing a range of tools for resourcing and containment to aid in the management of traumatic stress responses. When we did begin trauma processing, we avoided a lot of verbal discussion or interpretation, as that had not been terribly effective in the past. We used bilateral stimulation, eye movement desensitization and reprocessing (EMDR), graphic narrative from the Instinctual Trauma Response (ITR) and art therapy. We also integrated body-focused techniques from sensorimotor psychotherapy in our work. These tools and techniques will be described below.

## Challenges in the Work

Joanne presented as highly anxious and depressed and, in this state, would ruminate about her stressful situation. Her sleep was poor and she often felt overwhelmed with feelings of loneliness, grief and loss. Being childless amongst a group of similarly aged peers who had started raising families, Joanne had become increasingly detached and isolated from her previous supports of friends and neighbors. Despite attempts to get pregnant after the stillbirth, she and her husband had not had any success. Over the course of a year they froze her eggs, used donor eggs, and endured many months of invasive testing and IVF treatments in an attempt to get pregnant. Certainly, advanced maternal age was a factor in this difficulty conceiving and carrying a fetus, but I suspected the stress of the previous unprocessed traumatic losses was also playing a large role in the difficulty. Another issue that added to the complexity of the situation was that Joanne's husband had suddenly lost his job, putting the burden of financial responsibility for supporting the family squarely on her shoulders. Joanne had been successful and was financially rewarded for her work, but this was not even close to being the most important aspect of her life. Clearly, we had a sensitive timeline and an important agenda to face in our trauma-focused work together.

## Phase-Oriented Treatment for Trauma

Herman (1992) and others embrace a phase-oriented approach to trauma treatment with the initial stage being focused on establishing a sense of safety and stabilization. At this point, through our group work and intermittent individual meetings, we had laid the significant groundwork of stabilization and Joanne stated that she felt ready to begin "trauma processing" with me.

The second phase in trauma treatment, remembrance and mourning the loss, is the period for uncovering memories related to the traumatic experience (s). Traumatic events are often held with accompanying negative beliefs that can create faulty assumptions about both the individual's self-perceptions and assumptions about the world (Shapiro, 2001, 2012). While we cannot and do not aim to change the actual reality of what happened, we expect to revise the way the resulting beliefs inform and influence us in the present. For example, Joanne felt the loss of her baby was, in part, her "fault" and furthermore, she had come to believe that the medical community and all medical providers "could not be trusted." Rationally, she did not have any reason to believe that she, or even her doctors, had actually done anything wrong. However, Joanne's implicit, negatively held belief about this experience was that she was in part responsible for things going wrong and, ultimately, that the world was an unsafe place. Our work would focus on finding avenues that could revise these problematic assumptions without triggering a flood of overwhelming traumatic memory in the process.

## Mourning the Earlier Losses

Before processing the stillbirth, I felt it was necessary to address the earlier significant losses from her childhood including father's suicide and the even more fundamentally distressing experience of being emotionally cut off and neglected by mother (another ambiguous loss). Focusing on the sensorimotor experience of these losses brought increased awareness of the body's role in the traumatic experience (Ogden, Minton &

Pain, 2006). Being a devout yoga practitioner, Joanne was receptive to being prompted to "notice" the sensations in her body as she was guided to re-visit a disturbing experience of being shunned by her mother after the suicide of her dad. We incorporated a bilateral art therapy protocol (Tripp, 2016) that integrates sets of bilateral stimulation (tapping) with repeated body scanning. Observations about somatic experiences such as tension, tingling or warmth noted in the body, were recorded on a series of body template drawings. Between short sets of tapping (bilateral stimulation), I asked Joanne to focus on her body and, using a body outline template, mark the areas where tension, pain or any other body sensation was noted. At the end of the session, these drawings were reviewed as a visual representation of the somatic narrative related to the traumatic experience.

Similar to the standard EMDR reprocessing phase, we started the session with a "target" memory of the trauma of mother's neglect and her turning away from Joanne after father's suicide. We processed that memory with sets of alternating bilateral stimulation (tapping) and body scanning, noting feelings as they arose. Joanne produced a series of four simple drawings in a single session.

When we reviewed the body drawings at the end of the session, we could clearly see a somatic shift progressing from a held in, tight posture, moving to increasing expression of anger and then sadness to relief and, finally, resolution. Emotional changes and shifts in self-beliefs were also positively affected. The understanding that Joanne had held in so much rage that "mother was not was there" brought up an important, adaptive recognition that "no child should have been left without support." The relief she experienced was the recognition that her needs and feelings were valid. This allowed her to let go of some of the anger that kept her emotionally frozen. Although she may have known this intellectually, tracking the body's experience facilitated the resolution of the trauma.

We also discovered an interesting parallel between the earlier experiences of father's suicide, mother's neglect and the more recent trauma of the stillbirth. In each of these cases, Joanne felt she was essentially left alone without comfort or support from family. Mother's retreat after the suicide had been a traumatic loss without opportunity for resolution. Tears rolled down Joanne's cheeks as she recalled the related event of being in left the recovery room without a mother to comfort her and without a live baby to hold. Not having the opportunity to share the experience was almost as disturbing as the traumatic events themselves. The next question for us to face in our work was to determine if the unprocessed feelings of anger, sadness, grief, guilt, being left alone, etc. had been standing in the way of Joanne's current stressor: the inability to conceive or bring a pregnancy to full term.

## Processing the Stillbirth

I had prepared Joanne for processing the traumatic event of the stillbirth with weeks of resourcing and safe place imagery. We used two trauma treatment approaches: Eye Movement Desensitization and Reprocessing (EMDR) and the Instinctual Trauma Response (ITR). This work was intensive and sometimes required extended (90-minute) sessions that took place over a number of weeks. The two protocols worked in concert with one another to reduce the disturbance felt and revise the ongoing negative belief around feelings of helplessness and responsibility for the stillbirth. Both techniques were successful aspects in her healing journey and will be described in more depth in the following section.

## Brief Overview of EMDR Therapy

The EMDR protocol, as developed by Francine Shapiro (2001), is an 8-phase model that includes: 1. History; 2. Preparation; 3. Assessment; 4. Desensitization; 5. Installation; 6. Body Scan; 7. Closure; 8. Re-evaluation. For purposes of this chapter, I will focus on the desensitization phase where the reprocessing occurs. The client is asked to hold the image of the traumatic event (target) in mind, along with the negative self-referencing beliefs (negative cognition) and the associated body sensations. The therapist then begins bilateral stimulation (BLS) using either lateral eye movements or tapping (tactile stimulation) or some combination. The bilateral stimulation is posited to engage both hemispheres of the brain and thereby access adaptive information that has been blocked from availability due to the trauma (Tripp, 2007, 2016). The therapist provides the successive "sets" (usually lasting less than a minute each) of BLS, and then prompts the client to report what comes to mind in the form of images, thoughts, feelings or sensations. The therapist and client continue in this manner, processing whatever comes up until the disturbance has shifted to something neutral or positive.

We examined the negative beliefs about feeling helpless and out of control in relation to the birth experience. Our focus was to shift the self-referencing belief about the event from feeling helpless and out of control to recognizing that she "did the best she could" and "with time the trauma will heal." We kept in mind the important fact that her stillborn son would not be forgotten. We also kept a close eye on the somatic indicators of trauma and arousal noted in the body, so that the sessions did not become triggering or re-traumatizing. Also, as in any EMDR session, the client has the ultimate control to stop the processing at any time if needed with a simple hand signal.

## Processing the Stillbirth With EMDR

Joanne was 10 days past her due date when she went into labor. She described the events of that evening and the negative experience of feeling "out of control" and "unsafe" as her husband drove her to the hospital. Her body, neck and jaw felt "tight and weak" and she described experiencing extreme agitation while telling her husband to drive faster through the heavy traffic to get them to the hospital. Once at the hospital, the contractions were frequent and painful and she could feel tension in her chest and heart.

In describing the scenario leading to getting to the hospital, Joanne became tearful and her breathing was notably constricted. I instructed her to focus on deepening her breathing and provided her with some basic grounding techniques. This seemed to offer some relief as the first mental image shifted and Joanne now pictured herself lying flat on her back in a hospital bed, breathing more deeply. A subsequent negative belief came up as she remembered receiving an epidural for the extreme pain. Labor was not progressing and the negative belief (that we decided to use for our target) was "I can't do it right" (meaning I can't deliver this baby "right"). Again, somatic indicators of distress arose including tension in the jaw and some flushing or reddening in her chest and face. When I made a verbal observation about her body, Joanne acknowledged that she was experiencing some physical tension as she envisioned the frightening scene in the delivery room. To de-escalate the physical tension, I invited her to "just notice" the image and try to observe everything from a "safe distance" while we continued the BLS.

Joanne described a number of unfolding body sensations including a sense of overall physical numbness she felt while searching for the sensation to push. Staying with that numb sensation, another image arose of a dark grey cinderblock hovering above her prostrate body. When invited to picture "what happens next?" in response to the cinderblock, she described a sudden surge of energy and a desire to "smash it." This urgency to move to action seemed to signal a newly resourced state for Joanne. It may also have been the needed antidote to the feeling of numbness and corresponding powerlessness that had kept her frozen in a trauma response, unable to find the strength to push through the labor and delivery process. Joanne then described picturing herself smashing the cinderblock with a sledgehammer and watching the pieces fall to the ground. At this point there was a little glee in her voice and she described feeling both empowered and relieved.

When we looked back at the session and reviewed her earlier negative belief "I can't do it right" Joanne stated this feeling had now completely changed to "I am powerful, I can overcome it" and she even smiled a little as she shared this new insight. She stated she felt like giggling during the trauma processing as she pictured taking a sledgehammer and smashing a dense, grey cinderblock to bits. Her body was now relaxed and her breathing was steady and deep. She said she was feeling "strong and resourced."

In this session we did not get to the tragic image of the silent delivery room with the stillborn baby. What did happen, and perhaps what was most important, was that Joanne's negative, disempowered image of herself as a victim who was "unable to do it right," feeling weak and out of control, had shifted to a more resourced feeling of empowerment and strength. This was exactly the kind of belief that she would need to carry on into the present.

## Brief Overview of Intensive Trauma Therapy and the Graphic Narrative

The "graphic narrative" is an art-based element of the intensive trauma therapy approach developed by Linda Gantt and Lou Tinnin (2007, 2009). The graphic narrative protocol invites the client to create a drawing series that corresponds to the instinctual survival responses to threat that can be identified in the animal kingdom. Inherent in this undertaking is the understanding that trauma responses are naturally occurring. This can be helpful for reducing stigma and any remaining feelings of shame or guilt that may be present in the survivor. The intensive trauma therapy approach has been successful in bringing unconscious memories into awareness and processing preverbal trauma without causing overwhelming distress (Gantt & Tripp, 2016). Furthermore, trauma symptomatology can be eliminated through the creation of this drawing series when it is witnessed and processed through to the completion of the story with a trained mental health professional (Gantt & Tripp, 2016).

The Graphic Narrative series consists of the following nine drawings that are ideally completed in a single, extended session: 1. Before; 2. Startle; 3. Thwarted Intention; 4. Freeze; 5. Altered State of Consciousness; 6. Body Sensations; 7. Automatic Obedience; 8. Self-Repair; 9. After. Upon completion of the drawing series, the therapist and client review the images and story together, and then, the therapist invites the client to listen to her story while it is "re-told" by the therapist in sequence. This provides the client with an important experience of "being witnessed" and puts the previously disjointed trauma narrative into a coherent, visual narrative. This also brings an ending or bookmark to the story and helps the client come to the realization that the trauma is truly over.

## Reprocessing the Stillbirth With the Graphic Narrative

Joanne began her Graphic Narrative with a "before" image (Figure 8.1) of interconnected balls up in the air, calling it "the promise of my son" who is depicted as the small circle in the center surrounded by concentric rings.

The "before picture" depicts her belief that life would be "different" after this child was born, also suggesting the unknown element of how to juggle so many balls in the air. The "startle picture" (Figure 8.2) depicts the stress of going into labor and shows a shift

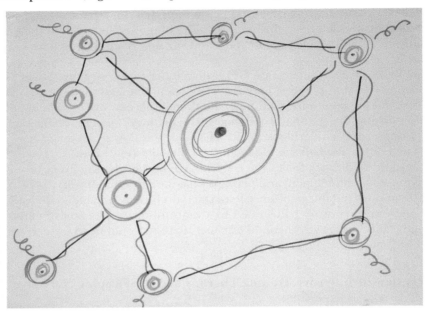

*Figure 8.1* The Promise of My Son

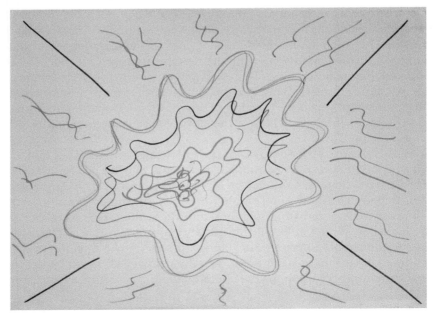

*Figure 8.2* Startle

in line quality depicting the panicked state of driving to the hospital. It is marked with agitated red, purple and blue lines. The picture of "thwarted intention" (Figure 8.3) is divided into two sides. The left side depicts one squiggly line essentially going from A to B, where B is a heart representing the birth of a healthy baby, and the expected course of events. The right side (which depicts the actual reality) contains the chaos of multiple intersecting lines and the sense of urgency Joanne felt knowing that "something was wrong." In the "freeze picture" (Figure 8.4) the page is divided into four segments

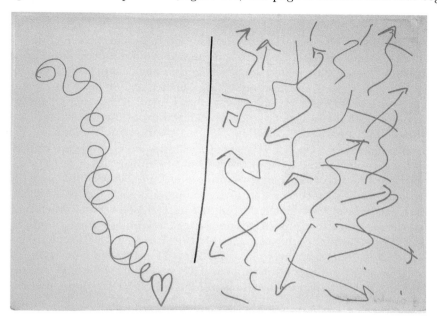

*Figure 8.3* Thwarted Intention

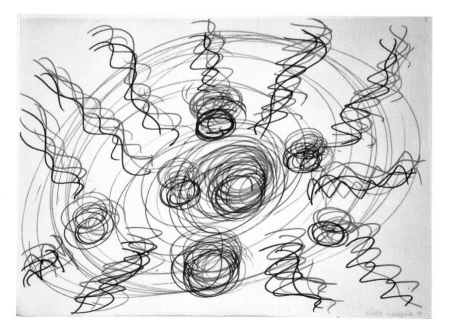

*Figure 8.4* Freeze

where various aspects of the hospital procedures are detailed such as getting an epidural, monitoring the fetal heart rate and other related medical testing. Joanne acknowledged that the medical interventions were frightening and she experienced a feeling of being frozen and even experiencing some dissociation as she felt herself to be was watching the process unfold from above. The neat compartmentalization and segments of experience further suggests a static, frozen state. The image of "altered state" (Figure 8.5) is the most agitated of the series where Joanne recalled the feeling of panic trying to "get him out" and fighting hard. Tears emerged as she drew this image and shared her accompanying thoughts and feelings. She expressed the anxiety that had been in her mind throughout: "What is happening?" "Why is no one responding" and ultimately the feeling of helplessness and defeat as she came to the realization that there was a problem. The line drawing that follows (Figure 8.6) is the "body sensation image" which depicts a tight band of tension across her chest and accompanying belief that her body was betraying her. The feeling she described was "I can't access what I need" which may relate to needing something more from medical personnel. The emptiness of the picture further suggests she is feeling alone and unsupported. The picture of "automatic obedience" (Figure 8.7) is another divided image. On the left she drew the desired, and expected, outcome: "I thought they would tell me what to do, it would be linear and it would make sense" and on the right, the actual outcome: "I am asking them, 'Is he OK?' and there is no response. I don't know what this means! I can no longer speak." Figure 8.8 is perhaps the most powerful picture of the series reflecting the state of "self-repair" which immediately followed the tragic stillbirth event. In this image that resembles some sort of solar system, connected circles represent both Joanne and her husband (she is the central circle, husband is the small circle connected to her by a line). The stillborn baby is represented as the largest circle surrounding both Joanne and her husband. She stated that his circle is the biggest because, on a spiritual level, his presence dwarfs everything else and "he has

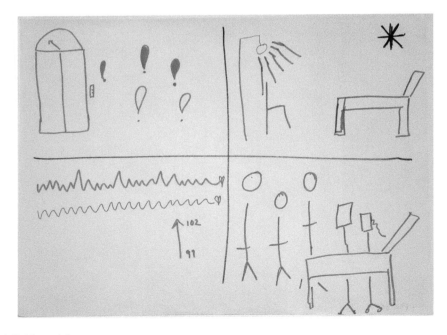

*Figure 8.5* Altered State

changed us forever." Joanne demonstrated great resourcefulness and resiliency in being able to depict the closely entwined family system as something positive and strong. There are other small circles on the page, more like dots along the outside of the system, that represent the friends and family that are secondary, but notably, present. The final image

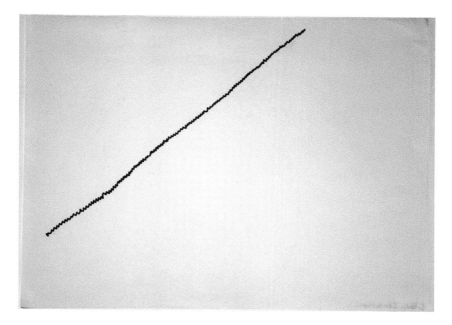

*Figure 8.6* Body Sensation Image

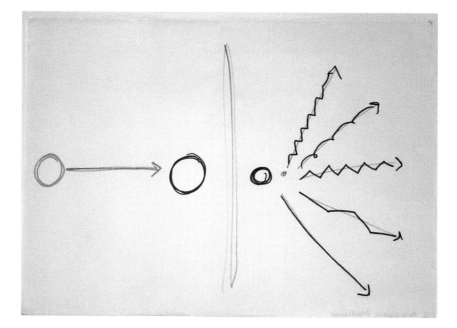

*Figure 8.7* Automatic Obedience

(Figure 8.9) is the "after picture" where many tight spirals form one small circle in the center of the page. Joanne recalled being in the recovery room with her husband, holding each other and embracing their lifeless son. The tightness of the circle may represent a metaphor of circling in of the wagons where everything stops for a moment and in that stillness and quiet, healing begins to take place. In this image she is distant, contained, but not alone.

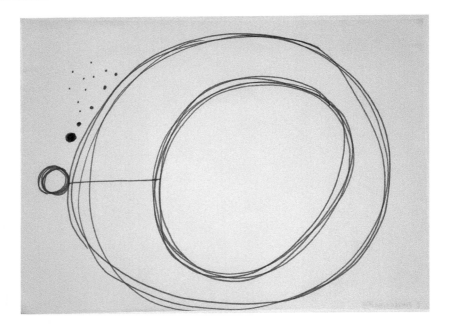

*Figure 8.8* Self-repair

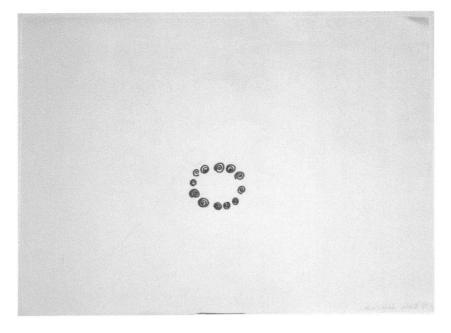

*Figure 8.9* After

## Discussion

Joanne effectively used EMDR, Bilateral Art Therapy, Sensorimotor Psychotherapy and the Graphic Narrative to work through her traumatic experiences. The early interpersonal trauma and neglect from her family of origin tied beautifully in to the ambiguous loss experiences associated with the stillbirth. The sensorimotor focus kept her in touch with the body's need to respond to the trauma that had been held inside. EMDR and Bilateral Art Therapy facilitated a shift in self-beliefs from a passive feeling of unimportance to an empowered surge of strength. The Graphic Narrative allowed us to reprocess the stillbirth experience and gave visual language to an event that had defied words and sequence.

A few months after completing these integrative therapy processes, Joanne and her husband were able to conceive and successfully deliver a healthy, baby boy. They could not have been happier to have an "earth baby" to join their "spiritual baby." Their love and commitment to the son they lost continues, in that they have created a memorial garden and 5K run in his honor as a way to keep his memory alive and to support parents with similar experiences of bereavement and traumatic grief.

## Post-Script

Approximately 8 months after the birth, Joanne and her husband and son are doing well and we are no longer meeting regularly. However, one afternoon, I did receive an urgent phone call from Joanne reporting that her son had taken a fall off an examining table at the doctor's office when she (Joanne) turned her back for a moment. Although the baby was not badly injured, everyone was understandably quite shaken, and Joanne felt extreme guilt and shame of "not being good enough" as a mother. We decided to meet a few days later for an EMDR session to address any residual trauma from this event.

Joanne told me that the most disturbing part of this experience was that after the fall she did not know what to do ("not good enough") and handed the baby over to the nurse. As the nurse held him in her arms, however, Joanne realized that she wanted to be the one to comfort him, and took the baby back into her own arms.

With tension noted in her jaw and neck, her self-referencing negative belief as related to the experience was "I am not good enough" and her desired positive belief was "I am more than enough." After only a few brief sets of BLS Joanne dropped the image of the scene in the doctor's office and pictured a bird, fluttering over her chest. Continuing to focus on the image of the bird, she recalled that she and her son had taken a walk along a nearby creek that morning, and they had come upon the nest of a blue heron. The beauty of this moment brought tears to Joanne's eyes as she said it told her unequivocally "everything's going to be OK!" She then pictured herself in the future, describing the magical shared experience with her son when he would be a little older. She appeared notably more relaxed at this point. She said she felt both she and her son were now in a more "intuitive" place, and recognized with some delight, that they both were growing and changing. She exclaimed, "It's not just his development . . . it's mine too!" With this realization, the power of their parallel process of growing together on their life journey seemed to strengthen. I invited Joanne to depict the experience with her son in a drawing so we could have a tangible ending to this story. The resulting image is of two similar mirror images of circles that are "parallel but different" of beings that she called "Cosmic Travelers."

## References

Barr, P. & Cacciatore, J. (2008). Problematic emotions and maternal grief. *Omega, 56* (4), 331–348.
Boss, P. (2006). Loss, trauma and resilience: Therapeutic work with ambiguous loss. New York: W.W. Norton.

Cacciatore, J. & Bushfield, S. (2007). Stillbirth: The mother's experience and implications for improving care. *Journal of Social Work in End-of-Life & Palliative Care, 3* (3), 59–79.

Cacciatore, J., Freen, J.F. & Killan, M. (2013). Condemning self, condemning other: Blame and mental health in women suffering stillbirth. *Journal of Mental Health Counseling, 35* (4), 342–359.

Center for Disease Control and Prevention. (2017). *Facts about stillbirth* (Data file). Retrieved from www.cdc.gov/ncbddd/stillbirth/facts.html

Gantt, L. & Tinnin, L.W. (2007). Intensive trauma therapy of PTSD and dissociation: An outcome study. *The Arts in Psychotherapy, 34* (1), 69–80.

Gantt, L. & Tinnin, L.W. (2009). Support for a neurobiological view of trauma with implications for art therapy. *The Arts in Psychotherapy, 36* (3), 148–153.

Gantt, L. & Tripp, T. (2016). The image comes first: Treating preverbal trauma with art therapy. In J. King (Ed.) *Art therapy, trauma and neuroscience: Theoretical and practical perspectives.* New York: Routledge Press.

Harr, N.D. & Thistlethwaite, J.E. (1990). Creative intervention strategies in the management of perinatal loss. *Maternal-Child Nursing Journal, 19* (2), 135–142.

Herman, J.L. (1992). *Trauma and recovery.* New York: Basic Books.

Lang, A., Fleiszer, A., Duhamel, F., Sword, W., Gilbert, K. & Corsini-Munt, S. (2011). Perinatal loss and parental grief: The challenge of ambiguity and disenfranchised grief. *Omega, 63* (2), 183–196.

Ogden, P., Minton, K. & Pain, C. (2006). *Trauma and the body: A sensorimotor approach to psychotherapy.* New York: W.W. Norton.

Seftel, L. (2006). Grief unseen: Healing pregnancy loss through the arts. London: Jessica Kingsley.

Shapiro, F. (2001). Eye movement desensitization and reprocessing: Basic principals, protocols and procedures. New York: Guilford Press.

Shapiro, F. (2012). Getting past your past: Take control of your life with self-help techniques from EMDR therapy. New York: Rodale Books.

Speert, E. (1992). The use of art therapy following perinatal death. *Art Therapy: Journal of the American Art Therapy Association, 9* (3), 121–128.

Tripp, T. (2007). A short-term approach to processing trauma: Art therapy and bilateral stimulation. *Art Therapy: Journal of the American Art Therapy Association, 24* (4), 176–183.

Tripp, T. (2016). A body-BASED bilateral art protocol for reprocessing trauma. In J. King (Ed.) *Art therapy, trauma and neuroscience: Theoretical and practical perspectives.* New York: Routledge Press (pp. 173–194).

# 9 The Empathic Mirror

## Healing Grief and Loss Through Portrait Therapy at End of Life

*Susan M.D. Carr*

The focus of this chapter is an exploration of the role *portrait therapy* plays in helping people living with life threatening or chronic illnesses to heal unresolved grief and loss. I examine the therapeutic implications of building 'continuing bonds' within the portraits, and argue that through a process of mirroring and attunement portrait therapy enables people to bring *closure* to painful experiences and find a sense of peace at end of life.

### Portrait Therapy, Illness, and Disrupted Self-Identity

The portraits discussed within this chapter were painted during a PhD project developing portrait therapy (Carr, 2014, 2015, 2017; Carr & Hancock 2017) as an innovative art therapy intervention for people who experience life-threatening or chronic illness as a disruption to their self-identity. This disruption is often characterised by statements such as 'I don't know who I am anymore,' or 'I'm not the person I used to be', and a general sense of disorientation, as Young (1988, p. 32) said 'to have one's identity disrupted is to travel without a compass [. . .]'. This sense of *disruption* and *disorientation* can cause increased stress, anxiety, depression and loss of meaning, as well as social isolation (Rodin et al, 1991; Falvo, 1999). I therefore developed portrait therapy as an intervention to help patients find 'health within illness' (Carel, 2008, p. 17), increasing their quality of life and develop a stronger, more coherent sense of self-identity.

Self-identity can be described as a kind of 'orientation' or way of 'knowing', something that Taylor (1989, p. 29) suggests is built through adopting 'frames' of identity, which serve to orientate us in moral space:

> To know who I am is a species of knowing where I stand. My identity is defined by the commitments and identifications which provide the frame or horizon within which I can try to determine from case to case what is good, or valuable, or what ought to be done, or what I endorse or oppose.
>
> (Taylor, 1989, p. 27)

Portrait therapy is a collaborative process within which the art therapist and patient co-design the portraits and the therapist then paints them *for* the patient, becoming their 'third hand' (Kramer, 1971). During a series of portrait sessions, the patient is invited to engage with a number of creative elicitation tasks designed to help them talk about their self-identity, and identify stories that suggest turning points, or moments of 'becoming' (Kinnvall, 2004, p. 748) in their lives. The therapist then reflects these stories back to the patient through collages and prose-poems as a form of response art

(Fish, 2012), and these are then used to negotiate a *statement of intention* (Carr, 2017, p. 218) for each portrait to be painted. (For a full portrait therapy protocol see Carr, 2017, pp. 209–222.)

Whilst this project does not enable patients to produce the artwork first hand, 'third hand' techniques are, I suggest, effective in enabling patients to co-design how they want to appear in their portraits, thus engaging in a process of intentionality and empowerment at a time when patients face an uncertain future. The 'third hand' process also makes portrait therapy totally *inclusive*, so that patients who are too unwell, disabled or fatigued to make art, or who find the process anxiety provoking, can also take part. Directing how they wish to appear in the portraits helps reduce the unequal hierarchy of patient/therapist relationship, and the therapist develops into more of a 'companioning-witness' and 'artist-therapist' role. Hardy (2013, p. 30) advocates that patients in palliative care require a therapist that will *accompany* them and demonstrate 'reciprocity', sharing 'more of themselves than they might do in another setting', and that 'the task of making sense of the inexplicable at a time of considerable stress [. . .] can only be realistically accomplished if the patient is accompanied in this way' (*ibid.*). Tjasink (2010) has also written about the need for therapists to establish a *mutual* or collaborative relationship with patients, especially for those whose sense of identity has been erased by medicalisation or invasive treatments.

One of the key theories underpinning portrait therapy is psychotherapist Kenneth Wright's (2009) theory of 'mirroring and attunement' through the art object. For Wright, the art object becomes a surrogate for the (m)other's mirroring and attuning face from infancy, becoming therefore 'that which they needed to see' (2009, p. 13). I have developed this theory to include (self-)portraits painted *for* the patient through the art therapist's 'third hand'. This means that the artist/therapist mirrors and attunes the patient's stories of self-identity and their preferred representation, through the portraits. This is a direct change from therapists who have 'written themselves out' of the creative process (Hardy, 2013, p. 35), or even the collaborative relationship, through adopting a 'blank screen' approach to therapy.

Stories of self-identity were once told to family and friends within the 'protective framework of the small community' (Giddens, 1991, p. 33), where they were *known* since childhood; however, the effect of globalisation on people in general has meant the breakdown of such communities. This has resulted in communities where people are more isolated than ever before (Kinnvall, 2004, p. 744), where you no longer know your own neighbour or General Practitioner and where opportunities for intersubjective validation of self-identity stories have largely disappeared. This means that for patients facing deep illness and the prospect of their own mortality, what is needed is the opportunity to tell their story and for empathic mirroring and attunement to take place, provided by a collaborative 'I-thou' (Buber, 2004 [1937]) relationship with the therapist.

## Death, Bereavement and Making Meaning

One of the common themes to emerge from my PhD research findings (Carr, 2015, 2017) was the way participants used the portraits to mourn their losses and bring a sense of 'closure' to previous bereavements. The inevitability of death, is the shadow under which all humanity lives; however, it is a distant fear for most people. The diagnosis of a life-threatening or chronic illness means that death can no longer be ignored, there is a demand to *understand life as finite* (Heidegger, 1962, pp. 276–277). People facing death often seek new ways to understand and express the range of feelings that arise (Heath & Lings, 2012, p. 106), and may be drawn to creative expression as a way to articulate these in a non-verbal way (*ibid.*, p. 116).

Bereavement and loss are part of life, and grief can be described as a 'universal response to loss' (Morycz, 1992, p. 545), however, the focus of this chapter is the *disruption* to self-identity caused by bereavement, and the sense of *disorientation* caused by this. If mourning practices and rituals are a way of dealing with grief caused by bereavement and loss, then a sense of disorientation may affect a person's ability to mourn effectively. The death of someone close to us inevitably strips away part of who we are; our self-identity in relation to that person is shattered. In Judith Butler's (2004) book about the 9/11 attacks on the World Trade Centre in New York, she examines the nature of mourning. We need to mourn, Butler suggests, as a way to acknowledge our 'ontological indebtedness' to each other:

> It is not as if an 'I' exists independently over here and then simply loses a 'you' over there, especially if the attachment to 'you' is part of what composes who 'I' am. If I lose you, under these conditions, then I not only mourn the loss, but I become inscrutable to myself. Who am 'I' without you?

> (Butler, 2004, p. 22)

This begins to explain the relationship people living with severe illness and disability have to lost aspects of their self-identity, highlighting the *intra*subjective nature of self-identity when asking the question 'who am I without you?' It seems, therefore, that without mourning such losses people risk becoming 'inscrutable' to themselves (Butler, 2004, p. 22).

In a relational view, self-identity is built through our relationships with significant others and what grief displays is the way in which their loss 'undoes us'. Bereavement challenges our sense of ourselves as separate, because 'we're undone by each other. And if we're not, we're missing something' (Butler, 2004, p. 23). This suggests that instead of thinking that bereavement causes a loss of 'roles' (Morycz, 1992, p. 546), the death of a loved one means the loss of, or disruption to, self-identity. Therefore, when working with patients to revision self-identity, it seems inevitable that this will resurrect previous unresolved bereavements.

Research evidence demonstrates that there is no single therapeutic approach to bereavement and loss that works for all (Beaumont, 2013; Mancini & Bonanno, 2006; Neimeyer & Currier, 2009; Stroebe & Stroebe, 1991), therefore it is important for interventions to be person centred, flexible and collaborative, understanding that people experience bereavement, loss and grief differently. I agree with Beaumont's (2013, p. 3) assertion that the approach with the most promise, from a portrait therapy point of view, is Neimeyer's (2000) 'constructivist theory of bereavement' with its inherent focus on the *meaning-making* process.

## 'Letting Go' Whilst 'Holding On': The Art of Continuing Bonds

In his book entitled *A Grief Observed*, the author C. S. Lewis writes eloquently about his feelings of disorientation following the loss of his wife:

> Thought after thought, feeling after feeling, action after action, had 'H' for their object. Now their target is gone. I keep on through habit fitting an arrow to the string: then I remember and have to lay the bow down.

> (Lewis, 2013 [1963], p. 55)

A theory that has received considerable attention in recent years in relation to bereavement is the idea of 'continuing bonds' (Klass et al, 1996), something that challenges the popular theory that an amelioration of grief requires the 'letting go' or detachment from the deceased. Beaumont (2013, p. 5) suggests that the ultimate goal of therapy should be to provide a safe space for grieving clients within which they can 'integrate their experience of loss into their self-narrative' in such a way that they feel 'a continuing bond with their deceased loved one, at the same time as experiencing a sense of renewed trust in their worlds'.

Maintaining a bond with the deceased was considered a normal part of the bereavement process in Western society up until the 20th Century, when the work of Sigmund Freud, highlighted in his paper *Mourning and Melancholia* (1917), suggested that the amelioration of grief was linked to the ability of the bereaved to detach themselves emotionally from the deceased. However, the idea of continuing bonds works on the basis that bereaved people often feel a need to maintain a bond with the deceased that entails the construction of a new kind of relationship, one that acknowledges a relationship with someone who is *emotionally present*, yet *physically absent* (Beaumont, 2013). However, studies have shown that a focus on continuing bonds may not be helpful in certain circumstances, particularly for those who 'retain strong ties' with their lost loved one, or who have experienced 'a sudden bereavement' (Stroebe et al, 2012, p. 265). That is, unless the bereaved person is able to *make sense* of their loss in 'personal, practical, existential, or spiritual terms' (Neimeyer et al, 2006, p. 715).

Making sense of bereavement, and making meaning, can be facilitated by rituals and ritualistic behaviour (Cohen, 2002; Turner, 1982, 1995); however, contemporary society has abandoned many historic ritual customs and behaviours around bereavement, meaning that mourners have little left to draw on to express their grief and respect for the deceased (Morycz, 1992, p. 546). This lack of ritualised behaviour can cause further hardship to the bereaved, as they have the additional burden of creating their own rituals at a time when feelings of personal disorientation and stress are prevalent (*ibid.*). A new form of mourning ritual has developed in the last two decades, which has seen the posting of images of the dead or missing, either in newspapers, on social media, or on walls and buildings around the site of the tragedy, e.g. the 'walls of the missing' that turned into spontaneous memorial walls following the September 11th attack on the World Trade Centre in New York in 2001 (Santino, 2016).

The use of photographs of deceased loved ones is frequently cited within art therapy interventions for bereaved clients (Beaumont, 2013, p. 4), and is used as an elicitation technique to help clients introduce and describe their story of loss (Kohut, 2011; Lister et al, 2008; Neimeyer & Sands, 2011). Gershman and Braddeley (2010) described the use of a 'prescriptive photomontage' as a way to help clients adapt their relationship bond to their loved one by rebuilding a sense of meaning through envisioning a future life story that includes a different, yet continuing bond with the deceased, that can then become a source of hope for the client. Portrait therapy works in a similar way, although photographs are used only as reference material, meaning that the painted imagery can truly reflect the patient's vision, with the only limit being the imagination of the patient and the technical competence of the therapist. The portraits therefore have the potential to integrate losses and attune them in a way that creates new meanings, and validate the patients' self-identity.

Bereavement also brings with it significant changes, both to the individual, but also to their 'world'. Volkan (1997, p. 36) suggests that in order to accept *change* people must first mourn what has been lost, and throughout history painted portraits have been linked to mourning rituals (Hilliker, 2006). As physical objects, portraits can play an important role in the development of mourning rituals, something that can help maintain the deceased's role within the life of the bereaved and the wider community, meaning that their *emotional presence* is recognised and brought into the *present*, rather than relegated to the *past*. If the deceased remains 'in the past' then so can the nature of a mourner's relationship, and the danger is that they also *live in the past*. Arguably relationships with significant others, both those absent and present, validate one's sense of self, and provide continuity between the past, present, and future. Without an understanding of how the *past* has informed the *present*, it is difficult to move forward into the *future* without feeling disorientated and lost.

From a constructivist view of bereavement (i.e. the belief that knowledge is built through reflecting on experience), grieving requires a profound effort to reconstruct or reaffirm a world of meaning challenged by loss (Neimeyer, 2006a). This means that people create their own meaning through drawing upon their own personal and cultural experiences; however death, be it one's own impending death, or the death of a loved one, can disrupt this process, as their worldview and sense of self-identity is shattered (Neimeyer & Currier, 2009, pp. 355–356). Such acute and painful losses can initiate 'a profound and protracted search for meaning in order to accommodate the self-narrative to painful new realities' (Neimeyer 2006b, p. 143). Therefore, interventions such as portrait therapy, which enable clients to reconstruct their self-narrative and worldview through the successful integration of these losses into their personal meaning systems, have the most positive outcomes and reduced grief symptoms (Neimeyer, 2012).

## Collaborating With Peter [& Mark]: Making Meaning Through Portrait Therapy at End of Life

When working with the patients involved in this study, I expected them to focus mainly on losses to their own self-identity caused by *illness*, and while they did do this, they also focused a considerable amount of time on previous losses and bereavements, some from many decades previously. This unresolved outpouring of loss and bereavement demonstrated how *new losses* bring to the surface and resurrect *past losses*, as Morycz (1992, p. 545) says, '[. . .] life can be a chain of losses, and the most recent loss can resurrect old, seemingly unrelated losses [. . .]'. Making sense of these losses became part of the task involved within the portrait therapy sessions, and these were often highlighted within the collages and prose poems prior to being included in the portraits. This is exemplified in the work Peter and I created together.

Peter was a 69-year-old gentleman diagnosed with chronic obstructive pulmonary disease (COPD), a progressive lung disease for which there is no cure and limited treatment. When I first met Peter, he was attending the day-therapy unit at the hospice where I worked as an art therapist. He was married with four grown sons, one of whom, his eldest son called Mark, had died of cancer over six months previously aged just 47. Peter's COPD had progressed to a point where his quality of life was severely compromised, requiring a constant supply of oxygen. Any physical movement would leave Peter exhausted and fighting for breath. Peter was identified by the multi-disciplinary team at the hospice as someone who may benefit from engaging with the portrait therapy project, and he agreed enthusiastically to take part.

It is important to recognise that there are gender differences in bereavement styles (Rathaupt, 2007, p. 10), however, due to the collaborative nature of portrait therapy and the opportunity within the portraits to communicate 'differently' (Liebmann, 2003, pp. 123–124; Tannen, 1992; Hodson, 1984), the process became a particularly useful way for men in particular to express emotion and vulnerability in a safe and non-threatening way (see Carr, 2014). When we began working together, it soon became clear that by working with Peter I was also working (by default) with his son Mark, which became evident through Peter's focus on the loss of his *father of Mark* self-identity. Together we co-designed, and I painted, six portraits for Peter, including two portraits of Mark, and two of Peter and Mark together, including one called *At the Races* (Figure 9.1).

This portrait shows Peter and Mark together again, in one of their favourite pastimes, watching horse racing together. The significance of the portrait was captured in the phenomenological essence statements developed through the analysis of the portrait:

*Statement of Emergent Knowing:*

I tell a joke, Mark smiles and laughs, we are there for the races, a small bet to place, not really for the winning but for being together and sharing our time, father and first-born son, united, relaxed. No oxygen required, your presence mends my broken lungs.

*Statement of Emergent Learning:*

Peter is happy in his treasured father of Mark role, reunited in the portrait, the relationship is remembered and validated and the magic is captured between layers of paint, together without illness and pain they rest in each other's enjoyment.

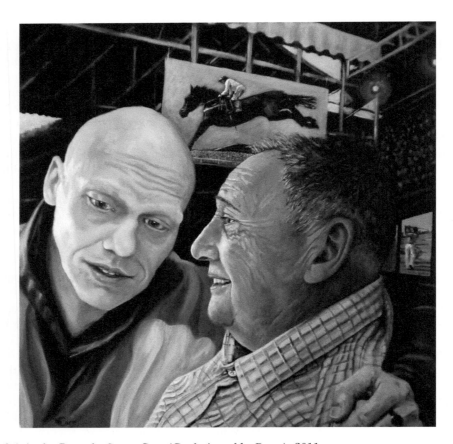

*Figure 9.1* At the Races by Susan Carr (Co-designed by Peter), 2011

Before his COPD became severe Peter had been an active member of the *Breathe Easy* support groups run by the British Lung Foundation, helping others to face their diagnosis with dignity and hope, giving talks to many different organisations explaining what it is like to live with breathlessness. When we began working together Peter was no longer able to take this active role, saying that his COPD had stripped away the majority of activities he had been able to do. I created the following collage for Peter, to reflect back this experience, when 'catching your breath' becomes your primary focus (Figure 9.2).

The psychological and emotional impact of bereavement is well documented (Parkes & Prigerson, 2010), however the physical impact or *embodiment* of bereavement is less often considered. Therese Rando (1991) talks of a lady who was both a bereaved parent and a widow who said. . . 'when you lose your spouse, it is like losing a limb; when you lose your

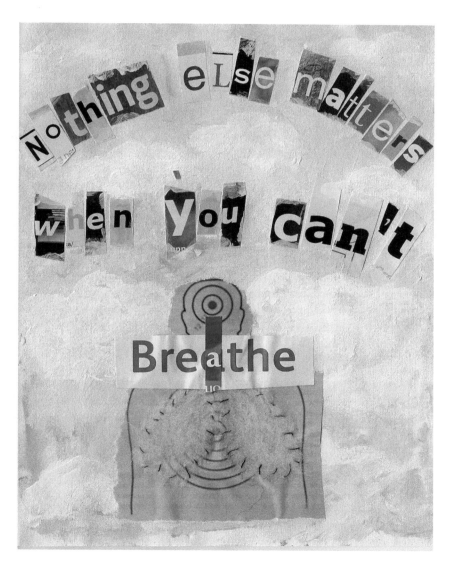

*Figure 9.2* Nothing Else Matters Collage, by Susan Carr, 2011

child it is like losing a lung'. Rando's quote seems to indicate that Peter had suffered a double blow where his breathing was concerned, living with both COPD and the recent loss of his son.

The author C. S. Lewis reflected on his own embodiment of bereavement after losing his wife:

> How often will the vast emptiness astonish me like a complete novelty and make me say, 'I never realized my loss till this moment'? The same leg is cut off time after time [. . .]. At present I am learning to get about on crutches. Perhaps I shall presently be given a wooden leg. But I shall never be a biped again.
>
> (Lewis, 2013 [1963], pp. 53–56)

Bereaved parents often express feelings of living in a void, or experiencing a sense of 'otherness' in relation to the people around them. In their study with parents who had lost a child, Riches and Dawson (1996, p. 145) quote a respondent as saying, 'This is a very exclusive *club*, I hope to God you never join it'. The idea of being an 'insider' suggests that their experiences are unique and exclusive, something that cannot easily be understood by 'outsiders' (Exley & Letherby, 2001, p. 119).

Although I couldn't physically meet Mark, I wanted to learn all I could about him, so I encouraged Peter to tell me what kind of person Mark was. I also went to visit Mark's grave, as a way of paying my respects to him, and to acknowledge his importance within the therapeutic relationship Peter and I had developed. Through the stories Peter told, I began to put together a picture of Mark in my mind, and through our discussions it was decided that I should paint a double life-sized portrait of him, to show the prominence of this relationship in Peter's life (Figure 9.3). Peter brought photographs of Mark to our portrait sessions and I made copies of these to use as reference, and one of the phrases Peter often used during our sessions was 'there was something about Mark. . . '. This then became the title of the portrait, adding RIP as a recognition and acknowledgement of his death.

By Susan M Carr (co-designed by Peter), 2011

Reflecting upon this portrait it seems that I situated Mark in a dark, empty space . . . with no distractions around him, which focuses the viewer's attention directly on Mark. A person removed from any kind of context is something rarely seen in daily life, and is potentially a disturbing way to view a person. This 'empty space' reminds us that we are all existentially alone, particularly when it comes to illness and death. Our own death and physical illness are something that are always 'our own', no other person can take on this burden for us, even for a moment. Interestingly when the portrait *There's Something About Mark RIP*, was exhibited recently in my 'Paint me this way!' portrait therapy exhibition (July—Sept 2017, at Swindon Museum and Art Gallery), the evaluation cards completed by visitors demonstrated that this painting was one of the portraits they 'most connected with'. Some of the reasons they gave were:

> 'Because of the depth in the eyes which express years of emotion'.
> 'Size & Impact. I feel like he is looking at me'.
> 'Such a direct gaze, you feel his mouth is ready to say something to you'.
> 'It's so moving—his eyes are full of sadness'.

In his end of project interview Peter anticipated how important this double life-sized portrait of Mark would be to both him and his family, saying '[. . .] I think when my sons and

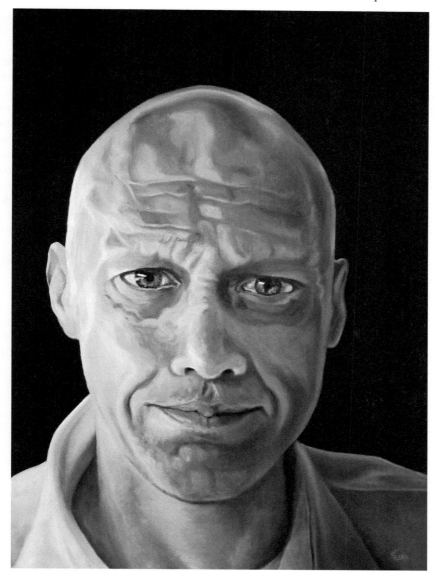

*Figure 9.3* There's Something About Mark, RIP

my wife see that [indicating *There's Something About Mark RIP portrait*] it will bring tears to their eyes. . . *it's as if he is there with us!* It's so wonderful. . . '.

The 'as if' quality inherent within portraiture, and the belief Peter speaks of, that Mark 'is there with us', does not mean he is *denying* Mark's death, what it does is bring Mark back, in a tangible sense, into the *present*, where his *presence* is a comfort to Peter and his family. Through the portrait, Mark becomes again part of a coherent life story, that equates to a seamless continuity between the past and present. The 'as if' quality means that Mark exists in two realities, the past and the present, and for a moment of 'suspended disbelief' Mark is brought before their eyes in a physical sense, closing the gap between someone who is *emotionally present* and *physically absent*. This works for Peter as an 'adaptive acceptance of separation and connection' (Carr, 2015, p. 192), and can therefore be seen as a reflection of Peter's ability to accept the loss of Mark.

All the patients involved in the project were given framed prints of their portraits, as the originals will be shown in exhibitions promoting portrait therapy, and Peter asked for small copies of his portraits to keep in his wallet at all times. Over the weeks that followed I noticed that whenever Peter met a new patient at day-hospice he would reach for his wallet and show them the portraits. It was a way to safely bring the conversation around to his lost son, perhaps a way into the private 'club' of the bereaved parent. I believe Peter did this, not to gain sympathy, but to be in his *father of Mark* identity again, and to have this validated by another person. The fact that these portraits were painted 'third hand' was also important, as it gave Peter another reason to show them . . . often to my own embarrassment, as he would point me out to the patient and say 'Susan painted these!' But the pleasure he derived from showing them was palpable, and because they were *painted* portraits and therefore considered 'works of art' it indicated a life *worthy* of being painted, and offered added interest for someone who hadn't met Mark. It would not have been so easy for Peter to show strangers photographs of Mark, it was somehow the fact that they were 'painted' and therefore 'made special' (Dissanayake, 1988), that gave him 'permission' to do so. As Dissanayake says:

> One intends by making special to place the activity or artefact in a 'realm' different from the everyday [. . .] Both artist and perceiver often feel that in art they have an intimate connection with a world that is different from if not superior to ordinary experience.
>
> (1988, p. 92)

In his end of project interview Peter talked about how the project helped him 'accept the loss of Mark', an acknowledgement of adaption and closure, saying:

> *what it has done is help me to accept the loss of Mark. It's helped me in that respect, I don't know why, but it has,* and I can talk about him now without filling up with tears, which I couldn't before. . .

For Peter, revisiting his 'father of Mark' identity through the portraits was an opportunity to reclaim his lost metaphoric 'lung' caused by bereavement, and a way to contain and visibly mend his feelings of helplessness over his inability to protect Mark from illness and death. Co-designing the portraits of Mark and himself, gave Peter something that he could still 'do' for Mark, a way of being in that caring 'father of Mark' role, and a way of honouring Mark's life. Sadly, Peter died several months after we worked together, but he was aware of how these portraits would become a legacy, part of his and Mark's *future* identity, through the exhibitions and publication of the portraits.

When these portraits were exhibited, it was an opportunity for his family to pay homage, and the importance of the portraits and the voice recording of Peter talking about being painted, were reflected within comments left at the gallery by his widow, she said:

> What a wonderful exhibition. I was so overwhelmed when I walked in and saw the amazing portraits of my late husband and son, and to hear my husband's voice again . . . I really didn't expect all this . . . thank you. . .

Peter's widow also left a message on my telephone answering machine to thank me, saying:

> This exhibition, and seeing the portraits of Peter and Mark has been wonderful . . . I have visited the exhibition *several times a week* during the three months it has been on . . . it has meant so much . . . thank you!

One of Peter's sons (Mark's brother) also left a comment in the book:

> Wow—Dad (Peter) and Mark (my Brother)! Emotional—I can't begin to tell you how grateful I am to you!

Peter's increased ability to 'accept the loss of Mark' may also have been linked to an increased feeling of 'control', through his active involvement in the co-designing process. This perception of control and autonomy served to reduce the intense feelings of helplessness, caused by uncontrollable losses such as illness and bereavement (Werner-Seidler et al, 2011). Within the portraits, metaphor and symbolic language were used to help patients develop a 'coherent life story' (Hass-Cohen, 2008, p. 290) and incorporate dualities such as 'presence and absence' into that story. The collages and prose poem were also important as they acknowledged the life stories and events that had both *made* and un-made Peter's self-identity.

Although the portrait therapy process helped Peter accept the loss of Mark, 'closure' can only ever be partial, with new losses such as illness bringing to the fore previous painful experiences, it seems that the 'door' of bereavement and grief is never quite 'closed' and can 'swing wide open' again with any new loss. However, it is clear that art and creative expression can be an empowering force which can 'voice one's darkest struggles. [. . .] Oppression can become vision. Despair can become determination' (Berger, 2006, p. 111).

### Afterward: Reflecting on Experience

Being close to and supporting someone who is dying, and accompanying them as best we can on their journey, inevitably leads to reflections on our own mortality and the complex processes of 'holding on' and 'letting go' involved in the grieving process. Throughout my 12 years working in palliative care, the existential shock and finality of death was something I found difficult to process, however I developed my own spiritual and artistic rituals to help alleviate these stresses and to enable a process of 'letting go' to begin. These included attending funerals of patients I worked closely with, both as a mark of respect for the patient, but also as a mark of solidarity with the families. I also created simple environmental artistic installations for each patient. These were small things that took very little time, but which highlighted for me, the personal significance of the patient (Figures 9.4 and 9.5).

I believe that, as Peter found, it is the process of *doing* and *being there for* that person one last time, that enables a sense of closure for the inevitable unfinished business which death brings, and stills the inner voice which asks. . . 'Could I have done more?'

The intensely personal nature of loss and bereavement highlights the importance of 'flexibility and innovation' when searching for new interventions to meet the diverse range of clients' needs, something that requires the therapist to step out of the shadows, and bring their own unique skills to the therapeutic encounter (Bocking, 2005, p. 222). Ultimately portrait therapy enables those living with severe illness who have unresolved

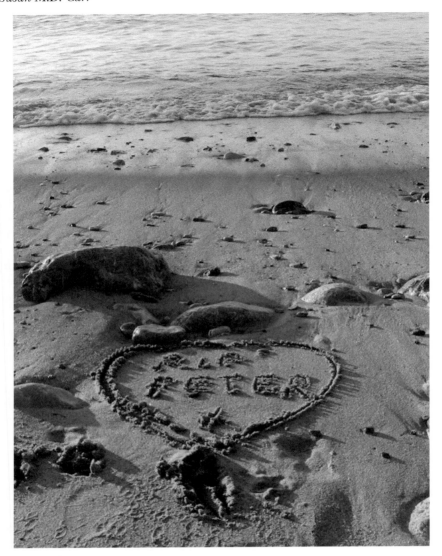

*Figure 9.4* RIP Peter (See Plate 8)

issues of bereavement to take time to rediscover the sense of self-identity they feel they have lost, and through co-designing the portraits, develop new meanings and connections, and begin the process of reconstructing and managing who they are (Exley & Letherby, 2001, p. 129). As McNiff (2004) says, 'Art adapts to every conceivable problem and lends its transformative, insightful, and experience-heightening powers to people in need. [. . .] The medicines of art are not confined within fixed borders' (p. 5). I hope therefore that this account of using my own artistic practice in the service of others, will motivate and inspire other therapists, to relinquish the ties that restrict the imagination and to continue to 'push at the edges of what the arts therapies might become' (Moon, 2002, p. 29).

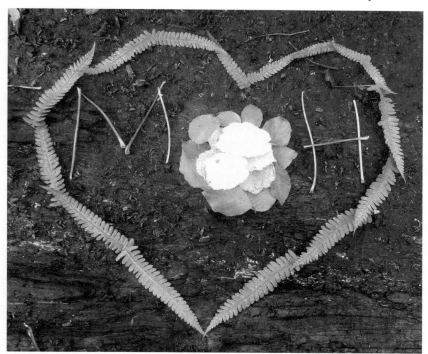

*Figure 9.5* RIP Mark

## References

Beaumont, S. (2013) Art therapy for complicated grief: A focus on meaning-making approaches. *Canadian Art Therapy Association Journal*, Vol. 26(2), pp. 1–7.

Berger, J. (2006) *Music of the Soul: Composing Life out of Loss*. Abingdon & New York: Routledge.

Bocking, M. (2005) 'A "don't know" story: Art therapy in an NHS medical oncology department'. In D. Waller & C. Sibbett (eds.) *Art Therapy and Cancer Care* (pp. 199–209). London: Open University Press.

Buber, M. (2004 [1937]) *I and Thou* (Second Edition). London: Continuum.

Butler, J. (2004) *Precarious Life: The Powers of Mourning and Violence*. London & New York: Verso.

Carel, H. (2008) *Illness: The Cry of the Flesh*. Stocksfield, UK: Acumen.

Carr, S. M. D. (2014) Revisioning self-identity: The role of portraits, neuroscience and the art therapist's 'third hand'. *The International Journal of Art Therapy*, Vol. 19(2), pp. 54–70.

Carr, S. M. D. (2015) *Enabling self-identity revisioning through portraiture, for people living with life threatening and chronic illnesses: Paint me this way!* Loughborough University Ph.D. Thesis.

Carr, S. M. D. (2017) *Portrait Therapy: Resolving Self-Identity Disruption in Clients with Life-Threatening and Chronic Illnesses*. London & Philadelphia: Jessica Kingsley.

Carr, S. M. D. & Hancock, S. (2017) Healing the inner child through portrait therapy: Illness, identity and childhood trauma. *International Journal of Art Therapy*, Vol. 22(1), pp. 8–21.

Cohen, M. (2002) 'Death ritual: Anthropological perspectives'. In P. Pecorino (ed.) *Perspectives on Death and Dying*. Online Textbook. Accessed on 8/3/2017 at https://goo.gl/RLjXlw

Dissanayake, E. (1988) *What Is Art for?* Seattle: University of Washington Press.

Exley, C. & Letherby, G. (2001) Managing a disrupted life course: Issue of identity and emotion work. *Health*, Vol. 5(1), pp. 112–132.

Falvo, D. (1999) *Medical and Psychosocial Aspects of Chronic Illness and Disability* (Second Edition). Gaithersburg, MD: Aspen.

Freud, S. (1917) *Mourning and Melancholia*. Online. Accessed on 6/10/ 2017 at www.english.upenn.edu/~cavitch/pdf-library/Freud_MourningAndMelancholia.pdf

Gershman, N. & Baddeley, J. (2010) Prescriptive photomontage: A process and product for meaning seekers with complicated grief. *Annals of American Psychotherapy*, Fall, pp. 28–34.

Giddens, A. (1991) *Modernity and Self-Identity: Self and Society in the Late Modern Age*. Cambridge: Polity.

Hardy, D. (2013) Working with loss: An examination of how language can be used to address the issue of loss in art therapy. *International Journal of Art Therapy*, Vol. 18(1), pp. 29–37.

Hass-Cohen, N. (2008) 'CREATE: Art therapy relational neuroscience principles (ATR-N)'. In N. Hass-Cohen & R. Carr (eds.) *Art Therapy and Clinical Neuroscience* (pp. 283–305). London & Philadelphia: Jessica Kingsley.

Heath, B. & Lings, J. (2012) Creative song writing in therapy at the end of life and in bereavement. *Mortality*, Vol. 17(2), pp. 106–118.

Heidegger, M. (1962 [1927]) *Being and Time*. New York: Harper & Row.

Hilliker, L. (2006) Letting go while holding on: Postmortem photography as an aid to the grieving process. *Illness, Crisis, & Loss*, Vol. 14(3), pp. 245–269.

Hodson, P. (1984) *Men: An Investigation into the Emotional Male*. London: British Broadcasting Corporation (BBC).

Kinnvall, C. (2004) Globalization and religious nationalism: Self, identity, and the search for ontological security. *Political Psychology*, Vol. 25(5), pp. 741–767.

Klass, D., Silverman, P. & Nickman, P. (1996) *Continuing Bonds: New Understandings of Grief*. London: Routledge.

Kohut, M. (2011) Making art from memories: Honoring deceased loved ones through a scrapbooking bereavement group. *Art Therapy: Journal of the American Art Therapy Association*, Vol. 28, pp. 123–131.

Kramer, E. (1971) *Art as Therapy with Children*. London: Schocken Books.

Lewis, C. S. (2013 [1963]) *A Grief Observed*. New York: Harper Collins.

Liebmann, M. (2003) 'Working with men'. In S. Hogan (ed.) *Gender Issues in Art Therapy* (pp. 108–125). London & Philadelphia: Jessica Kingsley.

Lister, S., Pushkar, D. & Connolly, K. (2008) Current bereavement theory: Implications for art therapy practice. *The Arts in Psychotherapy*, Vol. 35, pp. 245–250.

Mancini, A. & Bonanno, G. (2006) Resilience in the face of potential trauma: Clinical practices and illustrations. *Journal of Clinical Psychology: In Session*, Vol. 62, pp. 971–985.

McNiff, S. (2004) *Art Heals: How Creativity Cures the Soul*. Boston & London: Shambala.

Moon, C. (2002) *Studio Art Therapy: Cultivating the Artist Identity in the Art Therapist*. London & Philadelphia: Jessica Kingsley.

Morycz, R. (1992) 'Widowhood and bereavement in late life'. In V. B. Van Hasselt et al. (eds.) *Handbook of Social Development*. New York: Springer Science & Business Media.

Neimeyer, R. A. (2000) Searching for the meaning of meaning: Grief therapy and the process of reconstruction. *Death Studies*, Vol. 24, pp. 541–558.

Neimeyer, R. A. (2006a) 'Widowhood, grief, and the quest for meaning: A narrative perspective on resilience'. In D. Carr, R. M. Nesse & C. B. Wortman (eds.) *Spousal Bereavement in Late Life* (pp. 227–252). New York: Springer.

Neimeyer, R. A. (2006b) Complicated grief and the reconstruction of meaning: Conceptual and empirical contributions to a cognitive-constructivist model. *Clinical Psychology: Science and Practice*, Vol. 13, pp. 141–145.

Neimeyer, R. A. (2012) 'From stage follower to stage manager: Contemporary directions in bereavement care'. In K. J. Doak & A. S. Tucci (eds.) *Beyond Kubler-Ross: New Perspectives on Death, Dying and Grief* (pp. 129–150). Washington, DC: Hospice Foundation of America.

Neimeyer, R. A, Baldwin, S. & Gillies, J. (2006) Continuing bonds and reconstructing meaning: Mitigating complications in bereavement. *Death Studies*, Vol. 30(8), pp. 715–738.

Neimeyer, R. A. & Currier, J. M. (2009) Grief therapy: Evidence of efficacy and emerging directions. *Current Directions in Psychological Science*, Vol. 18, pp. 352–356.

Neimeyer, R. A. & Sands, D. C. (2011) 'Meaning reconstruction in bereavement: From principles to practice'. In R. A. Neimeyer, H. Winokuer, D. Harris & G. Thornton (eds.) *Grief and Bereavement in Contemporary Society: Bridging Research and Practice* (pp. 9–21). New York: Routledge.

Parkes, C. & Prigerson, H. (2010) *Bereavement: Studies in Grief in Adult Life.* Hove & New York: Routledge.

Rando, T. (1991) 'Parental adjustment to the loss of a child'. In D. Papadatou & C. Papadatos (eds.) *Children & Death.* London: Hemisphere Publishing Corporation.

Rathaupt, A. (2007) Literature review of western bereavement theory: From decathecting to continuing bonds. *The Family Journal: Counseling and Therapy for Couples and Families,* January, pp. 6–15.

Riches, G. & Dawson, P. (1996) Communities of feeling: The culture of bereaved parents. *Mortality,* Vol. 1(2), pp. 143–161.

Rodin, G., Craven, J. & Littlefield, C. (1991) *Depression in the Medically Ill: An Integrated Approach.* New York: Brunner/Mazel.

Santino, J. (ed.) (2016) *Spontaneous Shrines and the Public Memorialization of Death.* New York: Palgrave Macmillan.

Stroebe, M., Abakoumkin, G., Stroebe, W. & Schut, H. (2012) Continuing bonds in adjustment to bereavement: Impact of abrupt versus gradual separation. *Personal Relationships,* Vol. 19, pp. 255–266.

Stroebe, M. & Stroebe, W. (1991) Does 'grief work' work? *Journal of Consulting and Clinical Psychology,* Vol. 59, pp. 479–482.

Tannen, D. (1992 [1990]) *You Just Don't Understand—Women and Men in Conversation.* London: Virago.

Taylor, C. (1989) *Sources of the Self: The Making of Modern Identity.* Cambridge: Cambridge University Press.

Tjasink, M. (2010) Art psychotherapy in medical oncology: A search for meaning. *International Journal of Art Therapy,* Vol. 15(2), pp. 75–83.

Turner, V. (1982) *From Ritual to Theatre: The Human Seriousness of Play.* Performing Arts Journal Publication: New York.

Turner, V. (1995) *The Ritual Process: Structure and Anti-Structure.* New York: Aldine de Gruyter.

Volkan, V. (1997) *Bloodlines: From Ethnic Pride to Ethnic Terrorism.* Boulder, CO: Westview.

Werner-Seidler, A. & Moulds, M. L. (2011) Autobiographical memory characteristics in depression vulnerability: Formerly depressed individuals recall less vivid positive memories. *Cognition & Emotion,* Vol. 25(6), pp. 1087–1103.

Wright, K. (2009) *Mirroring and Attunement: Self-Realisation in Psychoanalysis and Art.* London; New York: Routledge.

Young, M. (1988) Understanding identity disruption and intimacy: One aspect of post-traumatic stress. *Contemporary Family Therapy,* Vol. 10(1), pp. 30–43.

# 10 Utilizing Tablet Computers in Art Therapy for Young People With Chronic and Life-Limiting Illnesses

*Amy Bucciarelli*

## Introduction

Art therapy is beneficial for a variety of hospitalized patients (Bucciarelli, 2016; Anand, 2016; Councill and Phlegar, 2013). However, sometimes traditional artmaking can feel intimidating, difficult to use, or even unrelatable. In these cases, art therapists have another tool in their toolbox: tablet computers. In this chapter I outline the therapeutic strengths of tablets according to ten years of clinical experience integrating electronic-based work into art therapy sessions. Within this work, my approach to art therapy has primarily originated from a humanistic theoretical framework (Garai, 2001). This chapter specifically focuses on tablets as appropriate and viable art tools for children, teenagers, and young adults who are hospitalized with chronic and life-limiting illnesses.

## Tablet Technology

Tablets are flat-screened mobile hand-held computing devices between seven and ten inches diagonally across their screen (Consumer Reports, 2016). Most tablets connect wirelessly to Internet and have built-in microphones and camera lenses. Tablets have touchscreens controlled by tapping, swiping, or pinching on the screen. They can also be controlled via pen-shaped stylus (for artists: a paintbrush-looking tool) offering further precision over screen-sensed marks. Tablets function on software called applications (apps). Thousands of downloadable apps simulate art activities such as drawing, painting, collage, sketchbooks, graphic design, photo editing, animation, filmmaking, and 3D modeling. A tablet strategically loaded with therapist-selected art apps expands the capabilities of art therapy and provides a tool that is accessible, easy to use, and adaptable to many patients.

## Therapeutic Advantages of Tablet Use

Art therapists have acknowledged that digital art is a viable twenty-first-century media adaptable to a variety of therapeutic settings (Alders et al., 2011; Orr, 2016; Thong, 2007). In particular, digital media is primed for work with children, adolescents, and young adults because it is an integrated part of how they navigate the world socially and physically (Malchiodi and Johnson, 2013; Orr, 2005; Kaimal et al., 2016). Authors have agreed that some of the most advantageous features of digital media include: adaptability, multimodal capabilities, and familiarity, leading to increased rapport (Choe, 2016; Orr, 2005; Thong, 2007).

Tablets are powerful tools for accessing digital media in hospital settings. Medical conditions and the hospital milieu can shift quickly, impacting both motivation and capabilities for art therapy engagement (Anand, 2016; Councill and Phlegar, 2013). Medical art therapists must be flexible and responsive to changing patient needs (Anand, 2016; Malchiodi, 2013; Ullmann, 2013). Tablets host a variety of art therapy possibilities within an easily available and compact tool that can help art therapists transform challenges of hospitalization into therapeutic opportunities. In particular, tablets can be used to: (1) increase accessibility to art, (2) provide an appropriate level of sensory stimulation, (3) ensure patient safety, (4) increase personal empowerment, (5) expand creativity, and (6) enrich the therapeutic relationship.

## Accessibility

### Adaptive

Traditional art processes can be too complex or cumbersome for people coping with medical conditions (McNiff, 1999; Ullmann, 2013). Tablets can serve as adaptive devices that facilitate artmaking for varied levels of ability (Barber and Garner, 2016; Malchiodi and Johnson, 2013; Orr, 2005; 2010). For example, people with brain injuries can drag a finger across a tablet without the fine-motor skills required to hold a pencil or paintbrush. Tablets also have assistive features such as text magnification, audio description, and voice recognition. People with significantly limited mobility can use tablet-compatible sensors to enable eye-control (Karamchandani et al., 2015) and brain-computer interface (BCI) features (Al-Taleb and Vuckovic, 2015; Tseng et al., 2015).

### Energy

The energy patients have for artmaking varies day-to-day (Anand, 2016; Councill and Phlegar, 2013). A patient can invest hours creating mixed-media work, but the next day, may not have enough energy to squish clay or pull paint across paper. Traditional art materials take time and effort to set up and later clean up. For some, simply watching the art therapist prepare the art space is exhausting or intimidating. Tablets can help patients self-regulate their art experience according to their energy level. A series of swipes across the tablet might be a patient's maximum available effort; however, s/he is still making art! The artwork can be effortlessly saved and then reopened when the patient has more energy.

### Space

Some hospitals in the United States have studios where patients can leave their rooms and visit a space designed for artmaking. However, more often, art therapists use communal spaces or deliver care at the bedside (Anand, 2016). Long-term and critical patients can have a lot of medical devices crowding their rooms. Additionally, the longer a patient has been hospitalized, the more likely the room is filled with personal items to help daily life seem as "normal" as possible. Medical art therapists cope with limited spaces. A table, tray, or easel is necessary for traditional artmaking but may be difficult to find a place for in hospital rooms. Space is also required to properly dry artwork and store materials. Tablets, on the other hand are fully self-contained. Patients can nest them in their lap, hold them in one hand, or even use them while lying down.

### Available

During bedside work, if patients run out of materials or desire additional art supplies the art therapist might have to interrupt the session to go gather the items. On the other hand, tablets theoretically contain limitless supplies of "art materials". Tablets also make art accessible even when the art therapist is unavailable. Tablet art is simple to initiate and tablets can be stored bedside for easy access. Backlit screens make it possible to use tablets in darkened rooms. If patients cannot sleep, they can make art to self-soothe without disturbing family members who might be resting. Because tablets are mobile, adaptable, and easily available, they are frequently the first art tool a patient can use after surgery and the last one they can use near the end of life.

### *Cost Efficient*

Art therapists have noted that technology can be expensive (Malchiodi and Johnson, 2013; Orr, 2005; Thong, 2007). Tablets require an initial financial investment, but then become cost-efficient tools for art therapy. The price of most apps is a one-time fee that ranges from $.99 to $5.00. The therapist's app account allows these purchases to be transferable to multiple tablet devices without repurchasing them. Art therapists should feel encouraged to seek donors or grants that could support tablet purchases.

## Sensory Stimulation

Art therapists who have used electronic-based art recognized that digital media, just like traditional art, should be selected with intentionality and an understanding of both the inherent benefits and challenges associated with its use (Carlton, 2016; Diggs, Lubas and De Leo, 2015; Parker-Bell, 1999). One of the top resistances to digital media is that it does not facilitate the same therapeutically important embodied experiences as traditional media (Choe, 2014; Klorer, 2009; Orr, 2005; 2012). Tablets, however, more than computers or cameras, re-engage the user with tactile sensations through the touchscreen (Carlton, 2016; Orr, 2016; Thong, 2007). Some apps even simulate body-based movements like shaking the tablet to erase the canvas (Radtastical, 2014) or tilting the tablet to roll a virtual paint-dipped marble across the screen (Shoe the Goose, 2013).

It is important to note that hospital settings can frequently be *over* stimulating (Councill, 2012). Art materials can add to an already saturated environment and can cause the patient to resist engaging in art therapy (Alders et al., 2011; Orr, 2005). Patients may be unable to articulate their resistance, yet it seems that at an unconscious level their bodies sense that the additional stimuli will be too much. A patient in critical condition might decline the opportunity to draw with markers on paper but agree to draw on a smooth, non-mess tablet. Sometimes, the tablet holds the art space until the patient is well enough to transition into traditional artmaking.

## Safety

### *Materials and Safety*

Art materials must be properly sterilized to prevent unintentional infection and to protect immune-compromised patients. For the most part, tablets are flat with only a few flush buttons, reducing potential places for bacteria to germinate. With a protective case, tablets are easy to wipe with hospital-approved disinfectants.

Some media cannot be used in medical settings because the environment needs to remain sterile, there is not proper ventilation, or the materials could negatively impact patients' health (Anand, 2016; Councill, 1999; 2012). For example, glitter is popularly requested but is usually not allowed in hospitals. It can be inhaled or clog IV lines. However, patients can be just as thrilled about a "glitter filter" on an app— and it is completely safe to use. Certain materials pose patient-specific health-risks. A patient on blood thinning medication should not use scissors because an accidental cut could be fatal. However, tablets can safely simulate the function of "cutting out" collage through image cropping. In fact, tablets can expand the collage experience by incorporating real-time photography and photo editing into the process. For example, a patient can create a personalized feeling-states chart (Figure 10.1). The chart is a fun expressive experience that can then be utilized in future art therapy session as a feelings check-in tool.

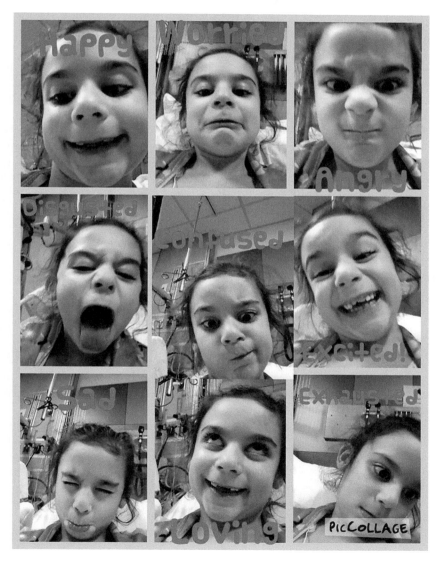

*Figure 10.1* Personalized Feeling-states chart

### Emotional Safety

In addition to physical safety, tablets can support emotional safety. Hospitalized patients have very little privacy, especially in critical or end-of-life care (Anand, 2016; Councill, 2012; Malchiodi, 1999). Intensive care units typically have hospital room doors made of glass, allowing the staff to constantly monitor the patient's health status, however, this means that during an art therapy session most anyone can watch the normally private therapeutic process. Additionally, family members might be in the patient's room and not want to leave. On a tablet, the screen space is small and the artist can exercise more control over whom the tablet is pointed towards and how public the artmaking becomes.

Many aspects of hospital care take precedence over art therapy. For example, an art therapy session might be interrupted so that doctors can examine the patient, a nurse can administer time-sensitive medications, or in the middle of a session, a patient might have a medical crisis that needs treatment. With most medical interruptions, traditional art materials have to be cleaned-up and put away. The likelihood the patient will wish to resume afterwards significantly drops because of the time and effort it takes to stop making art, clean up, and then re-set up. Patients using a tablet can pause their work at the press of a button and just as easily re-engage following medical care.

In bedside work, art therapists have to find ways to differentiate the therapeutic space from the place where scary, overwhelming, or traumatizing medical things happen. The boundaries of the tablet screen are literally a physical safety container for patient artwork. Unlike traditional art materials, the risk of excessive mess or extreme loss of control is minimal (Alders et al., 2011; Barber and Garner, 2016). Metaphorically, the tablet is a safe therapeutic space separate from the medical environment. The tablet creates a new dimension for therapy in the digital environment: a virtual safe place.

## Empowerment

### Control

Critically ill patients have very little autonomy during their hospital treatment (Anand, 2016; Councill, 1999; Councill and Phlegar, 2013; Malchiodi, 1999). Thong (2007) noted that choice is one of the most important things that digital media can facilitate. A single tablet loaded with a variety of apps empowers patients to make in-the-moment decisions about what type of art they prefer (painting, drawing, photography, etc.). Tablets allow patients not only to choose the creative processes appropriate for their current abilities, but also to regulate how many choices they wish to make. Patients can opt to fully control the app features or enable a *random* setting that uses computer algorithms to drive selections. Choe (2014) observed that digital media users are not solely creators, ". . . but also exert control over the development, production, and distribution of their own art" (p. 152). Patients can choose to keep their creations privately filed on the tablet, print and display them, or share them virtually on social media—when appropriate.

### Confidence

Digital media can increase artistic confidence through an intuitive exploration process that takes place as patients learn to navigate and master app software (Choe,

2014). Digital media facilitates creative experimentation while lowering the required technical skill and perceived risk of traditional artmaking (Kaimal et al., 2016). It is easy to undo a step, save iterations, and start over without wasting materials or time (Diggs, Lubas and De Leo, 2015). Practice with trial-and-error is valuable for developing problem solving skills that can eventually be translated to traditional artmaking processes and life tasks (Orr, 2010). Chronically ill patients can experience regressions or have developmental delays resulting from lifelong hospitalizations and medical complications (Anand, 2016; Councill, 1999). Apps that combine drawing with templates, forms, and collage features help artistic skill meet emotional expectations for self-expression. Tablets can help increase a sense of artistic mastery without leading to anxiety, frustration, or self-criticism (Choe, 2016; Diggs, Lubas and De Leo, 2015; Orr, 2005).

### *Normalization*

Hospitalized patients commonly make artwork as gifts for caregivers or as decorations for their rooms. There is a sense of meaning-making that becomes important in producing artwork that they are proud of during such a challenging time (Bucciarelli, 2016; Councill, 2012; Council and Phlegar, 2013; Malchiodi, 1999). Color-printed digital images look stunning on matt or glossy photo paper and they are easily replicated at a low-cost. There are many other options for printing digital images including fine art papers, specialty gifts, and 3D printed models. Digital work can also be virtually shared with loved ones who are not able to visit the hospital, fostering the potential for long-distance collaborations and social connections (Orr, 2010).

## Creativity

### *Creative Assistance*

Medications, fatigue, and discomfort can impair patients' abilities to think critically and creatively (Councill, 1999; 2012). Anxiety or depression resulting from the medical situation can further impact attention and focus (Anand, 2016; Councill, 1999; Malchiodi, 1999). People who are used to functioning at high cognitive levels might resist making art because they are embarrassed or frustrated by their current abilities. Tablets can boost creative confidence (Choe, 2016; Orr, 2012). Some apps will correct a shaky line to a straight line (FiftyThree, Inc., 2016). Other apps offer a combination of drawing, collage and virtual "stickers" that can help stimulate imaginative thinking (Shoe the Goose, 2014). A popular mandala app (Bendis, 2012) provides a circle form for the patient to use. Simple finger swipes elicit beautiful designs created in kaleidoscope patterns.

### *Creative Expansion*

Digital media enhances creative opportunities by expanding the boundaries of the art studio (Carlton, 2016; McNiff, 1999; Orr, 2005; 2016). Artistic expression has multi-layered possibilities when apps, Internet accessibility, and printing in 2D and 3D are combined (Choe, 2014; Kaimal et al., 2016; Orr, 2005; 2016). Digital media can be mixed with traditional media generating even more possibilities. If digital capabilities do not exist for what a user envisions, tech savvy patients can even design their own art apps with do-it-yourself mobile app builders.

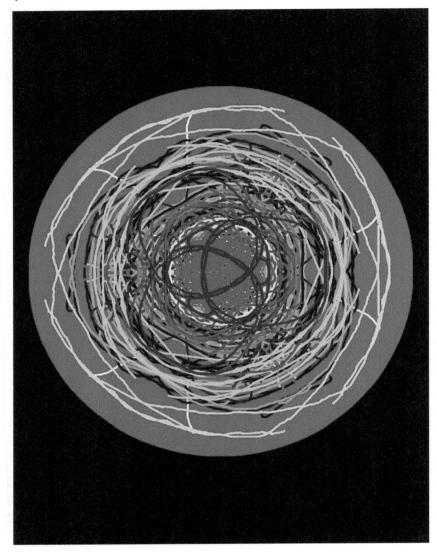

*Figure 10.2* iPad Mandala (See Plate 7)

### Creative Experimentation

Tablet artwork seems to be particularly symbolic for terminally sick patients contemplating questions about death. Patients nearing the end of life might make artwork with scenarios or symbols that represent relationships between this earthly life and the existence beyond it. Tablets can facilitate symbolic play between ideas of transition, transcendence, and impermanence. For example, a patient can create something in the liminal digital space, which is neither tangible nor non-existent. Then, the patient can choose to delete the image, make it tangible by printing it, or post it on the Internet (in which case it theoretically becomes transcendent, existing indefinitely on the worldwide web). Digital media facilitates the interplay between dimensions in a way that more traditional art media cannot do.

*Creative Legacy*

Artwork is frequently one of the only tangible things that families have left once a patient has passed away. The patient's artwork becomes archival treasures for loved ones (Malchiodi, 1999; Councill and Phelgar, 2013). With the appropriate permissions, tablet artwork can be printed, stored, or shared electronically as a lasting legacy. Many times, patients have clear and expansively creative visions for the artwork they want to leave behind. Examples of digital legacy projects include: a multimedia "bucket-list" movie (Beasley, 2015), a slideshow of digital artwork set to self-composed music (Medina, 2014), a book of poems about cancer illustrated with patient-produced artwork (Long, 2014), a life story designed with a combination of photographs and words (Williams, 2014), a book offering emotional education to teenagers who receive an artificial heart (Henderson and Bucciarelli, 2014), and an app to help educate young children about *How the Heart Works* (University of Florida, 2015).

## Therapeutic Relationship

In the United States, parents who work or have multiple children may have to leave their sick child alone in the hospital (Anand, 2016; Councill, 2012). Hospital staff work on rotating shifts with multiple patients, which makes it difficult to maintain schedules and monitor patient activities consistently. Television, movies, video games, volunteers, and visitors become distractions. Any one of these pastimes can be more appealing to patients than art therapy. Tablets can be used as a tool to overcome treatment resistance and build therapeutic rapport (Choe, 2016; Carlton, 2014; Diggs, Lubas and DeLeo, 2015; Orr, 2005; 2012; Thong, 2007). Patients may not be motivated to shift from playing video games to painting on paper but they might be open to use a tablet, which is a more similar media. In today's digital climate, a tablet might be *more* familiar to a young patient than crayons or paints. Familiarities with media can increase interest and creative capabilities (Orr, 2005).

Children and teenagers, who have experienced medical trauma, can sometimes "zone-out" on familiar electronics by watching movies or playing video games. Art therapy can help patients develop a healthier relationship with digital media: one that is positive, mindful, and constructive instead of reactive and sometimes destructive (Choe, 2016). Tablet art therapy facilitates the transition from passive to active electronic use. The tablet becomes a stepping-stone from non-arts activities to creative expression, then from digital to tactile artmaking. Confidence, trust, and functional skill are developed through the transitional process. Because young people can be more adept with digital media, it is possible that patients discover new techniques and capabilities that the art therapist did not know. Those instances should be celebrated. The patient is empowered to become the teacher and guide for the artmaking process, further building rapport and strengthening self-esteem (Kaimal et al., 2016; Thong, 2007).

Finally, tablets can serve as transitional objects between the therapeutic relationship and independent creative artmaking. Patients can easily access tablet art during nights and weekends when the therapist is unavailable. Many patients have their own tablets and will download their favorite art apps to use outside of art therapy sessions. As such, tablets can increase artistic independence and encourage self-initiated artmaking.

## Guide to Selecting Apps for Art Therapy

There are many art-based apps for free download or purchase in app stores. Table 10.1 is a list of recommended app characteristics I have found most helpful when choosing apps for art therapy.

*Table 10.1* Characteristics of Ideal Apps for Facilitating Art Therapy on a Tablet

| Feature | Description | Brief Rationale |
| --- | --- | --- |
| Active creation (NAEYC, 2012) | Requires active participation, creativity, and play. | Allows user to explore app functions and control the media/outcome of the experience. Might also allow user collaboration. This is a distinguishing feature for apps that are good for art therapy versus more passive art apps that are not. |
| Robust and simple (Choe, 2014) | Less than 10 main menu choices (ideally about 5). | Too many choices can be overwhelming, not enough choices can be limiting. |
| Intuitive / easy to use (Choe, 2014) | Can navigate without much instruction. | Interface is easy to learn and aesthetically nice. Allows time to be invested on artmaking process. |
| Responsive | No lag time for functions or saving. | Functions or saving that take a long time will frustrate and/or lose user interest. |
| Eraser or multiple undos | Able to erase or undo more than one consecutive time. | Some apps do not have an eraser or undo feature *or* they only allow backing up one-step. Patients prefer multiple erasures and undos/redos. |
| Levels of automation | Users can make all choices, or have the computer randomly make choices—such as change colors or patterns. | User may select different levels of independence or automation according to energy level and cognitive capability to make choices. |
| Intuitive assistance | Self-corrects a shaky line to straight line, wobbly circle to even circle, etc. | An assistive feature for patients with limitations. Helps increase esteem and success with artmaking. |
| Allows saving to the tablet | The work can be saved outside of the app and instead on the tablet's camera roll. | Some apps only allow saving work on the app's cloud. Artwork should be saved directly to the tablet for storage or future printing to protect user confidentiality. |
| Work is not lost if app is minimized | When app is minimized and then reopened artwork is saved and can still be edited. | Some apps lose data when they are minimized but not closed. User should be able to pause artmaking and continue working on it later. *Note: Most apps lose the data when the app is closed unless it is saved.* |
| Combination of media features | Drawing and also collage, stamps, stickers, etc. | Multiple features expand the creative potential. |
| Multi-finger drawing | More than one finger can draw on the screen at a time. | Patients w/poor motor control might unintentionally drag another finger. Some apps will not work and will be frustrating for user. Also, allows option for therapist to draw with patient. |
| Screen sensitivity (Choe, 2014) | Screen has appropriate responsiveness to touch that reflects pressure of finger/ stylus. | Marks are made without intention if overly sensitive. If app is under-sensitive it requires too much pressure from the user. Artwork will be disjointed or too hard for user to manipulate. |

| Kinesthetic features | Some apps include features like splatter paint, marble painting, or stamping. | Features encourage user to shake, move, or make kinesthetic movements with the screen. Simulates more traditional energy-releasing art experiences without the mess. |
|---|---|---|
| Playback feature (Choe, 2014) | Records the user's steps and then recreates the art at the prompt of a "play" button. | Not essential, but could be used as a tool for therapeutic reflection, feedback, and discussion. |
| Auto rotate sensitivity | Screen will rotate vertical to horizontal depending on how the screen is positioned. | Allows the screen space to expand if held horizontally. Too much sensitivity or not enough can be frustrating for users. |
| Runs without Wi-fi | The app is functional even when not connected to Internet. | User can work offline in case there's not reliable Internet or Internet is blocked for safety reasons. |
| Compatible with accessibility features | Accessible with text magnification, voice recognition, audio description, etc. | Users who need accessibility features are able to use them within the app. |
| Compatible with stylus pen or paintbrush | Detects stylus. Is responsive to stylus-made marks. | User can choose to use finger or stylus. |
| No advertisements | Free apps frequently have ads. Purchased apps usually have no ads and sometimes have more features. | Free apps have ads that might not be appropriate for young users. Hospitals may receive app store gift certificates that can be used to purchase apps. |

## Case Illustration

Lia was a fourteen-year-old girl with a complex medical history including congenital heart issues, spina bifida, hearing and language difficulties, and nutritional challenges. Lia communicated through a combination of speaking, sign language, and fingerspelling. She had poor grip strength and limited body mobility. Lia had been waiting for a heart transplant for nearly four years. Despite her medical issues, Lia was a spunky budding teenager. Occasionally, she became frustrated by her medical challenges, engaging in superficial self-harming behaviors and a passive desire to die.

Lia was referred to art therapy because she loved to make art. However, her work in outpatient art therapy consisted of quick simple line drawings that were concrete representations of the topics we discussed (Figure 10.3). Her art seemed more like a communication tool than an artistic outlet. I struggled to harness her creative and imaginative self-expression. Eventually Lia's health further declined and she was hospitalized to await transplant. I noticed that Lia's imagination flourished with more passive activities, but she nearly always declined to make art. For example, she loved to travel and would learn about foreign places through conversations with hospital volunteers. Then she would intricately imagine future dream trips to those locations. One time, a hospital musician came to play her cowboy songs and next thing you knew—at Lia's command— we were singing around a makeshift campfire (a cardboard box in the middle of the room). Her creativity was active but she did not seem to have the physical resources to make art.

I noticed that Lia used her iPad to stay connected to her life at home. One day, I brought the art therapy iPad to our session loaded with a menu of art apps customized for her use. I gave her a brief tutorial of commonly used apps and suggested that she give them a try. Lia openly and eagerly engaged. She most liked an app that had a combination of drawing, printmaking, and collage (Shoe the Goose, 2014).

The first image Lia made was an underwater scene filled with sea friends—a place she wished she were instead of the hospital (Figure 10.3). We saved the image and printed it on photo paper. The digital image transformed into a tangible reminder of her mental escape. We did sessions like this many more times. Each time, I would offer a pallet of traditional art materials and the iPad. She almost exclusively selected the iPad. Sometimes Lia worked on self-guided pieces, often exploring transcendent and subversive themes like starry nights and underwater explorations. Other times, I would offer prompts that related more directly to the indicated therapeutic goals such as helping Lia process the difficult emotions around hospitalization in a constructive way or, helping her develop her self-identity as a whole person beyond the sick patient. When Lia had less energy we worked together, each using a finger on the tablet to create the art. When Lia was feeling very ill she would direct me and I would navigate the tablet on her behalf.

One day when Lia was particularly frustrated and sad, I suggested she create a "vision board" to channel positive energies. Her vision was clear. Using the iPad she drew a big red heart. The work was simple and took only a few minutes to complete, but it was the most empowering artwork of her hospitalization (Figure 10.4). Manifesting her heart through the artwork empowered a sense of action over something that she actually had very little control over: getting a donated heart. She had me hang the image on her wall for daily inspiration. She would tell people who entered her room about it, which seemed to reiterate her powerful intention. Eventually, iPad artwork became such an important coping tool for Lia that she downloaded her favorite art apps to her own iPad. She could make art when I wasn't available, on weekends, or when she was feeling urges to self-harm.

During Lia's five-month hospitalization, we learned that she loved Claude Monet's artwork. Coincidentally, the local museum was simultaneously hosting a Monet exhibit. I worked with the treatment team to arrange a virtual visit to the museum via the Skype app and two iPads. We acquired confidentiality releases from her mother and her physicians to videoconference the museum into Lia's hospital room. A docent from the

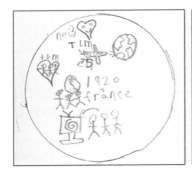
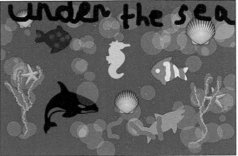

*Figure 10.3* Lia's Artwork

museum visited the hospital in-person and educated Lia about Monet's life and artwork (Figure 10.5). She even brought a sample of oil painted canvas so Lia could touch the layers she would eventually see on the gallery walls. A few days later, the docent "toured" Lia through the museum in real-time through the iPad screen. After the visit, Lia created her own artwork á la Monet style on the iPad. We used a combination of apps including an oil paint filter (Dezeustre, 2014) to create her personal Monet work. We printed the digital image on canvas-textured paper to give it an authentic look.

I attempted to use that experience to transition Lia from iPad work to acrylic painting that could mimic Monet's styles, but Lia still resisted using traditional art materials. The iPad required less technical precision while offering a sense of success and confidence. It took very little energy for us to create the therapeutic space and for her to actively engage

*Figure 10.4* Vision Board

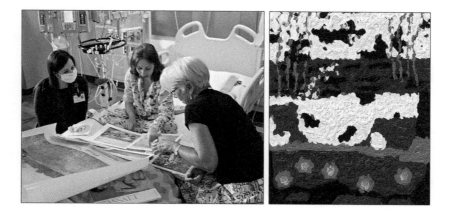

*Figure 10.5* Exploring Monet

with the digital art. The iPad was familiar and didn't require risky experimentation. It was the right tool for Lia to express herself in the hospital setting when she was critically ill.

I may have concluded that Lia simply preferred digital art to more traditional media. However, several days after she finally received her transplant, I walked in to her room and she was drawing on paper! In fact, she had an inch-thick stack of papers that she had drawn. Her hand-drawn characters were imaginative, playful, sophisticated, colorful, and detailed. The work was completely different than the images I had seen Lia draw before her transplant. Lia offers a valuable lesson to all art therapists. Sometimes patients do not resist artmaking because they don't want to engage in creative activities but rather, there is a mismatch between the tool being offered and the person's capabilities at the time. If I had not been open to using the iPad with Lia, I would have missed enormous therapeutic opportunities. Ultimately this may have denied a talented young artist the opportunity for positive coping and self-expression during the most difficult time of her life.

## Best-Practices for Tablet Use in Art Therapy

This chapter outlined many advantages and possibilities for using tablets in art therapy. Most authors have noted that art therapists should responsibly consider the safety and ethical issues of digital media work. Table 10.2 includes a suggested checklist for proper tablet use in art therapy sessions.

*Table 10.2* Checklist for Using Tablets in Art Therapy

- Art therapist is comfortable with digital media and seeks additional training when needed.
- Discuss preferred screen-time rules and social media boundaries with guardians.
- Guardians sign informed consent form outlining recognition of potential confidentiality risks with digital media and consent for future uses of the digital media, especially end-of-life.
- Encrypt tablet and configure for proper hospital-standard password protection. Consult appropriate safeguards with hospital IT team.
- Download a file-storage app to store patient artwork files with customized individual password protections (app store keyword: "secure files").
- Disable cloud storage and sharing features (Malchiodi and Johnson, 2013). Store files locally on the tablet.
- Transfer completed patient work to an encrypted and password protected hard drive for long-term storage.
- Enable parental controls. Block email and web-access according to age-appropriateness.
- Password protect app purchasing account. Keep password confidential from patients.
- Only load art-based apps onto art therapy tablet(s).
- Assess apps for developmental and cultural appropriateness.
- Customize app screen for current patient user. Deleted apps can be reloaded from the cloud without repurchasing.
- Review apps for inappropriate content or ads. Purchased versions usually do not have ads.
- Become familiar with app functions before introducing it in session.
- Conduct the session like a traditional art therapy session: actively guide, observe, and interact.
- Clear all stored files on tablet in between different patient users.
- Disinfect tablet between patient users.
- Use protective outer case and screen protector designed for withstanding drops and tolerating disinfectants.
- System for patient to access tablet and keep it safe. Consider bedside locking system, checkout system, or use it only with art therapist.
- Moderation. Always offer option for traditional art materials. Tablet art is one option within a range of art media.
- If tablet becomes limiting, stifling, or unhealthy for patient shift to more appropriate tool for therapeutic goals.

## Conclusions

Medical art therapists must be extremely flexible in their clinical approach in order to cope with the unique environmental, cultural, and physical aspects of hospitalization. Tablets are one more supportive tool that art therapists can use to meet the complex needs of patients. In particular, tablets are accessible to children, teenagers, and young adults coping with chronic and life-limiting illnesses. Tablet art can help these patients engage in empowering self-expression through a tool that is adaptable, easy to control, and safe to use. Tablets can expand creative capabilities and help build therapeutic rapport. Therapists are encouraged to use the guides in this chapter to select suitable digital apps as well as safeguard against the challenges of digital media. With informed conscious intention and open-minds, art therapists can use tablets to put limitless creative power—quite literally—into the hands of their patients.

## References

Alders, A., Beck, L., Allen, P. and Mosinski, B. (2011). Technology in Art Therapy: Ethical Challenges. *Art Therapy: Journal of the American Art Therapy Association* [online] 28(4), pp. 165–170. Available at: www.tandfonline.com/doi/abs/10.1080/07421656.2011.622683 [Accessed 23 December 2016].

Al-Taleb, M. and Vukovic, A. (2015). Home-based rehabilitation system using portable brain computer interface and functional electrical stimulation. In: *Proceedings of the Sixth International Brain-Computer Interface Meeting.* [online] Graz: Graz University of Technology, p. 100. Available at: http://castor.tugraz.at/doku/BCIMeeting2016/paper_100.pdf [Accessed 23 December 2016].

Anand, S. (2016). Dimensions of art therapy in illness. In: D. Gussak and M. Rosal, eds., *The Wiley Handbook of Art Therapy*, 1st ed. West Sussex: Wiley Blackwell, pp. 409–420.

Barber, B. and Garner, R. (2016). Materials and media: Developmentally appropriate apps. In: R. Garner, ed., *Digital Art Therapy: Materials, Methods, and Applications*, 1st ed. London: Jessica Kingsley, pp. 67–79.

Beasley, M. (2015). *Believe.* [video]. Available at: www.youtube.com/watch?v=CC8eoCPElK4 [Accessed 23 December 2016].

Bendis, J. (2012). *Mandalas 5.3.* [mobile software application]. Available at: https://itunes.apple.com/us/app/mandalas-free/id424903377?mt=8 [Accessed 23 December 2016].

Bucciarelli, A. (2016). The arts therapies: Approaches, goals and integration in arts and health. In: S. Clift and P. Camic, eds., *Oxford Textbook of Creative Arts, Health, and Wellbeing: International Perspectives on Practice, Policy, and Research*, 1st ed. Oxford: Oxford University, pp. 271–277.

Carlton, N. (2014). Digital Culture and Art Therapy. *The Arts in Psychotherapy* [online] 41, pp. 41–45. Available at: www.sciencedirect.com/science/article/pii/S0197455613001858 [Accessed 23 December 2016].

Carlton, N. (2016). Grid + pattern: Sensory qualities of digital media. In: R. Garner, ed., *Digital Art Therapy: Materials, Methods, and Approaches*, 1st ed. London: Jessica Kingsley, pp. 22–39.

Choe, N. (2014). An Exploration of the Qualities and Features of Art Apps for Art Therapy. *The Arts in Psychotherapy* [online] 41, pp. 145–154. Available at: www.sciencedirect.com/science/article/pii/S0197455614000033 [Accessed 23 December 2016].

Choe, N. (2016). Utilizing digital tools and apps in art therapy sessions. In: R. Garner, ed., *Digital Art Therapy: Materials, Methods, and Applications*, 1st ed. London: Jessica Kingsley, pp. 67–79.

Consumer Reports. (2016). *Tablet Buying Guide: Video Buying Guide.* [video] Available at: www.consumerreports.org/cro/tablets/buying-guide.htm [Accessed 23 December 2016].

Councill, T. (1999). Art therapy with pediatric cancer patients. In: C. Malchiodi, ed., *Medical Art Therapy with Children*, 1st ed. London: Jessica Kingsley, pp. 75–93.

Councill, T. (2012). Medical art therapy with children. In: C. Malchiodi, ed., *Handbook of Art Therapy*, 2nd ed. New York: Guilford, pp. 222–240.

Councill, T. and Phlegar, K. (2013). Cultural crossroads: Considerations in medical art therapy. In: P. Howie, S. Prasad and J. Kristel, eds., *Using Art Therapy with Diverse Populations*, 1st ed. London: Jessica Kingsley, pp. 203–213.

Diggs, L., Lubas, M. and De Leo, G. (2015). Use of Technology and Software Applications for Therapeutic Collage Making. *International Journal of Art Therapy* [online] 20(1), pp. 2–13. Available at: http://search.ebscohost.com/login.aspx?direct=true&AuthType=ip,uid&db=eue&AN=100776559&site=ehost-live [Accessed 23 December 2016].

Dezeustre, G. (2014). *Glaze 1.9* [mobile application software]. Available at: https://itunes.apple.com/us/app/glaze/id521573656?mt=8 [Accessed 23 December 2016].

FiftyThree, Inc. (2016). *Paper 3.6.6* [mobile application software]. Available at: https://itunes.apple.com/us/app/paper-by-fiftythree-sketch/id506003812?mt=8 [Accessed 23 December 2016].

Garai, J. (2001). Humanistic art therapy. In: J. Rubin, ed., *Approaches to Art Therapy: Theory and technique*, 2nd ed. New York: Brunner-Routledge, pp. 149–162.

Henderson, N. and Bucciarelli, A. (2014). *Taking Charge*. Gainesville, FL: UF Health Shands Arts in Medicine.

Kaimal, G., Rattigan, M., Miller, G. and Haddy, J. (2016). Implications of National Trends in Digital Media Use for Art Therapy Practice. *Journal of Clinical Art Therapy* [online] 3(1), pp. 1–12. Available at: http://digitalcommons.lmu.edu/jcat/vol3/iis1/6 [Accessed 23 December 2016].

Karamchandani, H., Chau, T., Hobbs, D. and Mumford, L. (2015). Development of a low cost, portable, tablet-based eye tracking system for children with impairments. In: *International Convention on Rehabilitation Engineering and Assistive Technology*. [online] Singapore: ICREATE. Available at: www.researchgate.net/publication/287817724_Development_of_a_low-cost_portable_tablet-based_eye_tracking_system_for_children_with_impairments [Accessed 23 December 2016].

Klorer, G. (2009). The Effects of Technological Overload on Children: An Art Therapist's Perspective. *Art Therapy: Journal of the American Art Therapy Association* [online] 26(2), pp. 80–82. Available at: www.tandfonline.com/doi/abs/10.1080/07421656.2009.10129742 [Accessed 23 December 2016].

Long, K. (2014). *Just a Journey*. Gainesville, FL: UF Health Shands Arts in Medicine.

Malchiodi, C. (1999). *Medical Art Therapy with Children*, 1st ed. London: Jessica Kingsley.

Malchiodi, C. (2013). *Art Therapy and Health Care*. New York: Guildford, pp. 1–12.

Malchiodi, C. and Johnson, E. (2013). Digital art therapy with hospitalized children. In: C. Malchiodi, ed., *Art Therapy and Health Care*, 1st ed. New York: Guilford, pp. 106–121.

McNiff, S. (1999). The Virtual Art Therapy Studio. *Art Therapy: Journal of the American Art Therapy Association* [online] 16(4), pp. 197–200. Available at: www.tandfonline.com/doi/pdf/10.1080/07421656.1999.10129484 [Accessed 23 December 2016].

Medina, B. (2014). *Brianna's Hope.* [video] Available at: www.youtube.com/watch?v=JRfPBuMXFCw [Accessed 23 December 2016].

National Association for the Education of Young Children (NAEYC). (2012). *Technology and Interactive Media as Tools in Early Childhood Programs Serving Children from Birth Through Age 8*. National Association for the Education of Young Children and the Fred Rogers Center for Early Learning and Children's Media at Sain Vincent College, pp. 1–15. Available at: www.naeyc.org/files/naeyc/file/positions/PS_technology_WEB2.pdf [Accessed 23 December 2016].

Orr, P. (2005). Technology Media: An Exploration for 'Inherent Qualities'. *The Arts in Psychotherapy* [online] 32, pp. 1–11. Available at: www.sciencedirect.com/science/article/pii/S0197455604001261 [Accessed 23 December 2016].

Orr, P. (2010). Social remixing: Art therapy media in the digital age. In: C. Moon, ed., *Materials and Media in Art Therapy: Critical Understandings of Diverse Artistic Vocabularies*. New York: Routledge, pp. 89–100.

Orr, P. (2012). Technology Use in Art Therapy Practice: 2004 and 2011 Comparison. *The Arts in Psychotherapy* [online] 39, pp. 234–238. Available at: http://dx.doi.org/10.1016/j.aip.2012.03.010 [Accessed 23 December 2016].

Orr, P. (2016). Art therapy and digital media. In: D. Gussak and M. Rosal, eds., *The Wiley Handbook of Art Therapy*, 1st ed. West Sussex: Wiley Blackwell, pp. 188–197.

Parker-Bell, B. (1999). Embracing a Future with Computers and Art Therapy. *Art Therapy: Journal of the American Art Therapy Association* [online] 16(4), pp. 180–185. Available at: www.tandfonline. com/doi/abs/10.1080/07421656.1999.10129482 [Accessed 23 December 2016].

Radtastical, Inc. (2014). *Splatter 2.0.* [mobile application software] Available at: https://itunes. apple.com/us/app/splatter!/id364895254?mt=8 [Accessed 23 December 2016].

Shoe the Goose. (2013). *Caboodle Doodle 1.03.* [mobile application software] Available at: https:// itunes.apple.com/us/app/caboodle-doodle/id486960795?mt=8 [Accessed 23 December 2016].

Thong, S. (2007). Redefining the Tools of Art Therapy. *Art Therapy: Journal of the American Art Therapy Association* [online] 23(2), pp. 52–58. Available at: www.tandfonline.com/doi/abs/10.1080/0 7421656.2007.10129583 [Accessed 23 December 2016].

Tseng, K., Lin, B., Wong, A. and Lin, S. (2015). Design of a Mobile Brain Computer Interface-based Smart Multimedia Controller. *Sensors* [online] 15(3), pp. 5518–5530. Available at: www. mdpi.com/1424-8220/15/3/5518/htm?ref=driverlayer.com/web [Accessed 23 December 2016].

Ullmann, P. (2013). Adaptive art therapy with children who have physical challenges and chronic medical issues. In: C. Malchiodi, ed., *Art Therapy and Health Care*, 1st ed. New York: Guilford, pp. 409–420.

University of Florida. (2015). *How the Heart Works.* [mobile software application] Available at: https://itunes.apple.com/us/app/how-the-heart-works/id1022001422?mt=8 [Accessed 23 December 2016].

Williams, C. (2014). *My Story.* Gainesville, FL: UF Health Shands Arts in Medicine.

# 11 Connecting and Belonging

## Using Technology for Art Therapy in Palliative Care

*Michèle J.M. Wood*

Digital technology, the Internet, home computers and portable digital devices have become everyday features of our lives. Almost all adults in the UK are internet users (ONS, Office for National Statistics, 2018), accessing it on our personal computers, tablet computers, smartphones, and wearable digital devices. Education, shopping, entertainment, banking, and health and social care are now reliant on this technology. It has opened up a 24/7 culture of constant connectivity and instant access to an infinite amount of information. A report of attitudes and usages of digital media in Britain found most adults valued the Internet as a way of maintaining their personal relationships, although they also recognised its disruptive impact on face-to face communications (OfCom, 2018). For example, the widespread practice of snubbing others in favour of our mobile phones has added a new word 'phubbing' to the growing lexicon of new terms to describe our digital behaviours. There is an increasing trend towards accessing the Internet on smartphones on the move, not only at home or work. This connectivity has its benefits but there are risks. Using the internet can lead to feelings of being overwhelmed, addictive behaviours, cyber-bullying, exploitation, anxieties related to technology, and the distribution of false, misleading or harmful information. These negative consequences of technology are likely to enter the art therapy room; either because the patient is seeking help to manage technology's impact on their lives, or as a disturbing intrusion and disruption to the boundaries of the therapeutic relationship. Thus, promoting critical thinking skills to support our patients' 'technoWellness' (Kennedy, 2014) is now considered an aspect of the art therapist's remit in the 21st century.

In this chapter I wish to explore the challenges and benefits of working as an art therapist in palliative care in this digital age. Using examples from my own practice and research I hope to illustrate some of the current discourses around technology. My aim is to highlight how patients are using technology to navigate their relationships, including those with healthcare professionals. I want to empower art therapists to think about how technology is changing people, and to consider how we may best work with these changes to drive forward effective interventions that support good palliative care.

## My Context

I work in a hospice run by a large UK charity, Marie Curie, who provide care and support to people living with a terminal illness and their families. The charity operates nine hospices, which are spread out across England, Scotland, Northern Ireland, and Wales. Additionally, Marie Curie provides a nursing service, and a volunteer helper service for those receiving palliative care in their own homes. It also offers a website and online community through which patients, relatives, and professionals can gain information and support. Hampstead Hospice, where I have worked part-time since 2002, provides care for patients and their families, and is situated in an affluent part of London, although its catchment area includes some of the city's least well off. For those needing rehabilitation, symptom control or terminal care the hospice has two inpatient units, with a total of 30 beds, most of which are individual rooms. There is also a day therapy unit for out-patients, informed by a rehabilitation model of care (Jones et al., 2013). There is a gym, garden, and hydrotherapy pool. Wi-fi connection to the Internet is available to patients and visitors throughout the building.

The hospice has a large staff team comprising doctors, nurses, physiotherapists, pharmacists, an occupational therapist, social workers, counsellors, chaplains, a psychologist, an art therapist and a music therapist, and volunteer complementary therapists. This multidisciplinary team (MDT) delivers holistic care to patients and their families and friends. Expectations of what it is to live well with terminal illness are explored, and by considering the things that matter most to each person and taking account of their immediate psychosocial, spiritual, and medical needs, packages of care are put in place and reviewed regularly as circumstances change.

Art therapy has been available at the Hampstead hospice since the mid-1990s as one service offered by the Patient and Family Support team. It is provided by a part-time art therapist and occasional art therapist trainees (interns) on placement. There is a dedicated art therapy room, and art therapy is delivered in a variety of formats, including at the patient's bedside (Wood, 2005). There is a weekly drop-in art therapy group open to all patients and their families and friends. Art therapy sessions for individuals, couples or family groups are arranged following an assessment meeting. Therapeutic contracts are usually short-term to accommodate the speed of health changes experienced by patients, and offered in blocks of six sessions, reviewed every fifth session. My therapeutic approach, informed by attachment theory, object-relations, and analytical psychology, enables me to engage with the range of interpersonal and existential issues brought by patients and their families.

One motivation that brings people to seek help is the need to make sense of the enormous changes that result from their physical illness, treatment, and prognosis. This is often described as a recalibration of identity. It can be a struggle for the patient relinquishing aspects of the person they felt they were before their illness, while letting go of who they had imagined they might become in the future. What is unique about art therapy's contribution to this process of psychological adjustment and sense-making, is the art form. In art therapy the affective, expressive, and metaphorical qualities of art materials can bypass talking to produce concrete artworks, affirming the person's sense of agency. Art therapy provides an embodied experience out of which a person can gain a new perspective. The process of making, under the gaze of the therapist's eye, can mobilise new insights, stimulate memories, and release emotions. The end product offers a tangible record of this 'journey', in its form as well as symbolic content. The safety of the therapeutic relationship is key.

A range of art materials are offered to patients from dry mark making through to paints, including air-drying clay, Modroc, textiles and found objects that provide a wealth of sensory experiences and affective associations. With the sensory qualities of the media, a person is thus able to evoke, communicate and even modulate their affective states. Harsh angry scratching of pencils or charcoal may give way to gentle stroking of pastels, or through dripping inks there may be a release of tears. Then there are the iPads. These portable tablet computers, with their smooth dark screens held in protective cases, sit alongside the other art media as additional tools with artmaking apps, a camera and access to the Internet.

## My Journey With Computers

I have never been very interested in computers, or gadgets in general. They seem to require a logical approach to life that sits uncomfortably with my 'scatty' disorganised intuitive thinking and natural tendency to feel uneasy around machines.

However, in the 1990s I was working in an HIV/AIDS hospice in London. We had recently received computers in the staff offices. This was a move forward for the Counselling and Social Care Team of which I was a member, where previously the team administrator typed our letters and took telephone messages. It was a new and exciting era for Information Communication Technology (ICT) in the hospice, and the Head of IT came to me with an idea. Could the patients benefit from using the basic artmaking software that came with the computers? It was an interesting thought, and I wondered if it might work for those with HIV-related brain impairment who found it hard to engage with the art materials.

With limited ICT knowledge and skills, I began facilitating sessions working individually with our HIV and AIDS dementia patients to test the feasibility of this new tool, supported by the IT manager and nursing staff. The patients were moderately responsive, but due to their deteriorating health engagement in the sessions was unpredictable. The head of IT moved to another job, and without him my computer skills were too basic to carry the initiative further. The organisation changed its delivery of services, and by 1997 the computers for patients were put away. In 1999 art therapist Barbara Parker-Bell was also considering the value of using computers with clients, recognising the increasing trend among the American population for home computers. She encouraged art therapists to consider becoming computer literate since 'Mastering computer arts is a daunting task for the uninitiated' (Parker-Bell, 1999, p. 180)—something my experience demonstrated.

Moving forward to 2012, this time working at the Marie Curie hospice and running a carers' art therapy group, I was intrigued to see my clients using artmaking apps on their personal tablet computers. Parker-Bell had predicted that pressure from clients would be the driving force for including computers in art therapy. In addition to the relatives using the carers group, I began noticing how patients came into art therapy sessions with their smartphones, not only to take important calls but to show me images that disturbed or delighted them. These portable digital devices became the source of conversations, and the starting point for artwork. Patients used their smartphones to photograph their paintings, to Bluetooth artwork to me, and send emails. I found these devices breaching my usual practice where I had sole responsibility for storage and safety of patients' images; instead this was shared with patients who were carrying their images in and out of the room on their phones. I found myself being nudged into new ways to engage with my palliative patients. Gaining a Winston Churchill Fellowship a few years later (Wood, 2015a), I was able to observe how other art therapists and healthcare professionals working in end of life care were responding to the challenges and opportunities of this new technology. Visiting a mental health facility in Brooklyn, New York, I witnessed the art therapist successfully engage a group of adult inpatients in spontaneous art making. They were using computers with the same artmaking computer program I had trialled in my HIV hospice 20 years previously. It was curious to reflect on how much had, and had not, changed in that time.

## 'NHS Digital'

Digital technologies are changing the way we do things, improving the accountability of services, reducing their cost, giving us new means of transacting and participating. This is more than an information revolution: it puts people first, giving us more control and more transparency.

(National Information Board, 2014)

The development of the internet has fundamentally altered the ways in which we interact with others and present ourselves. New forms of social media like Facebook, WhatsApp, and YouTube are being used to present and seek information, including health-related views. Social networking sites, online chat rooms, and the potential to upload text, images, and films to share with friends and strangers are now all possible. The Internet of Things (IoT) is extending this dynamic interplay to include the objects in our living spaces. Thus, data routinely collected from smart objects like wearable sensors are being used to monitor behaviour, calculate risk, and activate services.

Services and systems are being commissioned which utilise the dynamic arena of the Internet and the technologies that can enable people to meet through it. For example, Project ECHO (Zhou et al., 2016), and The Gold Line (Middleton-Green et al., 2016) are services comprising a hub of specialist healthcare professionals who support local doctors and nurses through telephone and video-conferencing to deliver palliative care to patients in their own homes. The idea of remote art therapy has been pilot-tested by Kate Collie and colleagues (Collie & Cubranic, 1999) and continues to be explored as an option in rural communities where access to in-person services is difficult (Wake, 2014).

There is evidence that tablet computers are increasingly being incorporated into art therapists' working practices (BAAT, 2015; Darewych et al., 2015; Choe, 2014). In a UK survey of art therapists' uses and views of digital technology, the digital device most frequently used with clients was the iPad (tablet computer) for art making, photography, animation, video recording, playing games and assessment (Wood, 2016). While art therapists responding to this survey came from a range of clinical settings, 12% identified as working in supportive and palliative care.

When my current hospice received a donation of four iPads for art therapy in 2012, I was excited to embrace this novel tool for its ease of making digital artwork. Once again, I could see the potential for these portable tablet computers to deliver art therapy for patients who found working with usual art materials difficult, such as the bedbound and those concerned about getting messy. But my enthusiasm was not matched by the organisation's IT system, which struggled to align two different operating systems (Windows and Apple Macintosh). The discrepancy between my patients' eager use of their phones for art making and photography, and the hospice's limited computer hardware was frustrating. This gap is gradually being filled as digital technology is becoming imbedded in all aspects of health and social care. This in turn is highlighting anxieties about the digital competencies of the workforce, and the potential for digital exclusion of some sectors of society. For example, the OfCom Report mentioned earlier highlighted lower income households and people aged over 54 years in the UK were less likely to have smartphones, laptops, and tablet computers. This digital 'divide' acknowledged in the art therapy community (Carlton, 2014) challenges practitioners working with all client groups to engage with the new digital systems to ensure they are able to meet the needs of their digitally competent clients and to advocate for those who are not.

## Why Digital?

There is a national strategy in the UK to use technology to meet the demand of an increasing ageing population of people living longer with multiple and complex health conditions (NHS England, 2017). The hope is that digital apps, devices, and digitally integrated interventions will support the entire population to take more responsibility for the consequences of their lifestyles, and help people manage their own care. With an ever-expanding push for digital technology to be integral to all health and social care services, it is important for art therapists to consider the meaning that digital technology has for the people who need their services and how best to work with them.

Focusing on healthcare in general, a report by the Nuffield Trust sets out a vision of the 'digital patient', and describes how digital tools may facilitate an individual to navigate their health trajectory (Castle-Clarke & Imison, 2016). From maintaining well-being by monitoring activity with the aid of apps and wearables (FitBit), checking signs of potential illness with online symptom checkers, and electronically arranging their own medical appointments, face-to-face or as remote consultations. This template for blending digital and face-to-face interactions is already being used to deliver art therapy services in mental health (e-Art Therapy) and elsewhere, as mentioned in this book (Chapters 10, 19, 23).

Examples from my own hospice patients indicate this has already begun in end of life care.

### Technology for Self-Care: Art-Making App

Jenny, a woman in her late 60s, told me how she coped with accompanying her terminally ill mother to her hospital appointments. She found this emotionally and physically draining at times, and so took to using her son's iPad for artmaking. She found this helped calm her anxiety, especially during lengthy periods waiting for procedures.

### Technology Bridging Hospice and Local Community: 'The Carers Field of Daffodils'

In 2012 I initiated and ran a project to raise awareness of the strain placed on family members caring for their loved ones with terminal illnesses. This involved collecting 365 digitally created doodles of daffodils (the hospice charity symbol) in order to highlight the fact that informal caregivers care every day of the year. Using an iPad, a team of art therapy volunteers invited all those family members and friends visiting the hospice during Carers Awareness Week to doodle a daffodil. Staff and patients were invited too. This project spread beyond the hospice building, with patients' families collecting digital doodles from their neighbours and staff members' children using their own iPads to collect doodles from their peers at school. Patients' children instructed their grandparents how to draw on the iPad, and patients with restricted mobility found ways to doodle, even using their feet.

Once collected, 365 individual images were printed and distributed across six canvases. Each canvas was taken to a public setting from school fairs, to large hospital foyers, and used as a focal point for distributing information about the hospice and resources for carers.

This project illustrates the ease with which iPads can be used creatively, bringing many people together in a collective project. The speed (it took only a few weeks) and scale of the activity (365 doodles) would not have been possible with traditional media of paper and pens. The final assemblage now hangs in the hospice cafe.

While the 'Carers Field of Daffodils' project serves to illustrate how technology helps to bridge the hospice and home environments, it also indicates how easily it was taken up by participants, facilitating connections within families and in communities.

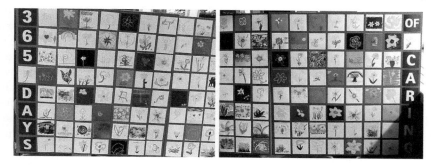

*Figure 11.1* Carers' Field of Daffodils (365 Digital Drawings)

## The Psychological Significance of Technology: Connectedness or Disconnect?

A study researching inpatients' experiences of connectedness while resident in a palliative care unit in Sweden, identified the importance of technology for participants to feel connected to friends, family, and events outside of the institution. Patients in this study still regarded their computers and telephones as important for maintaining a sense of connectedness, even when they were too unwell to use them.

> . . . having access [to a computer] had a symbolic value of 'still being able to go out there' and catch up with what was going on with significant people or with society.
> (Hakanson & Ohlen, 2016, p 51)

Maintaining connection to the familiar is a survival strategy learned early in life through interactions with our primary caregivers (Wallin, 2007). From these early experiences mental patterns of relating are laid down, forming the beliefs we hold about ourselves and our expectations of others, especially at times of stress and anxiety. Attachment behaviours from early childhood may be activated with increasing dependency as patients approach the end of their lives (Cherny & Catane, 2010; Tan et al., 2005). Understanding this can give art therapists a framework to think about their interactions with patients, especially those who feel unworthy of care, or who find it hard to trust others to meet their needs. The human impulse towards community and the sense of security felt in relationship with others is, according to Winnicott, at the core of all culture, the arts, and religions (Winnicott, 1971). Art therapists are familiar with Winnicott's concepts of potential space and transitional phenomena, as explanations for the psychological development of children, and ways cultural, artistic, and religious artefacts and experiences meet our need for psychological security long into adulthood.

Using insights from attachment studies and Winnicott's theory of transitional phenomena, we gain a lens to understand the value of the smartphones, tablet, and laptop computers in art therapy. Like the infant's rag doll, teddy bear or thumb-sucking sustaining a connection with their primary caretaker in her absence, these devices offer some value to individuals at the end of their lives. And like the rag doll they are small enough to be held close to the body and carried everywhere, helping the patient maintain a connection to those they love. It has been suggested by some that we protect ourselves against feelings of isolation and loss by maintaining a constant and close use of our smartphones (MacRury & Yates, 2017). MacRury and Yates point out that while the device can help us to maintain social connections, it also provides a means of regulating, inviting or avoiding experiences of intimacy with others. The mobile phone's easy access to all the resources of the Internet can offer instant gratification and pleasure without having to relate to anyone else. Or conversely the tracking and recording functions of mobile phones enable capture surveillance by others, including the faceless organisations gathering data for algorithms to 'enhance' functionality of digital tools. While MacRury and Yates point out how smartphone technology perpetuates feelings of disconnection and pathological attachments, they also warn against exaggerating its dangers; it may be a site of playfulness and creativity.

With digital technology now a central part of the health and social care landscape, and an ever-narrowing gap between technology at home and in the specialist environment of the hospice, how do we guard against what psychologist and psychoanalyst Sherry Turkle warns of—that mobile technology is undermining our capacity to be together (Turkle, 2011)? Like others (Balick, 2013; Weitz, 2014) she points out how being networked with online mobile devices feeds our desire for recognition, connection, and belonging. These feelings of connection and belonging are particularly relevant at the end of life, when illness dislodges a person from their usual status and roles in work and family life and changes their relationship with their own bodies. Psychotherapist Richard Frankel argues that digital technology and the internet are having a profound impact on our individual and collective capacities to experience, tolerate, and work through loss. Frankel argues that the features of the internet (instant access to infinite information retained indefinitely) support a regressive psychological position towards 'primary narcissism'. He proposes a narcissistic shadow hanging over the virtual world, where the frustrations of coming to terms with loss through not-knowing, forgetting, and the gap between self and another are removed and denied (Frankel, 2013). For art therapists working in palliative care, these aspects of loss are the focus of our work. The images made by those facing the end of their life are often imbued with a desire not to forget or be forgotten. This leads to the issue of legacy, and it is a standard part of my practice to discuss patients' intentions for their artwork once therapy has ended. Should the artwork be left with me? And in the event of the patient's death, who would they wish to have their work? When images are in digital format, it opens up the possibility of multiple recipients.

## Bridging Art Therapy Sessions: Caroline

'Caroline', a professional woman in her late 50s, joined my carers art therapy support group on the recommendation of her sister (the patient). On first meeting me Caroline confessed she was unsure how the group and its art therapy emphasis could help, especially since she 'could not draw'. I invited Caroline to tell me a little about herself and she reached into her bag and retrieved her iPad. With a finger she confidently drew a diagram of her home, highlighting how much of it had been taken over by her terminally ill sister (Wood, 2015b). Arguably there is little difference between the act of creating a visual representation on paper or on an iPad, yet Caroline's choice to use her own digital device was an important communication. Technology was her area of competence; her sister was the 'artist'. Caroline did join the group and regularly attended for many months until her sister died, and for some time afterwards. While her iPad continued to feature she also enjoyed working with a variety of other art media, often using her iPad to photograph the artwork so as to transform it using apps in the time between sessions. The art therapy group facilitated Caroline's creativity during a time of loss. The ease with which she could use her iPad to capture artwork made in the group then became very helpful in extending the group's support.

We can understand the 'playing' that Caroline did in her artwork and with her iPad in the Carers Support group as trying to make sense of the changing dynamics in her attachment to her older sister. This pre-bereavement work involved Caroline exploring possible consequences to her sense of self as her sister's health declined. The potential of the iPad with its transformative apps allowed her to share photos from the past, and then re-work them in paintings to create new visions of herself in the future.

A therapeutic alliance was built through Caroline's use of her iPad, which became the area of 'play' between us. Although Caroline's knowledge and skills outstripped my own, she was not fazed by my 'ignorance' of what this device could do; instead she appeared delighted to have the opportunity to hold an expert role.

## Technology Gets in the Way: Jon

Art therapy offers alternative and additional means for people to communicate thoughts and feelings, especially helpful when physical conditions compromise a person's ability to speak or use language. The mastery of using paints, pencils, clay, and other visual graphic media for self-expression also offers a satisfying and affirming self-experience; again, important for those re-adjusting to the physical changes that terminal illness brings. These features of art therapy prompted a referral of 'Jon', a man in his 70s. Jon came to our first art therapy session in a wheelchair with an iPad, wearing a headset that held a microphone close to his mouth, and a speaker to amplify his voice. He had experienced a recent onset of supraneural palsy with consequent difficulties in speaking. Despite communication difficulties I could see Jon was a warm and an engaging man who was keen to 'give art therapy a go'. Jon wanted to paint and draw, to foster some creativity. He also wanted to communicate the story of his life and affirm the wealth of experiences and knowledge that had hitherto given him meaning and purpose. However, two issues concerned me; the fact that Jon struggled to open his eyes, and because his voice was barely audible, his communication aids (headset, microphone, and iPad) were additional features to accommodate in the therapy.

In our early sessions, we sat together with two iPads (Jon's, for him to type out words and phrases that he struggled to say, and mine with the artmaking apps ready) attempting to get to know each other. Jon shakily tried to use pencils and pastels to draw a remembered landscape, while against his will his eyes lost their focus and shut. To counteract this symptom of his condition, Jon used a pair of spectacles with soft plastic spikes inside their frames, which on touching his eyelids prompted them to open. I would watch Jon struggle determinedly to reposition these spectacles, feeling something of his frustration and impotence.

The hope that the equipment serves its function by disappearing into the background, and thereby freeing its user to engage with the task at hand, is not always realised. While Jon's headset was to enhance his quiet voice, it also amplified Jon's breathing when he was not speaking. Since art therapy does not always involve talking, with the patient's attention being placed on being immersed in drawing and painting, the amplified sound of Jon's laboured breathing simply reinforced and highlighted his condition, providing another 'presence' in the room. I found I could lipread very well, and by matching his endeavours to communicate with my own struggles to understand, a relationship of trust built between us. Eventually the role of the headset was something we discussed, and in the end we both agreed that it was a barrier and distraction. The headset was removed. Jon continued in art therapy for a couple of years until his death. In that time, I supported Jon's choice to use a variety of art materials and techniques (from acrylic paints, modelling clay to monoprinting) all the while bearing with, and not rushing to alleviate, his faltering struggles to communicate and express himself through art making.

However, as Jon got weaker, he chose to work on the iPad. The size of the touchscreen was easier to navigate, and the undo function was also attractive, as it allowed him to correct errors resulting from his shaking hands. Jon was a highly intelligent and cultured man, and while he managed to retain a stoical humour about his failing health and capabilities, the technological challenge and novelty of the iPad kept him stimulated. Jon also enjoyed the fact that I was struggling to learn how to use my new iPads. Like Caroline, this work with Jon demonstrated that if a containing therapeutic relationship is established, the willingness of the therapist to follow the patient's choice in art making need not be hindered by the therapist's limited technical skills.

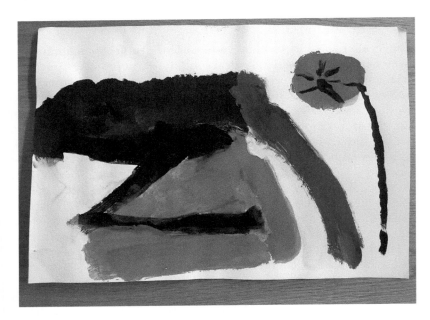

*Figure 11.2* Jon's Painting in Early Phase of Therapy (acrylic paints)

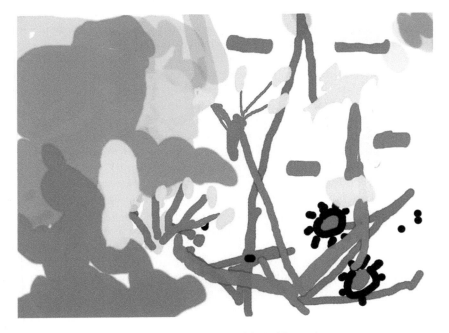

*Figure 11.3* Jon's iPad Art in Later Phase of Therapy (digital image)

While playful curiosity about art making on the iPad was an aspect of building a therapeutic alliance with Jon, I also had to navigate feelings of disappointment and frustration with regards to the technology. Disappointment, that despite its best efforts we could not bypass the realities of Jon's debilitating condition. It was important for frustration to be acknowledged, as it enabled us to explore Jon's feelings about his illness, and his way of coping with the responses of his family. However, I had to be careful that Jon's frustrations were not added to by my unfamiliarity with the iPad artmaking apps, so I worked hard on learning these.

Describing the benefits of art therapy Jon wrote:

> It has become a means of communicating the vitality of my inner life, which I cannot do in any other way now. It is as if I have left the depths of despair and climbed to a brighter, sunnier plateau.

## Conclusion

Eleven types of information and communications technologies used for patient care in the palliative stages have been identified in a recent systematic review (Ostherr et al., 2016). These digital tools (faxes, videos, telephones, compact discs and others) are being used for education, information, support with pain management, decision aids and help with advanced care planning. Communication through emails and by sending short message service (SMS) text messages are becoming common practice. The increasing interest around the world in telehealth is addressing the desire to support patients wishing to be cared for and to die in their own home, along with the need to support those living in rural and remote geographical areas.

It is obvious that for technology to transform health and social care for the better, there has to be an alignment of patients' and professionals' knowledge of and skills to use the technology, and the infrastructure supporting all parties. While inequalities in the provision of Wi-fi, the training of staff, and support for patients may be tackled by financial resourcing of equipment and education, it is vital to understand users' feelings about adopting digital technology. Concerns about cyber-security, fears of surveillance and digital exclusion of those not choosing to use technology must be addressed. Returning to the UK survey of art therapists' view of digital technology, there was a clear concern from participants that the detrimental effects of using technology in art therapy practice would reinforce avoidance and distraction in clients and would weaken the therapeutic boundaries and increase the client's vulnerability. Such concerns, however, should not prevent art therapists from using technology at all. Rather, understanding the motivations behind choices to use technology and supporting clients to manage their relationships with it is the therapist's ethical duty of care. The importance of all users of the internet gaining good critical skills to judge the authenticity and safety of the online environment has been highlighted by recent research. It is clear that digital technology, while solving a vast swathe of practical and economic problems is also changing how we think about ourselves and how we relate to others. Thus, technology opens up great possibilities for art therapists to extend their provision by develop digital art therapy interventions, and challenges us to think about the psychological needs that technology is servicing. The small examples from my practice presented in this chapter highlight the benefits of meeting our patients where they are; extending our creative toolkits to include digital devices and thinking about when and how best to use digital tools to maintain patients' autonomy, connection to others and ultimately, quality of life. With the huge financial investments in digital technologies being made by governments around the world, this is an area that demands our attention and participation.

## References

BAAT. (2015) *Digital Media Practice Guidelines*. London: British Association of Art Therapists.

Balick, A. (2013) *The Psychodynamics of Social Networking: Connected-up Instantaneous Culture and the Self.* London: Karnac Books.

Carlton, N.R. (2014) Digital culture and art therapy. *The Arts in Psychotherapy*. 41(1) pp. 41–45.

Castle-Clarke, S. & Imison, C. (2016) *The Digital Patient: Transforming Primary Care? Nuffield Trust.* London: Nuffield Trust.

Cherny, N. & Catane, R. (2010) 3.4 palliative medicine and modern cancer care. In: Hanks, G., Cherny, N.I., Christakis, N.A., Fallon, M., Kaasa, S. & Portenoy, R.K. (eds.) *Oxford Textbook of Palliative Medicine* (Fourth Edition). Oxford; New York: Oxford University Press. pp. 111–124.

Choe, S. (2014) An exploration of the qualities and features of art apps for art therapy. *The Arts in Psychotherapy*. 41(2) pp. 145–154. DOI: //dx.doi.org/10.1016/j.aip.2014.01.002

Collie, K. & Cubranic, D. (1999) An art therapy solution to a telehealth problem. *Art Therapy*. 16(4) pp. 186–193. DOI: 10.1080/07421656.1999.10129481

Darewych, O.H., Carlton, N.R. & Farrugie, K.W. (2015) Digital technology use in art therapy with adults with developmental disabilities. *Journal on Developmental Disabilities*. 21(2) pp. 95–102.

Frankel, R. (2013) Digital melancholy. *JungJournal*. 7(4) pp. 9–20. DOI: 10.1080/19342039.2013.840231

Hakanson, C. & Ohlen, J. (2016) Connectedness at the end of life among people admitted to inpatient palliative care. *American Journal of Hospice and Palliative Medicine®*. 33(1) pp. 47–54.

Jones, L., FitzGerald, G., Leurent, B., Round, J., Eades, J., Davis, S., Gishen, F., Holman, A., Hopkins, K. & Tookman, A. (2013) Rehabilitation in advanced, progressive, recurrent cancer: A randomized controlled trial. *Journal of Pain and Symptom Management*. 46(3) pp. 325.e3. DOI: //dx.doi.org/10.1016/j.jpainsymman.2012.08.017

Kennedy, S.D. (2014) TechnoWellness: A new wellness construct in the 21st century. *Journal of Counselor Leadership and Advocacy*. 1(2) pp. 113–127.

MacRury, I. & Yates, C. (2017) Framing the mobile phone: The psychopathologies of an everyday object. *CM: Communication and Media*. 11(38) pp. 41–70.

Middleton-Green, L., Gadoud, A., Norris, B., et al. (2016) 'A Friend in the Corner': Supporting people at home in the last year of life via telephone and video consultation—An evaluation. *BMJ Supportive & Palliative Care*. Published Online First: 05 February 2016. doi:10.1136/bmjspcare-2015-001016

National Information Board. (2014) *Personalised Health and Care 2020: Using Data and Technology to Transform Outcomes for Patients and Citizens a Framework for Action.* London: National Information Board.

NHS England. (2017) Next Steps on the NHS Five Years Forward View. London: NHS England.

OfCom. (2018) *Adults' Media use and Attitudes Report*. Office. Available at: https://www.ofcom.org.uk/research-and-data/media-literacy-research/adults/adults-media-use-and-attitudes (Accessed: 9/11/2018).

ONS, Office for National Statistics. (2018) *Internet Users, UK: 2018*. Available at: www.ons.gov.uk/businessindustryandtrade/itandinternetindustry/bulletins/internetusers/2018 (Accessed: 9/11/2018).

Ostherr, K., Killoran, P., Shegog, R. & Bruera, E. (2016) Death in the digital age: A systematic review of information and communication technologies in end-of-life care. *Journal of Palliative Medicine*. 19(4) pp. 408–420.

Parker-Bell, B. (1999) Embracing a future with computers and art therapy. *Art Therapy*. 16(4) pp. 180–185. DOI: 10.1080/07421656.1999.10129482

Tan, A., Zimmermann, C. & Rodin, G. (2005) Interpersonal processes in palliative care: An attachment perspective on the patient-clinician relationship. *Palliative Medicine*. 19(2) pp. 143–150.

Turkle, S. (2011) *Alone Together: Why We Expect More from Technology and Less from Each Other.* New York: Basic Books.

Wake, J. (2014) Finding time: An online art therapy group. *Australian and New Zealand Journal of Arts Therapy*. 9(1) pp. 41–52.

Wallin, D.J. (2007) *Attachment in Psychotherapy*. New York: The Guilford Press.

Weitz, P. (ed.) (2014) *Psychotherapy 2.0: Where Psychotherapy and Technology Meet.* London: Karnac Books.

Winnicott, D.W. (1971) *Playing and Reality* (Reprinted 1982). London: Penguin Books Ltd.

Wood, M.J.M. (2005) The shoreline: The realities of working in cancer care. In: Waller, D. & Sibbett, C. (eds.) *Art Therapy and Cancer Care*. Maidenhead, England; New York: Open University Press.

Wood, M.J.M. (2015a) *Art Therapy: Digital Devices, Tablet Computers, Palliative Care, Chronic Illness*. Winston Churchill Memorial Trust Fellow's Report. Available at: www.wcmt.org.uk/fellows/reports/art-therapy-digital-devices-tablet-computers-palliative-care-chronic-illness

Wood, M.J.M. (2015b) 4.11 the contribution of art therapy to palliative medicine. In: Cherny, N., Fallon, M., Kaasa, S., Portenoy, R.K. & Currow, D.C. (eds.) *Oxford Textbook of Palliative Medicine* (Fifth Edition). Oxford: Oxford University Press. p. 210.

Wood, M.J.M. (2016) *UK Survey of Digital Technology in Art Therapy 2016*. Unpublished report.

Zhou, C., Crawford, A., Serhal, E., Kurdyak, P. & Sockalingam, S. (2016) The impact of project ECHO on participant and patient outcomes: A systematic review. *Academic Medicine*. 91(10).

# 12  Snapshot of Practice

## Art Therapy in Hospice: The Florence Experience in Italy

*Stefania Romano*

## About Me

I completed my professional three-year training in art therapy in Italy in 2013. I am a member of the Italian Association of Art Therapists (APIArT). My background is in Counselling, Psychosynthesis and Psycho-Oncology. I have always been interested in meditation and in end-of-life care, and I have attended some courses run by Frank Ostaseski, the founding director of the Zen Hospice Project in San Francisco (USA). I have also attended professional courses in creative writing and autobiography. I have developed an approach of deep attention and respect for people, for their rights and for their different needs.

## About the Context in Which I Work

The beginning of art therapy in hospices in Florence goes back to 2008, when the first hospice was opened (S. Felice a Ema), within the National Health Service. There are no art therapists on the regular staff of hospitals or hospices, as art therapy in Italy is not recognized as a health profession. Roberta Cini, a senior psychologist in the hospice who had art therapy training, was able to incorporate art therapy into terminal care. At present, thanks to funding by the Association "La Finestra" (www.associazionelafinestra.com), I offer one day of art therapy in each of the three hospices in Florence.

Each hospice has ten single rooms. The Staff (doctors, nurses, physiotherapists, and psychologists) meet every morning for a 40 minutes briefing to discuss the patients' condition. I usually take part and, through reading the medical files, I try to form an idea as to which patients are most likely to benefit from art therapy. Of course the physical and emotional state of the patient may vary from day to day, or even from moment to moment. I have also learnt that often patients manifest to me a part of themselves that they may not have manifested to others. I keep my mind open and receptive. I am always aware that this may be the last session, or the only session.

I see the patients in their individual rooms. The objectives of a session range from providing relaxation, to helping patients to express their emotions and to find a form of serenity. There is a small table with two chairs. The time varies from 15 minutes to one hour. I am attentive to the patient's physical, emotional, and spiritual needs, and I am flexible about the use of modalities. In some cases, a session may become a profound spiritual experience.

## Case Example

During an art therapy session I may suggest "a free drawing", "colouring a mandala", "creative writing" or "the manipulation of a piece of clay"; but many patients are in a clinical state whereby handling a pencil, or a pen, or a piece of clay, is difficult. In such cases a receptive approach, at least for a start, may be better than an active approach. In the hospice I have a box containing a collection of postcards, laminated so that they can be sanitized regularly. Each postcard shows a landscape. Patients select a postcard and then we work on it. We call this intervention "the evocative landscape" (Cini 2009; Romano 2016). The medical team of the hospice asked me to see this patient, in part because they felt that she did not completely realize that her medical condition was terminal.

## R.T. — 39 Year-Old Woman, With Metastatic Colon Cancer

### 27/02 First Session

I ask R. what she needs at the moment, and she replies "energy and trust". I open the box of postcards, and she selects one with sea waves on the beach. I ask her to describe the image. She talks about "her sea" and I understand that she has already entered mentally into that picture. I ask her whether she wants to be guided to "be" in that landscape and she agrees and closes her eyes. With my voice, I help her to walk on the beach, and I ask her to focus on all the details of what she is seeing. The session includes long periods of silence. I use her words "energy" and "trust". She is obviously enjoying being in that space. At the end of the experience, she tells me she has seen a light and she felt free to walk towards that light. She felt moved by the experience, and she was surprised, as she regarded herself as a very practical and rational person.

### 01/03 Second Session

I see R. is upset. She tells me she has realized that "there is no hope" and bursts into tears. I ask her whether she wants to select another card, and she says she needs to go back to the same place where she was last time. She says she feels pain. I tell her she could imagine that the pain is a little child that she can take with her. She nods. I then invite her to imagine that the waves of the sea will bring to her an unexpected gift. When she opens her eyes, I invite her to draw the gift she has received. She draws a little box: she says it is similar to a gift she has received in the past . . . but she does not say what is inside it. She says she feels peaceful and she thanks me.

### 06/03 Third Session

R. asks me to go to the same place . . . I help her to be there, and this time I include the sounds of the waves, the light and the smell of the ocean. I encourage her to take this peacefulness into her mind and her heart. I suggest that this time she may shift her attention to the "essential" centre of herself, while at the same time looking at the ocean.

### 09/03 Fourth Session

R. tells me the work we do together is good. She talks about the relationship with her family. With her parents she has to pretend she does not know about her condition. With her brother instead she has to comfort him. She finds all this very tiring. She wants to continue with the same image, and this time I add the colours of the sunrise in the early morning. She says that is exactly what she needed.

### 13/03 Fifth and last Session

I know from the staff that there is not much time. R. wants to lie down and I sit on a chair near her. She wants to go to the same place. I take her to see the beach, the sea, the sky, and I connect the sounds of the waves to the rhythm of her breathing. I help her to distance herself from the beach, and to see everything from up in the sky, and then to come back. I can feel that her breathing is getting very slow and peaceful. She then tells me, with words and gestures, that she is OK, and I leave her. She will die two days later.

### Advantages of Art Therapy in My Context

I have noticed that the symbolic language of art therapy helps the patients to communicate their awareness of death and dying, to themselves and to others, and to process it. I have seen drawings of passages from one planet to another; trees that die and are reborn; boats sailing towards a distant island. Sometimes the patients ask me to place their images on the wall "so that my visitors can understand". On one side, they use these images to familiarize themselves with the great mystery of death; on another side, they communicate their awareness to relatives and to medical staff.

### One Idea That Shapes My Work

In art therapy an image can be a tool to contain the pain, to contact one's inner strength, to lead towards a spiritual path. A single idea that influenced my work is that there is no *a priori* reason why the image needs to be "made" by the patients: it may be an external image selected with the patients and used according to their needs. This idea has shaped my professional life and my activity in hospice. Art therapy at the end of life was a new area at the time in Italy. We were a small group of students and Paola Luzzatto was our mentor. We discussed this concept in length and breadth; and in putting together our collection of picture postcards we paid particular attention to the importance of being respectful of different cultural backgrounds. We tested images on patients one by one. It turned out that the most "evocative" images were always reflecting in some way one or more of the four ancient elements: Earth, Water, Air, Fire. Some images seemed to foster energy; others seemed to facilitate serenity and hope. They may all become precious "internal images" that may accompany patients until their last moments.

## Acknowledgement

I would like to thank Paola Caboara Luzzatto who has always encouraged and supported me with her great heart and experience during the work.

## References

Cini, R. (2009) "Sulla Soglia", Thesis for the Diploma in Art Therapy, Art Therapy Italiana, Bologna.
Romano, S. (2016) Art Therapy in Palliative Care: Acts from the International Conference "Complementary Therapies in Oncology: Dance, Yoga, Music and Art: What Evidence of Efficacy?" October 6–7. Brescia, Italy.

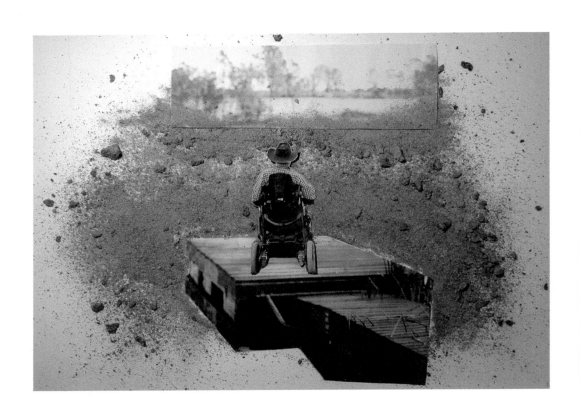

# Section Two

# Art Therapy for Groups, Families and Communities

Death, dying, grief and loss not only impact one person at a time; they leave a profound impression on entire families and communities. In Section One we considered specific instances of art therapy with individuals. In Section Two we present authors working with groups, families and communities, supporting patients in a more collective and systems-focused manner. Art therapy offered to people gathered together can look quite different from art therapy offered to individuals alone, enabling healing and meaning to be found in shared experiences. The following chapters, while offering different perspectives, all indicate that connecting with others can be beneficial for the healing process.

Family and community-based art therapy may be held in a medical institution, a public space, outdoors, or in many other settings. Art therapists are equipped to be flexible in how they work and in how they create a safe, therapeutic and creative space, considering structure, guidelines and boundaries before the first session begins. Within these boundaries a number of approaches are possible, the two most frequently used in art therapy are:

- an "open studio" approach—where art materials and the therapist's non-judgemental attention are provided, but not specific instructions
- a directive art therapy approach—where the art therapist will present a theme, question, or specific materials

Claudia McKnight (Chapter 18) outlines a closed art therapy group for children diagnosed with a chronic illness, siblings of children diagnosed with cancer, and bereaved siblings. The cohesiveness and safety of the group is maintained by ensuring only one member of each family attends any given group. McKnight's model of groupwork sits between a fully structured and open studio format, with a fixed membership, and time for spontaneous art making. Annalie Ashwell and Hannah Cridford's chapter (14) focuses on a large-scale art therapy project, combining the use of therapeutic arts activities, community engagement arts, and art psychotherapy. This example shows how a more directive project helped to promote greater understanding of palliative care by engaging the community at large as well as those receiving and delivering hospice care. This resonates with the digital art project mentioned by Michèle J.M. Wood in Section One (Chapter 11).

Innovation in models of art therapy and the development of partnerships are strong in this area of practice, overcoming barriers to engagement. Jones et al's chapter (23) describes the process of piloting an art therapy intervention delivered at distance for those living in rural Wales, where travelling to cancer services can be an onerous task. In this group the therapist and patients connect using videoconferencing. McMahon et al (Chapter 22) discuss another pilot project implemented within a public area of an inpatient palliative care unit in Ireland. A collaboration between art and music therapy, this chapter details how the creative arts were able to ensure a safe, secure and therapeutic venue for group members.

Several chapters focus on the support art therapy interventions provide for carers and family members, both pre- and post-bereavement. Ofira Honig and colleagues, working in Israel (Chapter 15), present an innovative art therapy intervention for carers of people with dementia. The support art therapy offers to caregivers facing the challenges of looking after their relatives with dementia is outlined throughout the chapter. Heidi Bardot and Jean McCaw's (chapter 20) focuses specifically on the use of art therapy within a grief camp for bereaved children and the impact it had on those who participated. In Chapter 21, Kayleigh Orr provides a view of art therapy with families, differentiating art therapy with patients, bereaved relatives and siblings.

In addition to these contributions from professionals working in the field, Lynda Kachurek (Chapter 25) provides a moving account of her experiences as a service user. She discusses how joining a bereavement focused art therapy group after the death of her husband greatly benefited her healing process. Personal narratives are examined further by Judy Thomson (Chapter 17), whose research inquiry offers the reader valuable insights into the Australian palliative care system. The roles and experiences of several art therapists working in palliative care are explored through the research methodology of immersive visual analysis. These accounts illuminate the anger, frustrations, enthusiasm and passion of art therapists working within this field. The chapter draws attention to the power of stories that art therapists encounter and participate in as they go about their work, and emphasizes the unique properties of visual art making as a tool for healing.

# 13 Snapshot of Practice

## Art Therapy in Paediatric Oncology

*Urania Dominguez*

## About Me

I studied my master's and got my training in art therapy in Barcelona, Spain. I mostly worked in multicultural educational settings and I specialized in cultural sensitivity within art therapy. Upon arriving in Puerto Rico, after seven and a half years living and working in Spain, my focus in art therapy changed since Puerto Rico is not culturally diverse. I did some training for teachers regarding the creative process in the classroom and related to working with special needs children.

However, when I began to work in a children´s hospital setting, I focused my work on pediatric cancer and the different aspects this entails such as grief, loss, trauma and emotional support during chemotherapy. I combine art therapy goals with child life goals to provide better psychosocial care. Both art therapy and child life professions are unknown in Puerto Rico; it has been challenging for me to be taken seriously and for other professionals to understand how my work helps them do theirs.

Currently, I work in the Oncology, Intensive Care, Pre-Op and Mental Health units of a local children's hospital as an art therapist and child life specialist.

## About the Context in Which I Work

The island of Puerto Rico is the smallest island of the Major Antilles, settled between the Atlantic Ocean and the Caribbean Sea. Its 100 × 35 mile span holds over 4 million inhabitants, almost one million of those live in the metropolitan area. Puerto Rico is a self-governing commonwealth in association with the United States. The chief of state is the president and the head of government is an elected governor. Puerto Rico has authority over its internal affairs. The United States controls interstate trade, foreign relations and commerce, customs, control of air, land and sea, immigration and emigration, nationality and citizenship, currency, maritime laws, military service and bases, legal procedures, treaties, communications, agriculture, highways, the postal system, Social Security and other areas generally controlled by the federal government within the USA (Welcome. topuertorico.org, 2019).

There are only three free-standing pediatric hospitals on the island. I work as an art therapist and child life specialist in one of these hospitals, San Jorge Children's hospital, and my work is mostly with pre-surgical, mental health and oncology patients, including at their end of life stage. It is the most complete privately-owned children's hospital.

A pediatric cancer diagnosis can bring serious distress to the whole family because of the implication that the child may die. However, depending on the type of cancer, 5-year survival rates can be as high as 75–85% (CureSearch for Children's Cancer, 2019). The most common cancer in children is leukemia, but I have also worked with osteosarcoma (with and without amputation), neuroblastoma and patients with Hodgkin's disease. The oncology unit has strict guidelines for visiting hours and number of visitors allowed; therefore, my interventions are much anticipated and provide emotional support for the patients and the family as well.

## Case Example

Oncology patients often have long and repetitive hospitalizations. Being in the hospital for long periods of time may cause serious emotional distress to children of all ages. Many may feel sad, fearful, nervous and angry, and their physical, social and emotional development can also be affected by their circumstances.

Interventions in the oncology unit may vary in purpose and procedure depending on the needs of each child. One of the objectives when working in this unit is helping the children express their emotions and adjust to the clinical setting. As an art therapist, I understand that expression comes in many forms; knowing that children nowadays enjoy picture taking, I decided to plan a therapeutic photography activity as an alternative means to accomplish my goals.

> The pursuit of photography as a form of self-help is usually done as a means to gain personal insight or a better understanding of oneself. It could also be used to gain mastery over a certain element of a person's life.
>
> (Natoli, 2011, p. 2)

The photography activity consisted of providing a professional grade digital camera to children individually and inviting them to take pictures, in and out of their rooms, of things and/or people they liked, found interesting or that were important to them. Ten children participated in the activity from ages 6 to 16 and their subject choices varied.

Everyone took pictures of their surroundings and of people that mattered to them. Some of the photographs taken showed aspects of the hospital; details of the play room, the movie theater, the intravenous bags and medications, empty beds or simply the water fountain in the hallway. Some pictures showed their personal belongings such as coloring books, crayons and stuffed animals. In other pictures, we saw how the children viewed themselves within their hospitalization, taking pictures of their shadow, their feet, their IV and IV stands and even their blood transfusion bag.

Though not a conscious process, taking photographs allowed them to view the hospital and their hospitalization in another light, as if from the outside looking in. They depicted objects and people that were part of their hospital routine and that they were accustomed to. It also allowed them to explore familiarity and communication with these objects and people. The pictures also established their passage through the oncology unit, evidencing it as an important part in their life's story.

Furthermore, the activity of taking pictures in itself allowed for a process of normalization. For example, a boy who had a recent amputation wished to take pictures of different things in the unit. There were no wheelchairs available that I could quickly grab, so I used a rolling office chair and pushed him wherever he wanted to go. This chair gave him more liberty than a wheelchair because it would roll and turn in every direction. He was free from the constraints of a wheelchair, which helped him feel like any other person on a rolling office chair and not a patient with an amputated leg.

## Advantages of Art Therapy in My Context

Though the creative process is a beneficial tool to exteriorize inner conflicts and express emotions, in my experience many patients in a clinical setting welcome art activities, mainly as a means of distraction and as a normalization process. Their artwork expresses the things they like or like to do. They use art to decorate their hospital rooms and make their space feel more like home. This form of creative expression provides the hospitalized child a means to control their environment and give their personal space a less clinical feel.

The mere process of creating helps children to focus on more pleasant issues, helping their mind to relax and be able to manage difficult emotions such as anxiety, fear, anger and sadness, while at the same time the body also relaxes, helping them cope with pain associated with their condition or treatment.

Furthermore, creative activities provide patients with the opportunity to make choices, giving them a sense of control and empowerment in a place where they have lost all control of what they can do, how they can dress, what they can eat and when they are going to be tested, prodded or pricked.

Lastly, the artwork made in medical art therapy can help patients communicate their understanding and feelings regarding their condition, treatment and hospitalization. This allows the therapist to correct any misconceptions and address the patient's concerns and fears while at the same time helping them to develop their motor and communication skills.

## One Idea that Shapes My Work

Often, I have been told: "I couldn't do what you do", or I have been asked: "How are you able to work with patients who are sick or dying?" My answer is that my patients are first and foremost children, not their condition or their medical situation. I have to keep in mind that my job is to help them have quality of life in their time in the hospital. It is important to remember that children understand the world around them through play and communication with others; creating art is a form of play and a form of communication. Therefore, providing art opportunities helps patients in their healing process, continuing their healthy development. Thus, when I provide medical art therapy to these patients the first thing I ask myself is if what I am doing is beneficial and therapeutic, and whether it provides tools for managing stress, anxiety, pain and fear? And lastly, I ask myself if the child is being a child and if not, what can I do to support them in their process? I believe that children need to play, create and express themselves to develop properly and heal quicker.

## References

Natoli, Adam, 2011: *The Psychologically Beneficial Aspects of Photography*. Bachelor of Arts. Available at: https://www.researchgate.net/publication/297731083_The_Psychologically_Beneficial_Aspects_of_Photography [Accessed 25 Mar. 2019].

## Online Resources

/CureSearch for Children's Cancer, 2019. 5-Year Survival Rate|CureSearch. [online]. Available at: https://curesearch.org/5-Year-Survival-Rate [Accessed 25 Mar. 2019].

Welcome.topuertorico.org, 2019. Government of Puerto Rico. [online] Available at: http://welcome.topuertorico.org/government.shtml [Accessed 25 Mar. 2019].

# 14 Art Therapy, Community Engagement, and Living and Dying

*Annalie Ashwell and Hannah Cridford*

## Introduction

This chapter will focus on a large-scale art project, offering individuals connected to a hospice the opportunity to create a piece of artwork and contribute it to a public exhibition. Exhibiting the creativity, thoughts and feelings of people in touch with illness, loss, death and dying attempts to bridge the gap that exists between those supported by hospices and mainstream society. Each artwork created in the project is like a pebble that, when dropped in water, creates ripples that flow on to influence others in ways that cannot be fully known at the time of making (The 14th Dalai Lama, 2018). This chapter will explore the impact of such ripples on the communities in which we work, the field of art psychotherapy, and societal responses to living and dying in the UK in the 21st century.

As two qualified art psychotherapists sharing one full-time job, our remit is to develop a creative therapy service across two hospices in one county in England, UK. The hospices are very different from each other—one is purpose-built and located in large rural grounds, on the outskirts of a largely affluent small town; the other, an historic building in the centre of a multicultural town. Each hospice has developed services in response to the needs of their local community, and together have established a partnership to deliver a range of innovative outpatient services, including rehabilitation, wellbeing and therapeutic interventions, bereavement services and palliative care. In this chapter, we will explore the community engagement aspect of our role. To contextualise this, it is important to briefly outline how hospice care sits in relation to the wider healthcare system.

Hospices in the UK are charitable organisations, rooted in their communities and largely financed by fundraising activities. They are also partially funded by the National Health System (NHS). As medical advancements mean that many people recover from serious illness, or live with life limiting conditions for longer, our healthcare systems are stretched and continually face new challenges. In response, an overarching move to a 'self-management agenda' has developed. This agenda regards the patient and their carers as experts, requiring them to work in partnership with professionals to choose and access appropriate treatments to effectively manage their condition.

Arguably, this partnership has always been the approach of the hospice movement; multi-disciplinary teams work thoughtfully and compassionately alongside the patient and their family to address complex circumstances, and apply Dame Cicely Saunders' concept of 'Total Pain' (Saunders, 1990), which encapsulates the physical, emotional, social and spiritual suffering that may be present at the end of life. However, in the last 15–20 years, end of life care has faced a number of criticisms, including inequity of access (Sims, Radford, Doran and Page, 1997); limited understanding of holistic care, at the expense of social and spiritual needs of service users (Kearney, 1992); and increased dependency on professionals rather than encouraging individual resilience and self-management (Kellehear, 2013). In response to such criticisms hospices have been diversifying the services they offer, with many transforming the traditional 'day care' model into innovative community hubs, operating more like an outpatient system than a day centre. Community engagement projects and open access groups have also become commonplace, as they have the potential to increase accessibility of services and nurture self-management. The focus of this chapter is on a part of our service that aims to increase accessibility and independence, drawing new people into the hospice and supporting those already involved to live creatively alongside their illness.

## Creative Practice in the Hospice Environment

Hospices in the UK have always hosted a diversity of art practice. Arts in health initiatives, community arts activities and art psychotherapy may all take place in the same institution, and may be facilitated by a variety of practitioners, both paid and unpaid, qualified and unqualified. Our creative therapies service is reflective of this, and is made up of three types of activity:

- **Community Engagement Arts**: events, projects and drop-in activities open to the whole community
- **Therapeutic Arts Activities**: a series of workshops, including dance/movement, music, visual arts/crafts
- **Art Psychotherapy**: available on a referral basis to people who identify as needing emotional or psychological support; delivered by qualified Art Psychotherapists

We see this model as enabling people to access different intensities of activity, according to their needs, thus providing a person-centred, holistic service.

The Art Bag project, which we will explore in detail in this chapter, comes under the Community Engagement category. As the project has developed, the richness it offers in terms of its versatility, therapeutic possibility, and power to connect people has become increasingly apparent. We have come to think of it as the foundation of our service, a flagship project and fundamental to how we, as art therapists, both contribute to and creatively challenge the organisations in which we work.

## Art Bag Project Overview

### *"Create, Contemplate, Connect"*

The Art Bag project offers people the chance to: *create*, by completing a small, straightforward craft activity; *contemplate*, by considering choices within the making process, or ruminating on other thoughts that may occur during making; and *connect*, by making alongside others or by contributing to the end of project exhibition.

The Art Bag itself is a little paper bag (Figure 14.1) containing:

- Materials needed to complete a simple craft activity
- Ideas and inspiration
- A summary of the history and symbolism of the activity
- Feedback and consent card
- A flier for our service

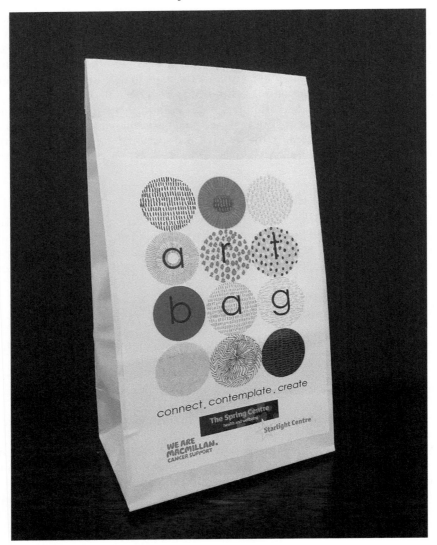

*Figure 14.1* The Art Bag

Bags are available in the reception, inpatient ward and outpatient areas of each hospice, and are presented alongside a box where participants can return their completed activity.

The project has an annual life, launching during Hospice Care week in October, running through the autumn and winter, coming to a natural end in late spring and culminating in an exhibition at the beginning of summer. This life cycle complements seasonal changes in the UK: the launch offers an injection of creativity at a time when leaves start to fall, nights become shorter, and thoughts turn to endings; the exhibition synchronises with the rebirth of nature, marking connections between life and death, creation, creativity and rebirth.

In our first year, each bag contained a small, weaving loom, a selection of yarn and a pre-threaded, plastic needle. The weaving loom was made from a recycled CD and was therefore circular. The circle, a profound, universal symbol, provides a visual component that draws connections with wider, existential issues, commonly explored within hospice care. The circle or 'Mandala' (1967), in relation to Jungian theory, is one of the most common archetypal images, and "signifies the wholeness of self, representing the wholeness of the psychic ground or, to put it in mythic terms, the divinity incarnate in man" (Jung, G. C., 1967, p. 367). Some writing on the powerful symbolism of the circle was therefore included in the bag, as was a short piece on the rich tradition of weaving:

> Weaving is an ancient and universal craft dating back to Neolithic times; it is a practical skill that also holds ideas of protection and shelter. The activity of weaving is one of balance, where warp and weft, and over and under, are used in equal measure to progress the work.

The tactility of weaving provides a sensory experience for participants and is simple and achievable, suitable for people of varying ages, abilities and strength (Figure 14.2). The repetition of interlacing yarn, over and under, can calm the mind, alleviating stress and anxiety, as one participant remarked:

> Have yarn, keep calm.

For some, the activity brought similar benefits to mindfulness practice:

> A very good way of bringing you into the here and now. Very soothing.

The choice of craft consequently has the potential to proffer powerful symbolic meaning, and plays a large part in setting the tone each year. At the time of writing this chapter, the choice of activity is soap carving (Figure 14.3), providing an opportunity for participants to "carve out a space and time for themselves". Each bag contains a bar of soft, malleable soap and the materials needed for carving. The ancient practice of carving has traditionally been used to create artefacts that can hold many meanings. Ideas of change

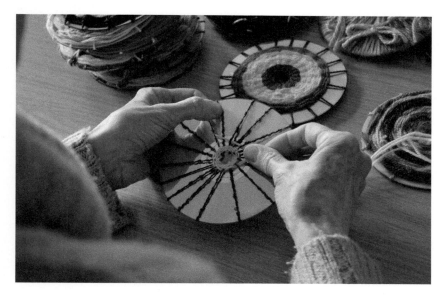

*Figure 14.2* Weaving

and transformation are bound up within the carving process as through manipulation of the material, shapes begin to surface. This echoes the process of personal exploration and discovery that may be seen in those who are diagnosed and living with a life limiting illness.

As outlined earlier, one of the main aims of the Art Bag project is to encourage participants to be as self-sufficient as possible. All necessary materials are included so that participation can take place either at the hospice or elsewhere. Participants may choose to complete their bag individually, or with family or friends, or they may take part in an

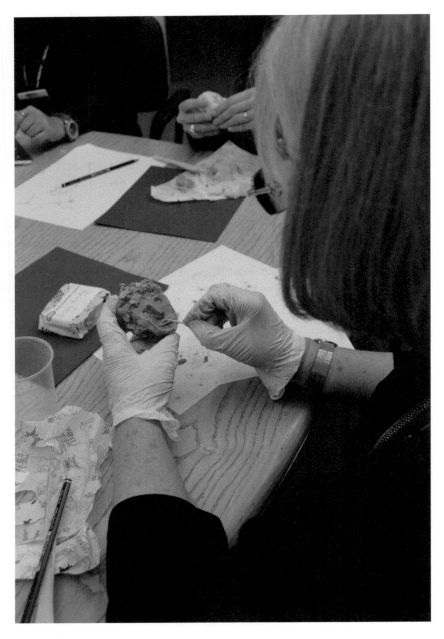

*Figure 14.3* Soap Carving

organised group experience where the art bag is the central activity. Staff members and volunteers can access the project as participants, and can also use the art bag as a 'toolkit', enabling non-arts practitioners to employ creative methods in engaging with patients and families in their care. For instance, a volunteer and patient might sit together and complete an art bag at the same time; this shared activity supports the building of relationships, encourages relaxation and a sense of achievement, and may also lead to meaningful conversation. The versatility of the project means that people can participate according to their own needs and desires, resulting in a range of 'levels' of engagement, highlighted in participants' feedback:

"I nearly tore my hair out as the yarn kept tangling. But, am happy with the end product". (patient)

"Participating in the art bag project re-connected me with how calming and satisfying it is to sit quietly and create something with my hands". (patient)

"It made me sit and relax but, at the same time made me concentrate in a constructive way". (patient)

"It was fun to have permission and encouragement to create something". (volunteer)

"It does what it says on the bag—connect, contemplate, create. This is from someone who does not have a creative bone in her body. I have explained as I have gone alone to my husband who is very poorly and I am sure he smiled inside at the thought of me doing something like this and finding it very calming and therapeutic. Thank you for the opportunity to take part". (carer)

"My Japanese daughter-in-law made this whilst we listened to football on the radio, thank you for the pretty colours". (unknown)

"Not enough wool for both sides". (unknown)

## The Art Bag Project as Community Engagement

In order to understand the relevance of the Art Bag project in the wider context, it is important to define what we mean by 'community engagement'. In relation to hospice care, the term can refer to engaging *with* a community and also *in* the community, i.e. service delivery that takes place away from the hospice building (Paul and Sallnow, 2013). Morgan (2001) has clarified this divide into two models: '*utilitarian*' and '*empowerment*'. The use of community resources (such as volunteers and existing service delivery) is deemed as '*utilitarian*', whereas engagement which aims to give communities responsibility and the potential to change situations, beliefs and understandings is deemed an '*empowerment*' model. These definitions are helpful in exploring the Art Bag project as it encompasses both models. The development and delivery of the project is heavily reliant upon our team of volunteers and makes use of community spaces for the exhibition of artworks, and thus is indicative of Morgan's '*utilitarian*' model. However, the overall aims and objectives of the project are more in keeping with an '*empowerment*' model, by encouraging the hospice communities to engage in a creative platform that supports personal exploration of death, dying and loss. In addition, the project culminates each year in a public exhibition that aims to gently reintroduce these subjects to the collective conscious, whilst also increasing awareness of hospice care and the range of support available.

As art therapists we utilise our knowledge and experience as a way of framing the activities we have on offer; our professional identities as art therapists are central to providing a safe and effective service. We also draw upon these skills in recruiting, training and supervising volunteers, who make up the vast majority of our team and whose skill and commitment are critical to the development and delivery of the service as a whole. Our volunteer team are involved not only in delivering our service, but also in developing initiatives from the outset via individual and group consultation. Many of our volunteers have personal connections to the hospice through experiencing their own complex illness or through bereavement, and are 'creatives' in their own right with a wide range of skills. The team are driven to support our art bag project due to personal experiences and their understanding of wider local need and thus, in a reciprocal relationship, the community both informs and benefits from the service we provide. Sallnow and Paul (2014) describes this as collaborative community engagement, whereby "communities are supported to develop alternative models of care and to deliver these jointly with the service" (p. 235), raising the quality of engagement. Sallnow and Paul (2014) explains that this method is more likely to lead to long-term outcomes than services that aim to raise awareness and educate without involving the community in the work. It is the amalgamation of both 'utilitarian' and 'empowerment' models that generates such rich community engagement, garnering benefits for both hospices.

## The Exhibition

Societal responses to death and dying are culture specific (Clark and Seymour, 1999; Evans, 2005). Within the last 100 years of western European culture, the responsibility of supporting those with chronic and terminal illness has increasingly fallen upon the immediate family and healthcare professionals, with a growing disconnect between the family unit and the wider community (A. Kellehear, 2013). In addition to this, modern western societies tend to experience death obliquely, through the media 'filter', which brings news of war, natural disasters and famine (Clark and Seymour, 1999, p. 8), meaning that everyday death is, paradoxically, further removed from everyday life. Ken Evans (2005) powerfully describes how people diagnosed with terminal illness become changed in status and alienated from the healthy populace; with our ubiquitous emphasis on material and commercial values—on 'getting ahead' (Yalom, 1998, p. 217)—there is a psychological and institutional 'void' when it comes to dying that results in despair (Evans, 2005, p. 7) and an unpreparedness for the death of our loved ones, or ourselves. Dying is essentially a social act, Evans says, and in our society it is set apart from life and living, left in the hands of specialists (2005, p. 7).

*Ars moriendi*, or 'the art of dying', refers to the rituals that surround dying that enable the individual and society to better deal with death. In traditional societies, these rituals might include the bereaved not cutting their hair or fingernails, or providing food for the newly deceased, and serve to "[blur] the lines . . . between the living and the dead" (Evans, 2005, p. 10). In our society, with advancements in technology and research, the prevailing emphasis is firmly on preventing and curing illness, seemingly in pursuit of ridding society of serious diseases such as cancer. Patients have more information available to them via the Internet; they can become masters of their illness, picking and choosing what treatments they wish to have. These influences may offer us empowerment, a sense of gaining control over our mortality, but may simultaneously be contributing to a cultural distraction from death itself.

An important aim of this project is to reconnect the wider community with the 'art of dying'. Through exhibiting the artworks and related thoughts of people who are seriously ill, those caring for them, and the bereaved, the exhibition offers an opportunity for the viewing public to consider aspects of illness, loss and death, gently challenging the viewer to confront 'the final taboo' (Evans, 2005, p. 4). From the outset participants are invited to hand their artwork back to the hospice for it to be part of a public exhibition. A feedback card is included in the art bag; thoughts and reflections on how people felt when completing their craft activity are encouraged and have become an integral and emotive part of the exhibition. In the first exhibition, reflections on the making process were inscribed on mirrors (Figure 14.4), encouraging visitors to see themselves in the comments. In viewing our own reflection, we connect more tangibly with those who might have experienced the death of a loved one or be experiencing the loss of their own health. In that moment, symbolically, viewer and participant become as one: one community, experiencing losses and triumphs together.

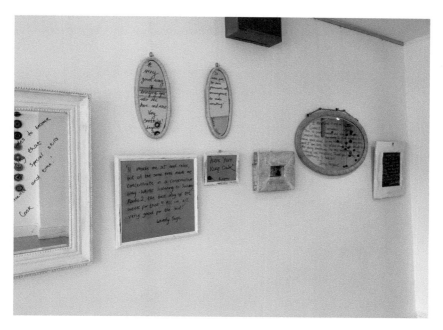

*Figure 14.4* The Exhibition—Reflections

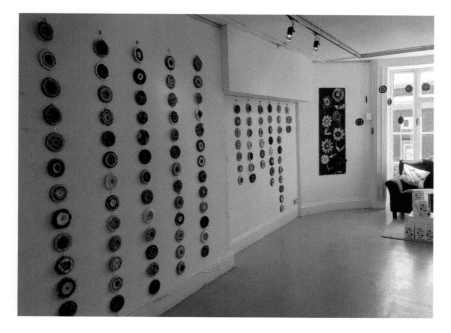

*Figure 14.5* The Exhibition—Numbers of People in Touch With Hospice Services

The completed Art Bag artworks may also have a powerful effect on the viewer. Over 200 completed artworks were submitted for the first Art Bag project exhibition (Figure 14.5); the sheer quantity serves to represent the numbers of people in touch with hospice services, who are thereby in touch with serious illness, death and dying. This effect may be heightened by the diversity of colour, texture and design within the uniform shape and size (Figure 14.6): each artwork represents a human being, each one unique and distinct. For the participants, the artwork may provide the opportunity to share a part of themselves with other people, both known and unknown. In considering the exhibition at the

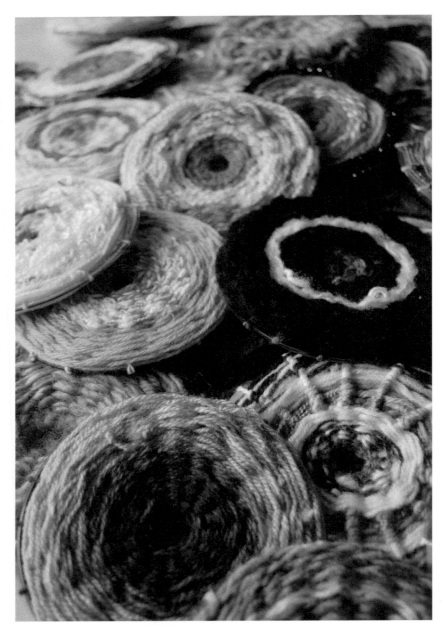

*Figure 14.6* Diversity

time of making, the object may perform the act of projecting aspects of the maker into the future. For some participants, this future may exist beyond their death; the art object thereby blurring the lines between living and dying much like the aforementioned death rituals. For those that remain, the experience of having made the artwork is often vividly remembered—as in art therapy sessions, we can trace our emotional journey through viewing images we have made along the way, so powerful is the mind-body connect during making. And so, like death rituals, the artworks in the exhibition may serve to ". . . strengthen attachments between surviving members of families and friends and the deceased person" (Evans, 2005, p. 10).

The exhibition also hosted a mock-up 'living space' (including a sofa, coffee table, and lamp), which encouraged visitors to engage more fully with the project by taking the time to complete their own Art Bag activity and hang their completed artwork alongside the others. This 'living' component facilitated a shared experience, provided an opportunity for the audience to connect more directly with the hospice community, and has led to partnerships with other community groups. One such partnership is with a local centre for adults with learning disabilities, who came on a group visit to the exhibition. Verbal feedback from this group indicated their immediate connection to the exhibition; many of them had felt deeply moved, having experienced the death of their own relatives at the hospice. The group continued to engage with the exhibition, creating artwork in response. A subsequent conversation with the centre co-ordinator revealed that the exhibition had connected with feelings of isolation and loss that service users may experience as a result of their disability, and that having a public exhibition had enabled them to feel less alone. From this small example, we see the power of the exhibition to ignite a dialogue between individuals and agencies, enabling a deeper level of connection and assisting thoughts and feelings, that may be previously unheard, to find voice. It is in the exhibition that the ripples of the individual can be seen and felt by others, ". . . bridging the space between the personal and the public" (Evans, 2005, p. 10) and offering an alternative *Ars Moriendi* for the present-day.

## Reflection—The Art Bag Project and Art Therapy

The Art Bag project is versatile, with shoots of actual and potential development reaching into a range of areas relevant to hospice care, all rich topics for exploration and consideration. For the purpose of this chapter, we will focus on how and why it has proved valuable to those who have participated, exploring this in relation to contemporary art therapy practice.

One of the forebears credited with developing art therapy in the UK was Adrian Hill (Case and Dalley, 2006)—a professional artist, who re-embarked upon personal art making during a prolonged period of hospitalisation due to physical ill health. Interest amongst fellow patients grew and at a later date he was formally invited by the occupational therapist at the hospital to support others to create artwork, mainly painting and drawing. Hill's developments ran in parallel with forerunners in other settings, but a shared belief at this time was that art making had the potential to be healing, in and of itself:

> . . . in the early years of pioneer work . . . most art therapists emphasised the process of art and its inherent healing properties.
>
> (Case and Dalley, 2006, p. 3)

In more recent times, art therapy has increasingly developed to incorporate aspects of psychoanalysis, making use of the therapeutic relationship that exists between therapist, client and their artwork. As art therapy has become more aligned with the psychotherapies, the inherent healing properties of art making may now be more commonly regarded as 'arts in health' activity; that is, activity which recognises that participatory arts and personal creativity is beneficial for wellbeing, but tends not to explore unconscious processes. Participation in the Art Bag project does not take place within a strictly psychotherapeutic frame, and oftentimes not in the presence of a qualified art psychotherapist, but nonetheless the project has been developed to facilitate therapeutic benefit and may therefore be regarded as art therapy.

## Adapting Practice to the Palliative Care Setting

Adaptability and innovation have long been the domain of art therapists working in palliative care. In the midst of the uncertainty and change brought about by serious illness, people who may benefit from taking part in art interventions may feel wary of involvement, perhaps fearing the unknown aspects of a creative opportunity or of reviving deeply held beliefs about lack of ability. Accessing opportunities may also be problematic for practical reasons connected to declining physical health or diminished cognitive capacities related to drug regimes. Flexing the traditional boundaries of art therapy to enable people to take part therefore becomes a necessity.

In "The search for a model which opens" (1998), Camilla Connell talks of minimal understanding of art therapy in the cancer care centre where she works. She refers to the surprise that is often expressed, by patients and professionals, that a creative psychological service should be provided where people are primarily receiving medical treatments for physical symptoms. Connell states that "most people are not looking for 'therapy' as such" (1998, p. 78) but may nonetheless be in need of support during the 'emotional disturbance' (1998, p. 79) that a cancer diagnosis may bring. She explores the sensitivity that is therefore necessary in approaching and enabling patients to engage in art therapy and outlines a number of activities that have worked well in opening up the possibility of participation. These include a 'Group Notebook' (1998, p. 77)—an on-going and now substantial collection of artwork by patients in Connell's setting, including imagery, poetry and prose—and hanging exhibitions within the setting itself.

The Art Bag is our response to the need for an opening. The project informs the workforce and service users about the existence of our service as a whole, lightly educating on the possible benefits of engaging in creative therapies. The activity can be picked up whenever the patient feels able or motivated, contending as they are with fluctuating health and levels of energy, as well as periods of enforced inactivity and boredom. It is not always possible for patients, or indeed carers, to access groups made available at specific times or in specific places, and yet the need to feel connected to others remains, as stated by Connell: ". . . in developing a model of art therapy which is relevant to the situation of patients, the value of shared experience becomes evident" (Connell, 1998, p. 78). The large scale of the Art Bag project provides a sense of being connected—participants are aware that other people are similarly working towards completing the activity, with the same start and end point. The aim of contributing to an end point (the exhibition) may mirror some aspects of a group art therapy session, which might include a period of looking and thinking together about the images that have been made. In this way, the project could be seen to be echoing the process of a slow, open group.

For many, the invitation to be creative brings a mixture of feelings—intrigue and excitement may be present, alongside apprehension and fear of humiliation. As an art bag can be accessed privately and independently, feelings of doubt or embarrassment about 'giving it a go' are minimised, and the project may therefore offer a gentle entry point into creative therapies.

## 'Re-Purposing' Creative Activity

Arts and crafts activity have always been present in hospice care. A creative practitioner (sometimes paid, sometimes voluntary) may frequently be found within day hospice provision, offering a range of accessible arts and crafts activities, for example card making, mono-printing, knitting/crochet, drawing and painting. These practitioners are often very accomplished, creatively and with interpersonal skills; they will encourage people to participate, bringing a group of people together to discover or re-discover creative interest, offering richness of activity and engagement to the setting. Sadly, however, this sphere of activity is sometimes regarded as 'diversionary' and seems at times to be deemed of secondary importance to other aspects of care—medical, nursing and pastoral/spiritual—that also take place within the setting.

As discussed earlier, the historical and cultural qualities found in crafts such as weaving and carving provide powerful metaphors for exploring existential issues. With careful use of language and visuals we aim to make use of this symbolism, harnessing the potential for craft to support a deeper exploration of feelings and emotions that relate to living, dying and death. We have therefore come to view the Art Bag project as 're-purposing' the craft activity traditionally found in palliative care settings, accentuating their therapeutic values rather than diminishing them, and challenging the notion that crafts activity is merely diversionary. Taking part in creative activity may enable 'flow'; "a holistic sensation experienced when one is totally involved in an activity" (Sibbett, 2005, p. 28). Such experiences may offer absorption, reverie, and the potential for respite from pain, and may also focus the mind, enabling thoughts and feelings that may be previously unrealised to take shape. We have witnessed this in the feedback obtained from people participating in the project. Some people engaged in a very profound way, processing the death of loved ones:

"By making this circle of life, I call it, I think I turned a corner and I now realise my daughter is happy now, and I feel she is at peace. To my lovely Sarah".

Others found the opportunity to process anxious feelings, seemingly absorbing them through embodied practice, which supported them to release pent-up emotion:

"I really enjoyed taking part in this project. I have a bad habit of pulling my hair out (weird I know!) and I found that whilst my hands were busy weaving, I didn't pull any out. So thank you".

## Conclusion

In this chapter, we have explored how a large-scale, community project may be a relevant and important facet of art therapy practice in contemporary hospice care in the UK. Much of the work of an art therapist is in supporting people (both colleagues and clients) to understand the benefits that creativity may bring. As professionals, we know that the arts are pivotal to good mental and physical health and overall wellbeing; as a sector, art therapists have an important role to play in educating and enlightening others, particularly in times of tight funding. The model of the Art Bag project enables aspects of art therapy to be seen and experienced by larger numbers of people, gently promoting both the work of hospices and the role that the arts has to play within it. It showcases what the creative therapies can offer, shedding light on the often shielded, private nature of art therapy.

Through our training as art psychotherapists, our understanding of the complexities involved in art making and exhibiting enhance and harness the therapeutic nature of the project. The language used in the art bag itself, the choices offered within the activity, the choice of participating in the end exhibition, and the authentic request for feedback, thoughts and feelings, serve to retain core principles of art therapy, offering a certain type of therapeutic alliance that enables those participating to feel safe in engaging. The project is not rigid in how, when or where it is delivered, but is available and flexible to meet the needs of individuals, offering accompaniment on their individual journey. It is not uncommon for therapists to describe their role in this way too—as a companion, travelling alongside their client.

Just as a pebble creates ripples when dropped into water, individual contributions to the Art Bag project facilitate ripples of change. In connecting with one another through this project we acknowledge our shared experiences, particularly in relation to loss, death and dying. In doing so we shift towards becoming an 'empowered' community, with an increased responsibility to care, acknowledge and support those living with a life limiting illness, their family and friends. In a culture that segregates death and dying, handing it over to 'experts', the project aims both to promote pro-active creativity amongst the patient and carer cohort, and bridge the gap between those involved in hospice care and the wider community, thereby reviving aspects of the *Ars Moriendi*.

## References

The 14th Dalai Lama. (2018). *The Office of His Holiness The Dalai Lama | The 14th Dalai Lama.* [online] Available at: www.dalailama.com/news/2013/a-meeting-of-faiths-and-concern-for-the-outer-and-inner-environment-in-portland-oregon/amp [Accessed 18 December 2018].

Case, C. and Dalley, T. (2006). *The Handbook of Art Therapy.* London: Routledge.

Clark, D. and Seymour, J. (1999). *Reflections on Palliative Care.* Buckingham: Open University Press.

Connell, C. (1998). 'The search for a model which opens', in Pratt, M. and Wood, M. (eds.) *Art Therapy in Palliative Care.* London: Routledge, pp. 75–87.

Evans, K. (2005). 'On death and dying', in Waller, D. and Sibbett, C. (eds.) *Art Therapy and Cancer Care.* Maidenhead: Open University Press, pp. 1–11.

Jung, C. (1967). *The Collected Works of C.G. Jung.* London: Routledge & K. Paul.

Kearney, M. (1992). Palliative medicine—Just another specialty? *Palliative Medicine,* 6, pp. 39–46.

Kellehear, A. (2013). Compassionate communities: End-of-life care as everyone's responsibility. *Q J Medicine,* pp. 1–5.

Morgan, L.M. (2001). Community participation in health: Perpetual allure, persistent challenge. *Health Policy and Planning,* 16, pp. 221–230.

Paul, S. and Sallnow, L. (2013). Public health approaches to end of life care in the UK: An online survey of palliative care services. *British Medical Journal: Supportive and Palliative Care,* 3, pp. 196–199.

Sallnow, L. and Paul, S. (2014). Understanding community engagement in end-of-life care: Developing conceptual clarity. *Critical Public Health,* 25(2), pp. 231–238.

Saunders, C. (1990). *Hospice and Palliative Care: An Interdisciplinary Approach.* Sevenoaks, Kent: Edward Arnold.

Sibbett, C. (2005). ' "Betwixt and between": Crossing thresholds', in Waller, D. and Sibbett, C. (eds.) *Art Therapy and Cancer Care.* Maidenhead: Open University Press, pp. 12–37.

Sims, A., Radford, J., Doran, K. and Page, H. (1997). Social class variation in place of cancer death. *Palliative Medicine,* 11, pp. 369–373.

Yalom, I.D. (1998). *The Yalom Reader: Selections from the Work of a Master Therapist and Storyteller.* New York: Basic Books.

# 15 A Chorus of Angels, The Ripple of Water, and The Weight of Stone

## Art Therapy and Artwork Which Cradle Both Family Carers and Their Relative With Dementia

*Ofira Honig, Aya Feldman, Shlomit Rinat, and Shahar Gindi*

## Introduction

In his book, *The Pure Elements of Time*, Be'er wrote,

> After all the merciful Madonnas carrying an adorable baby on their lap, Madonnas that have populated Christian art for twenty generations, here is a reverse Pieta: an adult with the plump and impassive face of a baby carrying in its arms a diapered baby with the face of a grownup woman. He means me, I am the one cared for by a sick old mother. The stinking fruit of modern medicine which extends a person's life but can't grant him a minimal quality of life and which throws into the arms of the sons sick and stumbling parents who need somebody to help them on their shoulders.
>
> (Be'er, 2003, p. 278)

The extension of life expectancy in the 21st century and the resulting increase in the size of the elderly population as a whole and of elderly persons with dementia in particular, requires us to prepare to provide more assistance in both institutional and domestic contexts, and to remember that the primary caregivers will continue to be family members.

The importance of training these family members, which the research reported here proposes, received timely validation on September 21, 2016, when the Alzheimer's Association (comprising 73 non-profit organizations worldwide) published its annual report on the state of the disease and its forecasted trends. The key new findings were the disease's projected costs and the general unpreparedness around the world to contend with increasing numbers of patients with dementia. In other words, the brunt of care will still fall on the families, who will perforce provide the 'primary carers'. And the reality of family carers is harsh: they feel removed from their own lives.

In light of this we propose an intervention and support model comprising two major components:

(a) **Training the primary family carer** (individually or in a group), to introduce tools and materials of artistic expression into the time they spend with the family member with dementia. This will help build a bridge to the relative who is being robbed of their faculties. The artwork constitutes a third object which widens the space of the encounter to a three-dimensional container of new memories, for both carer and cared for, just as occurs in art psychotherapy.

(b) **Supervision sessions with an art psychotherapist** are proposed as a place both where the carers can express their own selves creatively and where they can draw mental, practical, and emotional support for the journey with their loved ones to the loved one's oblivion and death. The role of the art psychotherapist/supervisor in these sessions will be to contain and cradle the exhaustion and helplessness which the carers will inevitably feel. This cradling will help the family carer in his/her turn use the power of art to cradle their relative with dementia.

The central emphasis of the intervention proposed here is the coming and being together of carer and elderly relative (without the presence of a therapist or supervisor). In this our proposal crucially differs both from art therapy provided by a professional art therapist to an elderly person with dementia (Abraham, 2005, see Figure 15.3) or to an elderly person's relative (Dasa, 2016, see Figure 15.2), as well as from occupational therapy's use of artwork to occupy and/or maintain the remaining skills of an elderly dementia sufferer. Essential to our model's design is that it takes into account that many of the carers who will seek its help will be seriously depressed and feel their creative energies to have been battered into muteness. Our intervention is designed to re-open and redevelop a carer's capacity for containment and empathy. The supervision sessions provided to carers within this project (see Figure 15.6) provide a very necessary cradling environment for the by no means easy intervention envisaged.

The three demonstrated outcomes of the proposed model are that (a) carers spend more time with their relative with dementia, even when the relative has descended into a severely 'emptied' state, (b) that the time spent with their relative causes the carers less stress and guilt than before they entered the project, and (c) that in many instances they renew their sense of involvement and connection with their relative. As an unlooked-for bonus, the project unplugged an outflow of creativity, the fruits of which include a book of poems by Rama, (all participant names are invented) who read them to her father; Ariel resuming writing her doctorate; and Noa, who began taking art lessons at a recognized school of art.

Jung (1983) declared that his aim in therapy was that the therapeutic process emerge from the personality of the patient/client, so that its effect might be all the deeper and more long-lasting. Our project took a similar approach. In training carers to use artwork to revive their connection to a relative with dementia, we invited the carers to use their knowledge of their relative and of their own tastes to select the type of art they felt would best suit the both of them. And most of the participants indeed found ways to steer their relative into working with art materials suited to their physical and mental state. The professional supervisors (all with Israel Art therapy Association certification), carefully keeping in mind the carer's limitations, remind them to be attentive to their own feelings as well as to their relative's, as a way of helping them sense and identify moments of communication and alertness when the relative with dementia is trying to cooperate.

Currently the psychotherapeutic approaches deployed in Israel with dementia patients comprise:

(a) Emotional Therapy for One or More Family Members (Figure 15.1):

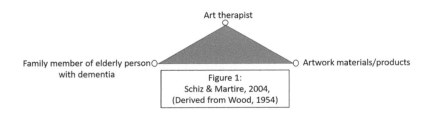

Art therapist

Family member of elderly person
with dementia

Artwork materials/products

Figure 1:
Schiz & Martire, 2004,
(Derived from Wood, 1954)

(b) A Support Team Works With the Person With Dementia via Artwork (Figure 15.2):

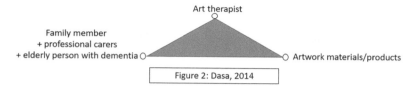

Figure 2: Dasa, 2014

and (c) Art Therapy for the Person With Dementia (Figure 15.3):

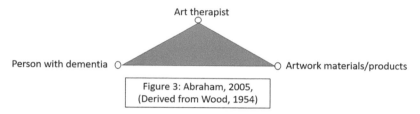

Figure 3: Abraham, 2005,
(Derived from Wood, 1954)

The four authors of this chapter are all senior staff in the art therapy department of the Faculty of Arts at Beit Berl Academic College. Dr. Honig is director of the department and the head of the M.A. programme in art therapy. She, Ms. Feldman and Ms. Rinat, all art psychotherapists and senior art therapy supervisors, are experts in a "transformative dynamic experiential artwork-based teaching mode" (Honig, 2014) developed for student art therapists and are senior lecturers on the Beit Berl programme. Dr. Gindi is a clinical psychologist and senior supervisor whose specialism is work with children and adults on the autism spectrum. In 2015 discussions with colleagues on certain dilemmas in field practice led Dr. Honig to set up a research team at Beit Berl Academic institute with the aim of examining whether artistic expression (Robbins, 1987, 2000)—of whatever kind—could make it easier for family members to take care of a relative with dementia, could relieve their stress and guilt feelings, could—and this would be the ideal—help create a shared and enabling space for both carer and cared for.

The motivation for the research reported here emerged gradually from a number of sources—from our own art therapy work with clients coping with caring for a parent with dementia (especially second-generation Holocaust survivors), from our supervision of art therapists working with patients descending into dementia, and even from the personal experience of some of us whose own parents had set foot on the same slow descent. We had discovered that our own professional training and work as therapists had not prepared us for coping with the situation. Shlomit Rinat and Aya Feldman, two of the present authors, and several of our supervisees all told us that the first great coping challenge presented to them by a family member with dementia was the steady succession of large and small losses and the sense that they were losing their loved one piece by piece. At the same time, they felt themselves losing elements of their own capacity for creativity and the joy of life.

Consultation within the research team convinced us to explore the ideas, approaches, and techniques we had each come up with to cope with this challenge. We had all also noted that over recent years public awareness of dementia and Alzheimer's and the hardships it brought had grown significantly and that family carers were more willing to seek mental/emotional assistance and support, and both acknowledge their hardships and ask for help (Regev & Bar-Tur, 2015), tools and advice in the face of their growing unwillingness to maintain the caring relationship they had been thrown into.

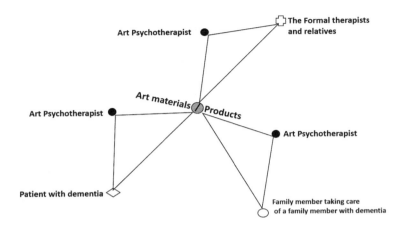

*Figure 15.4* A Co-Presentation of the Three Approaches

*Stage One* of our research work was a programme of joint study, theoretical reading and interpretation. As soon as we had constructed Figure 15.4—as a co-presentation of the three established therapeutic approaches deployed in Israel with dementia patients—we realised that all these approaches centred on the art materials and that this positioning had to be re-examined: at the centre instead had to be the patient.

Underlying our thinking were the following five premises:

1.  **The need to identify avoidances** (the defence mechanisms family members resort to avoid seeing the reality of their situation): Family carers of a relative with dementia who seek therapy are often looking to extract themselves from their significant bond with that relative in order to avoid seeing the disease and the 'absence' it is making in their relative.
2.  **Artwork can bond**: The authors of this paper believe profoundly in the power of artwork to create a sense of togetherness, uniting carers in shared meaningful being and doing.
3.  **This very painful family situation presents an opportunity**. We also have great faith in Kubler-Ross's concept that contending with cases of extreme illness offers the family the rare gift of closeness and openness (Kubler-Ross, 1973). This is why we pursued the added value and secondary gain which come from family members sharing artwork with the relative with dementia.
4.  **Expanding the 'potential space'**: An art therapist must look for ways to expand and enrich the 'potential space' (Winnicott, 1982) between the main family carer and their relative with dementia, in this case space for (a) greater emotional closeness and (b) for enquiry.
5.  A person deteriorating into dementia experiences a series of **losses which need to be confronted** (Amichai, 2004), but at the same time family members are experiencing a comparable sequence of losses. As the person with dementia suffers loss of memory, of orientation, of identity and the ability to recognize the unique presence of close relatives, the family members around them have to contend with their own emotional response to this progressive loss and departure.

*Stage Two* was to assemble a supervision group of eight art therapist colleagues from across the country who either worked with clients who were caring for a parent with dementia or were themselves in the situation of caring for a mother or father with dementia. Two of these recruits were former students of the present authors who were working in old age homes. The four researchers and our eight art therapist colleagues held long discussions on the design of an intervention model that, founded in our five premises, could achieve our therapeutic aims. The decision we came up with was to borrow the combined supervision and emotional support model that the Beit Berl art therapy programme applied to its first-year students. Under this model, the students were required to maintain a supportive relationship, mediated through plastic or other artwork, with two clients and which featured no interpretation but was designed to develop the students' capacity for containment—of both the clients and themself. Weekly supervision sessions helped the students work through the experiences of these encounters with clients and expand their capacity for containment and empathy.

*Stage Three* was to test our model in the field, that is to examine in practical terms whether training main family carers in the approach and techniques of art therapy could render the carers significant help and support in caring for their relative with dementia over the long term. This stage lasted twelve months.

Our twelve study participants were all women aged 55–65 from a variety of religio-ethnic populations, all of them the main carer for an elderly first-degree relative with dementia. All were born in Israel and some are second-generation Holocaust survivors. All share feelings of great loss, both personal and other loss (Goldstein, 2012). Socioeconomically they are middle-class. Some live in the same town as their relative with dementia, some in a neighbouring town. They are unanimous in wanting to take responsibility for the care of their elderly relative, seeing this as an unshirkable duty. This duty comprises supervising the professional carers, paying the bills, driving, maintenance work, shopping, and providing their relative companionship, occupation, and entertainment—activities which constitute for them little less than 'a second career' (Even-Zohar, 2015, p. 113) They belong to the 'sandwiched' generation (Hantman & Berenstein, 2000). They have children, a professional and social life, hobbies, and the full range of regular family commitments. Some are grandmothers and caught in an intra-family struggle between the demands of their younger generation for help with their own children and jobs and their own commitment to their elderly mother or father.

Each project participant was appointed an art therapist-supervisor from the supervisor group to provide them (a) the same supervision and close emotional support as student art therapists received and (b) guidance in the art therapy techniques which they might deploy in their meetings with their relative. Carer and supervisor met once a week. The eight members of our supervisor group played a multiple role within the research project—they helped design it, they recruited family carers (often from among their own former clients) as project participants, they trained these participants in the project's techniques, and some of them were, as noted, themselves main carers of a parent with dementia. These supervisors attended regular individual and group support sessions with the research project's four leaders and senior investigators.

*Stage Four* of our project was to conduct a formal evaluation of the care model we had field-tested. Both the eight supervisors and the twelve main carers were interviewed twice, at the start and end of the project. The supervisors were interviewed by the four project leaders and each carer by their supervisor. Both interviews measured the carers' 'wellbeing' (Diener et al, 1999) when they were in the company of their relative with dementia. The second interview was based on the in-depth and wide-ranging first interview. It both revisited the open-ended questions posed in the first interview and also invited the family carer to describe how they had experienced their participation in the project.

## A Review of the Situation in Israel, 2016

In Israel there are currently over 117,000 patients diagnosed with Alzheimer's, the most prevalent form of dementia (Alzheimer's Association, 2012). A 2010 survey conducted for International Alzheimer's Day showed that one in every five Israeli senior citizens was afflicted with Alzheimer's disease and also warned that by 2030 this number would climb to 120,000 (Gal, 2010).

Among all Israeli ethno-religious groupings (Jews, Moslems, Druze, and Christians) the value of the family is central and the sanctity of life is paramount. This means that almost all families will want to nurse sick parents in their old age. Since 2006, approximately one-third of the adult population (aged 20+) have been taking care of a close relative, of whom 43% have been elderly parents and/or parents with dementia (Central Bureau of Statistics, 2014). The brunt of the care burden falls on the 45–64 age group, who give an average of 12–20 hours per week of care and support and do so for an average period of four years. Around one-third do so for ten years or more, and a third of these for over fifteen years, all without any financial compensation or institutional recognition. Most of these family carers must also work for a living (Brodsky et al, 2013).

Despite this high level of need among both persons with dementia and their family carers the issue is totally absent from public discourse, reflected in the fact that neither Hebrew nor Arabic even has a word for family members who care for other family members. English calls them 'caregivers' or 'carers' but in Hebrew the most common term is '*metapel*' which is the term for a professional salaried staff person. Some have tried to introduce the term '*metapel karov*' (a carer-relative) but at the 2016 Bar Ilan conference No'a Vilchanski proposed—with bitter irony—that this be replaced by '*karov makriv*' = "a self-sacrificing relative" (Reisfeld, 2016).

According to Bowlby's attachment theory (1969) there is a strong correlation between the type of parenting a child receives and the care the child returns his/her parents in their old age. This is vividly illustrated by participants in our study:

*BINA:* "My mother was the only one of her family to survive the Second World War and made me a gift-surrogate for her mother and sisters killed in the Holocaust. I imbibed this message with my mother's milk—that I was in some way her mother and sister. She would say that my smell and touch brought her mother back. She was a good mother to me and at the end of her life I tried to be a good mother to her".

*YAFIT:* "Throughout my childhood my mother used to call me 'the snake' and I still see myself as a 'bad girl'. I could have visited her more, even if only for 10 seconds. I seemed to see in her eyes, when I did come, that she knew it was me. But I was always 'too busy'. It's quite obvious to me that I avoided making that window of time for her. And now I try not to think about it because when I do I feel bad".

## Let this Nightmare Be Over: The Study Participants' Mental-Emotional Predicament

*ARIEL:* "That's all I can do for her. I don't have the time or the emotional availability. I'm mother to two young daughters who need me. This caring for her takes time I don't have. I visit her once a week and phone her every day for a few minutes".

Many of our participants, like Ariel, report guilt feelings, some so painful as to drive them to extreme responses, such as wishing their demented father or mother dead.

Rama has been taking care of her father for 10 years: "I find myself holding my father. He is no longer strong, can no longer take me in his arms. I hold his hands so that he won't break anything in a fit of anger. My father—that gentle, polite, explainer, listener, interested person—who would look deep into my eyes, as if studying my soul beyond the stories I was telling—is not there in this confused, angry and fragile person I now hold".

As the dementia worsens the family carers pass through different stages: At first, the personality changes taking place in the relative as part of the dementia process are bewildering, leaving their family dumbfounded in face of the no-longer-familiar. This is a difficult stage where it is not yet always obvious that it is the disease that has brought about the change and family members are filled with mixed feelings of sadness, confusion, and rejection (Schulz & Martire, 2004). One of our study participants told us in her interview how, having recognized her father's condition, her mother announced that she was leaving home and wanted a divorce because "this was not the man she knew".

Later comes a sense of alienation in the carers, anger at the helpless relative and at the need to provide support without the reciprocity of being recognized by the relative. In their frustration they say that their "relative is no longer his or herself" (Rubinstein, 2012, p. 45). Edna, who has been taking care of her mother for five years, described her feelings before participating in the study: "It is no longer my mother, my mother left the house and her body long ago . . . now it is someone else who I am getting used to, and pain is sharp and continuous".

A third stage arrives when the situation deteriorates into having to move the relative to an assisted-living institution, or bring in a live-in carer. At this stage, our study participants reported, the family carer tends to shorten the time spent with the relative with dementia, to visit rarely, or even avoid visiting altogether. This adds to their guilt feelings the sense that the professional carers are viewing them with critical eyes and that any potential for a dyadic relationship with their relative has been further impaired.

No'a, who has been taking care of her mother for two years: "I find it very difficult to talk to my mother when the nurse is around. I feel as if she is listening and judging me on the sparseness of the conversation".

Rubinstein (2012) reports that carers' attitudes change when they become aware that it is the dementia speaking out of, and motivating, the patient. They come to see the patient not as an individual but as 'someone else' (Rubinstein, 2012, p. 32).

Amnon Shamosh, interviewed in 2015 about his book, *Good Morning Alz Heimer*, explained that he made a separation between his wife Hannah, whom he loved, and the dementia, he called "the bastard that has come between us". This is to be interpreted as Shamosh allowing himself to feel anger and vent his frustrations: "Fuck you! You will not get me into an asylum!" . . . "I tell myself, it's him, it's Alz. Rage and swear at him in every language you know".

Breaking up the disease's name Alzheimer into two short words: 'Alz' and 'Heimer', not only breaks it up, it also belittles the gravity of its ramifications. This is using humour creatively to form a direct relationship with the disease. In this way Shamosh makes the separation between his beloved wife Hannah, with whom he has a shared past and who is now sick, and, over against her, the disease. The separation helps Shamosh be angry at elements of Hannah and not at all of what she represents. Like him, both Rama and Noa, participants in our study, drew a distinction between their parent living in his/her familiar body and another 'unfamiliar' being also now sharing it with them.

These examples illustrate that there can simultaneously co-exist a beloved memory, anger at the current situation, a sense of guilt at experiencing that anger, and the encoded wish lurking behind it for "this nightmare to be over" as phrases it Dr. Meitar in the Epilogue of Kubler-Ross's book (Meitar, 2000, p. 181).

Like Gila, who has been taking care of her mother for five years:

"I feel terrible with myself when I understand that I would prefer for this situation to end".

## The Barriers to Carer Creativity

Our survey of the dementia literature shows that in family carers of Alzheimer patients the care commitment creates a heavier burden than in other groups of informal carers for other diseases, and that the carers' degree of physical and mental vulnerability is also significantly higher. Caring for an Alzheimer's patient is a prolonged process and as the disease progresses communication problems worsen because of the increasing failure of language and memory. Behavioural problems, such as aggression and severe restlessness, may add to the burden. As the memory of the person with dementia is wiped away so a sense of helplessness and of 'deletion' takes over the space between the primary carer and their family 'patient', and also between the carer and themself. Eisen and Werner (2015) report that main carers get more and more depressed and at the same time come to feel that any creativity they had has been killed off. Even the desire for creativity withers. "Removing the barriers to creativity and treating the damage caused by these barriers can be the key to change . . . particularly among primary Alzheimer carers" (p. 93). As Ruth Abraham (2005) puts it in *When Words Have Lost Their Meaning* (Abraham, 2005), togetherness during a visit becomes oppressive and an effort, time stands still and the void is omnipresent. The elderly relative loses the connection between verbalising and reality and ceases to speak. In response the carer loses patience and starts trying to help the old person find a word, complete a sentence. The carer tries to fill the void which has opened up between them and her effort lasts until she too 'contracts the disease' of silence.

Among the participants in our study, those who had ever had any involvement in artwork told us how they used to be creative, could think flexibly, but that the stress of caring for their relative had stifled all that. This is an important point for the therapy model we propose here. Over the course of our field project we noticed that family carers, who had observed the first steps in our art therapy work with their relative with dementia as a mechanical care element or as a mere exercise, then began to take a student's interest in it. The artwork gradually became a fixed ritual and, as such, a phenomenon we felt merited investigation. As a result, our sessions with main carers moved into a dynamic supervision mode (Naumburg, 1987), the outcomes of which we examined by observing the artwork created and its effect (as reported by the carer) on their dyad with their relative with dementia.

Storr (1991, p. 7) defines creativity as the desire to create and as the creation of something new, even if it was there before unknown to the creator. Published studies have shown that art therapy usually has the power to revive a withered creative instinct (Rubin, 2011; Malchiodi, 1998; Dalley et al, 1987; Gonen et al, 1992) and the present authors deem this power to be a key resource for the carers of patients with dementia. Eisen and Werner's recent study (2015) emphasizes this by showing how contact with these patients withers the carer's spirit and depresses any creative instinct.

Understanding from our review of current approaches to work with dementia patients in Israel (see Figures 15.1–15.3) that art therapy both with dementia carers (Dasa, 2016) and with dementia sufferers (Abraham, 2005) can bring them moments of creative experience on the very brink of the chasm of loss, we designed our project to (a) offer primary carers an intimate creative space with their relative with dementia and (b) give their power of creativity a chance to re-emerge.

Carers who have been through our project and drawn strength from it reported that even being able to fashion their relative's fragmented words into a complete sentence has been like building a bridge over all the impossibilities of communication, and inspired them to feel they could create again. As for the artwork generated, this had the capacity to provide a space in which they and their relative could come closer and hold together. It revived their will to create—to be, not to give up being.

Before finding this creative space family carers felt spending time with the relative with dementia to be totally draining. After artwork was introduced into the space between patient and carer our participants reported experiencing moments of cradling which gave comfort to both carer and cared for. Rama reported that when visiting her father there were no words said, so depleted were his mental powers, but that words emerged which she dared to read aloud into the silence:

*Exchanges*

A poem by Rama
As you are steadily robbed of your powers
So I contemplate accretions,
fortify my body with gratifying toys and graceful ornaments
So that the two of us in a shared rhythm
bring two voids into balance—
as you lose so I accrue

Nira attested to a similar experience: "I needed someone to tell me to pick up a soft paintbrush so that I could at least make a spot". Even a soft spot on a sheet of paper constituted a cradle and anchor for void states.

## The Model

Our intervention model (Figure 15.5) is an expansion of the conventional triangular (Wood, 1990; Case & Dalley, 1992; Schaverien, 2000) models (see Figures 15.1–15.3) into a pyramidal intervention model whose four vertices are:

- The primary family carer
- The relative with dementia
- Artwork materials and the creative process
- The art psychotherapist/supervisor who serves as guide and companion, cradling the interaction from outside it.

The pyramidal support and intervention model is designed, as stated earlier, to revive and reinforce the primary family carer's creative caring powers and rebuild their capacity for containment and empathy. The art therapist as supervisor takes on the role of 'environmental mother' (Winnicott, 1992). She/he teaches the carer some of the techniques and 'trade secrets' of art therapy and provides dynamic supervision, both as an alternative to the lost means of communication, and as an act of support and empowerment to the carer.

In this three-dimensional space, the family carer is both therapy client and apprentice therapist, learning how to be and behave with an elderly family member with dementia. The pyramid shape is formed by adding a fourth vertex (Honig, 2014) to the former triangular space composed of main family carer, relative with dementia and artwork materials/product. The art therapist uses dynamic[1]—supervision to advise, instruct, hold, and support the carer (Bar-Tur 2010). And the group supervision sessions enable the art therapist to 'hold' the triangle of family carer, relative with dementia and artwork. This holding, the present authors believe, is analogous to the father holding the unit of 'mother-infant' (Winnicott, 1992), where the relative with dementia is the 'infant' the carer is the 'parent/therapist', and the art therapist/supervisor is the parent/father holding the dyad.

Underlying this model is the understanding that the family carer is in a constant state of alienation in a world that is losing its logic. The model takes into consideration the panic and loneliness such a situation can evoke.

The pyramidal model (Figure 15.6) represents the experience of being with an elderly relative with dementia and illustrates that the potential space formed between the four vertices is a 'holding environment' or, in Winnicottian terms, a 'holding circle' (Winnicott, 2011).

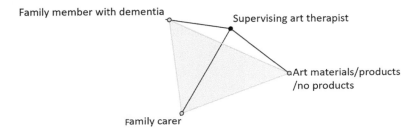

*Figure 15.5* The Pyramidal Schema of the Expanded Intervention Space

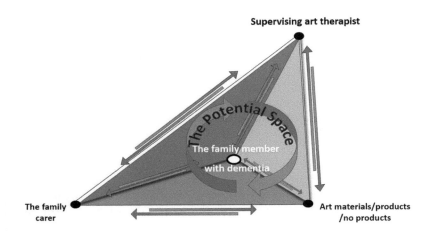

*Figure 15.6* A Pyramidal Model of Holding

## Implementing the Pyramidal Model

Edna told her supervisor that visiting hours with her mother were long, filled with despair and empty of any content: "My mother has nothingness and even the nothingness is gone". The therapist suggested Edna buy some water-colours "with the understanding of the cradling powers these materials have" and showed her how to offer the paints to her mother. Edna returned and recounted with excitement how she had felt an intimate closeness with her mother as she tried to introduce her to water-colour painting, together with a deeper understanding of her mother's awesomely demented state:

> My mother could not even remember the colours' names. . . . There was an incomprehensible rift between the title or name of the painting and what mother painted." 'Look', said Edna, taking out her mother's artwork, "my mother called this painting [no. 2, in Figure 15.9] '*Time Worn Out*', which is a high-level title compared to her usual communicative ability.

Another participant reported the effect the art therapy intervention had on her own capacity to spend time with her mother, turning it into a meaningful experience for her (Figure 15.7). She said that when the entire family got together she brought along the paints, and while everyone else sat around chatting, she sat on the porch with her mother, painting.

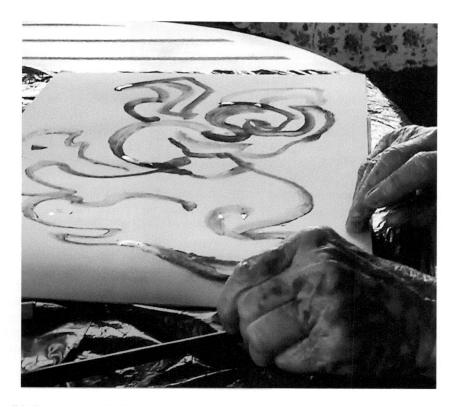

*Figure 15.7* Grandma Bracha Painting

"I started by putting before her three little pots of paint and with considerable effort got her to choose one. She pointed to the pot of purple. I took a brush and drew a semi-circle in the middle of the sheet of paper and then put the brush in her hand. I helped her curl her stiff fingers around the brush and she gripped it and began painting". (Image 1) ". . . She was so proud of herself, like a child succeeding with a first painting. Her face shone from all the attention around her and she laughed. . . . It had been such a long time since I had seen such pure pleasure on her face . . ."

When the young members of the family saw the connection that had been made, they all asked to 'paint with grandma' and there was great joy, unlike on previous visits. The grandchildren photographed their grandmother painting and everyone had a sense of happiness. Grandma seemed particularly proud of herself.

## Artwork Generates Movement

Both the family member with dementia and the carer move between representations of death and life. Artwork materials—such as watercolours and a paintbrush moving across paper, music, and movement in space—serve as alternative representations of life. Stranded before a language void, barriers to creativity, and depression, under the guidance of the supervisor the family carer summons his/her life force to enlist artistic tools as a means to enable them to not only survive their close relative's dementia but even make their last moments together meaningful.

Painting, music, and dance serve as means of communication, a small window of connection and mutual satisfaction moments before the blanket of forgetfulness and neurological damage make bodily movement impossible. The dementia sufferer will often respond to the effort at shared activity (Arieli-Kelm, 2016). The artistic tools of music, painting, and dance become mediators in a twilight zone before the 'curtain falls'. One main carer said of her experience with her mother:

*RINA:* "I wanted to speak to her, do something with her, to feel that I was holding on to the last drop, that I was not letting go—but I had no strength. I felt drained, like a dry shell empty of life juices. And then, hesitantly, I tried to introduce artwork and the experience filled me with affection for her. Teary-eyed, I felt as if I were showing her how not to sink, that I was succeeding in communicating with her. . . "

In their supervision sessions project participants (main carers) were invited to recount their current experiences in caring for their parent, how they coped with the disease process and their parent's changing state, their reactions to being with their parent. Then the supervisor would suggest how they might introduce artwork into these caring sessions. In the following example we see how one participant experienced this (from the interview with the supervisor):

Ariel, (reports her supervisor), was a client of mine who had sought therapy because the deterioration of her mother's dementia had overwhelmed her with painful guilt feelings, deriving from the multiple burden of contending with wordless sessions with her mother and at the same time with the demands of her own children. In one of her therapy sessions with me before she joined the project, Ariel asked for water colours, and painted the picture on the left of Figure 15.8. This is what she then said about it:

*ARIEL:* "The horizontal lines—very faint, almost invisible black lines underneath the white remind me of the lines on an old-style thermometer, not a digital one: perhaps they are signs of life or perhaps lines of routine duties, of the 'have to', 'do it', 'get there' kind".

Ariel had left three-quarters of the page empty. A year later, after I had got her agreement to enrol in the project, I suggested that she work with her mother in water colours as I remembered her love and pleasure in working with this medium and also remembered the painting she had made the year before. In few months, over the course of the new intervention, Ariel reported a significant change in her ability to spend time with her mother.

I could sense the empathy and warmth emanating from the stories she told of the sessions with her mother, feelings that had not been present a year earlier and I asked her if she wanted to paint these new feelings. She asked me if I still had the painting she had done the year before. I fetched it and put it on the table and she began working (right-hand image in Figure 15.8). When she was done Ariel said:

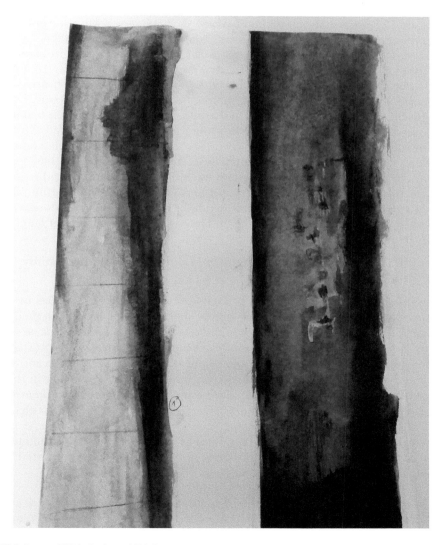

*Figure 15.8* Image With Left and Right

It's only now that I can see that the previous image I made was the shadow of me, her and the disease. Today I can see that I have given the shadow a new place, I have let the void of disability become something else, exist between us here on the page without me panicking. I can see that I have allowed some colours to show through, I have let in droplets of light. I can feel it in the moments that we spend painting together.

As she painted in front of me, for me . . . I feel moved by it even now when I see that feeling appear here as well.

Ariel looks at the space between the two pictures and says of it: "And here, the space between me and her raises the question of the meaning of my life in this space". Ariel was actually asking herself who she was in this space facing her mother, and our conversation developed into her asking if there is life outside the disease, or in her own words: "outside the shadow of my mother and her disease. . . . Will I be able to leave the shadow and get to a place where the disease, the void and the burden that goes with it have no effect?"

The story told by Ariel and her supervisor, in the example above, shows that the initial image (Figure 15.8, Left) refers to doing (*'have to'*, *'do it'*, *'get there'*), while the graphic depiction of the disease (*'the black blot'* in her words) is narrow. The second image, on the other hand, (Figure 15.8, Right) depicts the disease as a larger and more powerful blot, while at the same time *"glimmers of colour are allowed to shine through"*. We see and hear from the therapist/supervisor that the family carer working with her mother through artwork connected both to herself, to the materials, and to the moment with her mother and even allowed herself to enjoy the sessions with her mother. In therapeutic terms, we would say that the therapeutic process had made room for observing the white space as a graphic expression of connection and separation between past and present, as well as for questions about herself. Being with an elderly person with dementia, especially a close relative, is hard emotional work and a difficult experience. "The space between us has narrowed", said Ariel, having experienced the disease's invasion of hers and her mother's lives and its infiltration into her mother's and her own mind. The introduction of shared artwork had done want it was intended to—expand the space between the relative with dementia and her family carer.

### The Artwork That Allows a Family Carer to Make Contact With a Family Member with Dementia

The intervention model seemed to bring notable reinforcement to families in enabling them to cope with a relative's degenerative illness, spend longer periods with their relative, and even provide meaningful experiences to the relative. *Most important of all, we felt that the family carers' depression lightened, which in turn allowed them to reach acceptance of what they were losing.* The intervention model encourages and enables family carers to enliven and stimulate a space of torpor and degeneration. Project data reveal significant changes in the carer's experience of and with the family member after artwork is introduced into their meetings. This is how she described the state of affairs before her participation in the project:

SARA: "Going home after visiting my mother, I would get lost on the way. I would tell myself that I had got like my mother, I too knew nothing, I too was disoriented like her. I would arrive home afraid it was contagious".

Sara's words show that the experience of spending time with an elder with dementia combines elements of identification, enmeshment, and the blurring of boundaries. The quote below, however, is typical of how project participants reported the effect of introducing various forms of artwork, how it created the possibility of being sensitively aware of a shared experience:

*SARA:* "My parents loved dancing. My mother's body responds to the music I play, her weak, measured steps allow me close physical connection with her. Arm touching arm, one movement following another, these were intimate moments that I could appreciate and they pleased us both . . . I remember the experience as one of love and continuity".

Others felt that these hours of grace (Amichai, 2004) generated a sense of togetherness and an active space for the long process of separation. They all found themselves clearly and markedly spending more time at their relative's home and the visits cost them less strain and stress. Malchiodi has said about the language of visual art: "colors, shapes, lines and images speak to us in ways which words cannot" (Malchiodi, 1998, p. XIII).

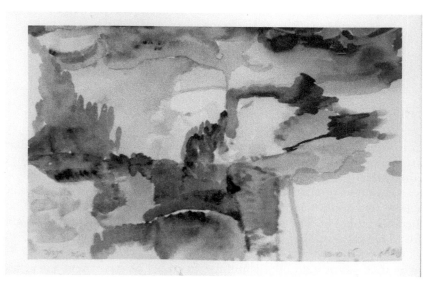

*Figure 15.9* Paintings by Edna's Mother (Image 1) (See Plate 3)

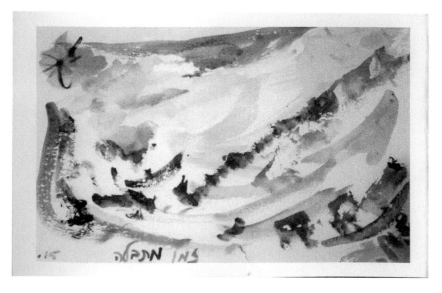

*Figure 15.10* Paintings by Edna's Mother (Image 2)

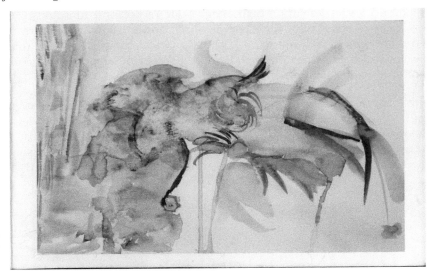

*Figure 15.11* Paintings by Edna's Mother (Image 3)

We also made a careful study of the artwork products themselves and talked to our participants about them. This analysis of the artworks demonstrated that they held importance in themselves, as reflections of the family member's achievement and victory, as testimony to moments of intimacy and coherence, and as souvenirs which would remain with the family. As Edna affirmed: "Mother finished the painting (Figure 15.9) and a process reached its fulfilment. The sheet of paper was full like a fruit basket of references to movements in hers and my life".

EDNA: "My mother was proud of the paintings we made. We gave them a central place on the entrance table (Image 3), and whenever guests came, she or the person with her would proudly show them off. It was a ready and interesting topic of conversation and a source of amazement. I tell you, those paintings really did take the place of the family photograph albums full of pictures she could no longer identify and which were therefore of no interest to her. Mother asked me to write what she said about the paintings on them 'so that you won't forget'".

In the language of art therapy to work with artwork materials is, in essence, to dip one's brush into one's soul (Honig, 2014, p. 183).

We analysed the artworks that emerged from the present project in several ways, both the works that the carers participating in our study had made themselves during sessions with their supervisors and the works they had made together with their relative with dementia. Looking at the artworks together with them, we asked them to describe their creative processes (Naumburg, 1987; Rubin, 2011; Schaverien, 2000)—how they used the materials, created their composition, the application of the paint, the role and place of the artwork in their relations with their relative and in their meetings with them. We urged them to say how they understood the artwork products, the connection between the product and its title (if it had one), how the process and its products had influenced their understanding of and relations with their relative. Listening to the tapes of the interviews, we paid close attention to how the carers interpreted the connections and disconnections between the artwork and the process of their care for their relative.

The overall approach to the analysis of these interviews between researcher and carer was the Socratic method (Kvale, 2009; Colley, 2010) "which holds that analysis is open to the insider researcher working together with his/her interviewees, provided that all are deeply versed in the theory of the field". (Honig, 2014, p. 173). This approach enabled us to see how the artwork products became transition objects between the patients' periods of lucidity and disconnection; how they gifted the patients' moments of felt connection with themself or with an intangible transient something in themselves. We watched and listened as artwork helped weave a tissue of relationship between carer and patient. We saw how the task of the art therapist was to provide the carer a tool and a means for surviving the period of their care for their relative with dementia.

There was even the bonus that the artwork product sometimes briefly reconnected the parent with dementia to their surroundings. Occasionally they could also reconnect to their family and these moments, we realised, were critical to the sense of connection between the patient and their family's desire to care for them. Recall, for example, how deeply moved Edna was by her mother entitling her multi-layered water-colour '*Time Worn Out*' (drawing no. 2 in Figure 15.9). What struck and moved her most was that "Mum was connecting both to me and to her own situation". True, to some extent this was Edna's 'interpretation' of what was happening in her mother's mind but, for all that, it was undeniable that the process and experience of joint creativity with her mother redoubled Edna's capacity to look at her mother with eyes that could still dream, to

*Table 15.1* Applying the Model

How to identify the right moment to suggest artwork to an elderly patient with dementia and how to seize such moments repeatedly. Here are key pointers:
- Have the materials to hand.
- The content of each visit will be governed by how alert the patient is and when they are capable of communication.
- The size of the paper, the type of paints and what is done with them will also take account of where the patient is—in bed, armchair, at a table, in their own space or a public space.
- The materials: can be broad felt-tip pens using a water-based ink, or finger paints, or brushes and water-colours which leave a mark even when contact with the paper is feeble.
- Weak muscle tone makes for weak contact with the paper. Paint and brush must be of a length, width, and weight so that hands and arms with weak muscle tone can feel and hold them.
- The availability of paints and paper open up new opportunities for the carer and their relative.
- For artwork activity to start the carer must say: "Here are paints and paper" and put them into the patient's hand.
- If the patient does not respond the carer can sit down next to them and begin painting, describing in words what they are doing—a low steady commentary.
- Knowing that a painting can be a container of memories of a shared past, at the same time as it brings into being a 'continuous present' or 'memories in the making', makes a painting into a 'time capsule' of a particular visit.
- If the carer feels alone in their bleakness, despondency, and despair these are the emotions which will transfer to the paper. In the words of Eckhardt Toll's *The Power of the Moment*, "He is the conductor of the moment". Painting in the present moment becomes a transitional object into the carer's next session with the supervisor which will provide him/her the strength and resilience to survive the invading and unstoppable oblivion.
- When these joint efforts result in a visible product it should be shared with the people around the patient. This filling of a shared experience with meaning and potency gives both partners a sense of fulfilment and satisfaction.
- Make a mantra of such a shared experience and achievement with the aim of creating a habit, a pattern of activity.
- Make painting/dance/music into a shared ritual repeated like a mantra. Maintaining such a ritual is like maintaining the possibility of togetherness and this closeness to another and oneself is like sharing prayer.

'understand' that her mother had opened for her perhaps a last window of connection as her life faded away.

Compare this to Edna's reaction to another artwork product of her mother's (Figure 15.9, painting no. 3) which consisted of abstract blue splotches and which her mother had entitled '*Africa*'. Her mother, said Edna, had never been to Africa and she could find no connection between the artwork and its creator. Indeed, the disconnect brought her to tears. Yet this response provided more evidence of Edna's capacity to absorb and cope with the process of her mother's fading away. A year earlier, reported her supervisor, Edna would have responded with anger and just gone home to '*sleep off her pain*'.

Indeed, this '*Africa*' serves as a vivid metaphor or representation for the strange world, the Alzheimer land, inhabited by people like Edna's mother. Winnicott's concept of a 'transition object' is very apt here to characterize the role played by the artwork products which emerge from this land: they serve as transition objects between periods of disconnect and moments of lucidity. They also help the carer get through the successive stages of slow separation and loss. The artwork products are also both reminders and objects which help the carer talk through their feelings with the therapist. As both transition object and reminder of what once was, they provide some comfort and help carers through moments of loss of control.

## Afterword

After what we have evaluated as the project's successful conclusion, the authors are now expanding their repertoire of interventions. Together with our advanced students we are supervising groups of main carers in order to pass on to them the techniques and approach applied by this research and intervention project. Our supervision combines elements of dynamic containment (Naumburg, 1987) and personal instruction/guidance, with the intention of creating for the carers a space in which they can look at and into themselves and from there find the empathy and compassion (Brill & Nahmani, 2014) that will enable them to pass more time with their relative. The instruction given them in the use of artwork materials helps them 'contain' both their relative with dementia and themselves.

## Note

1  In individual psychotherapy, by the patient's (client's) psychodynamics we mean the conflict between their inner forces which gives rise to certain patterns of feeling and behaviour. Since Freud the premise is that these forces clash at different levels of awareness, some operating entirely within a dynamic unconscious.

## References

Abraham, R., (2005), *When words have lost their meaning: Alzheimer's patients communicate through art*, Praeger, Westport, CT.

Alzheimer's Association, (2012), 'Alzheimer's disease facts and figures: Alzheimer's & dementia', *Journal of the Alzheimer's Association*, vol. 8, no. 2.

Amichai, Y., (2004), *A touch of grace*, Shocken, Jerusalem. [In Hebrew].

Arieli-Kelm, D., (2016), 'Talking to dementia: Characteristics and patterns of a unique form of communication', *Gerontology and Geriatrics*, vol. 43, no. 1, pp. 29–47. [In Hebrew].

Bar-Tur, L., (2010), 'Who cares for the carers? Professionalism and emotionality among carers for the elderly', *Practical Gerontology*, vol. 37, nos. 2–3, pp. 69–85. [In Hebrew].

Be'er, H., (2003), *The pure elements of time*. Translated from the Hebrew by Barbara Harshav, Brandeis University Press, p. 279.

Bowlby, J., (1969), *Attachment and loss* (vol. 1), Basic Books, New York, NY.

Brill, M., & Nahmani, N., (2014), 'The role of compassion in care', *Gerontology and Geriatrics*, vol. 41, no. 1, pp. 51–64. [In Hebrew]. UPNE.

Brodsky, G., Bentor, N., Laron, M., & Shuni-ben-Yisrael, S., (2013), 'Nationwide plan for coping with Alzheimer's and other dementias: Multi-organizational and multi-professional expert group', *Summary Statement*, Myers-Joint-Brookdale Institute, Jerusalem. [In Hebrew].

Case, C., & Dalley, T., (1992), *The handbook of art therapy*, Routledge, London.

Central Bureau of Statistics, (2014), *Statistical abstract of Israel*, available at www.cbs.gov.il/reader/cw_usr_view_Folder?ID=141

Colley, H., (2010), 'There Is No Golden Key, Overcoming Problems with Data Analysis in Qualitative Research', in P. Thomson, and M. Walker (eds.), *The Routledge Doctoral Student's Companion: Getting to Grips with Research in Education and the Social Sciences*, Routledge, New York, N.Y. (Chapter 15, pp. 183–199).

Dalley, T., Case, C., Schaverien, J., Weir, F., Halliday, D., Hall, P.N., & Waller, D., (eds.), (1987), *Image of art therapy: New developments in theory and practice*, Routledge, London.

Dasa, A., (2016), 'Project for teaching carers and family members to use music in the daily care of dementia sufferers', *Gerontology and Geriatrics*, vol. 33, no. 1, pp. 11–28. [In Hebrew].

Diener, E., Suh, E.M., Lucas, R.E., & Smith, H.E., (1999), 'Subjective well-being: Three decades of progress', *Psychological Bulletin*, vol. 125, pp. 276–302.

Eisen, G., & Werner, P., (2015), 'Imagination and artistic creativity as a care-stress coping strategy for main carers of Alzheimer's sufferers', *Gerontology and Geriatrics*, vol. 42, nos. 3–4, pp. 75–101. [In Hebrew].

Even-Zohar, A. (2015), 'The connection between the sense of caretaking pressure and the quality of life of offspring caring for their parents and the parents membership in a "supportive community"', *Gerontology*, vol. 42, no. 2, pp. 109–140. [In Hebrew].

Gal, I., (21 October 2010), 'The forecast for the state of Alzheimer over the coming 20 years in Israel', Report in honor of the International Alzheimer Day —*On-line Health Report*, [In Hebrew], available at www.ynet.co.il/articles/0,7340,L-3958113,00.html

Goldstein, D., (2012), 'The meaning of caring for Alzheimer's sufferers: The perceptions of adult children caring for their parents and the association between the meaning of their care and the depth of their depression', *Gerontology and Geriatrics*, vol. 39, nos. 1–2, pp. 15–36. [In Hebrew].

Gonen, J., Ring, H., Stern, M., & Soroker, N., (1992), 'Art therapy with stroke patients', *NeuroRehabilitation*, vol. 2, pp. 36–44.

Hantman, S., & Berenstein, M., (2000), *The sandwiched generation: How can we learn to resign ourselves to our parents' aging and adapt to it?* Modan Publishing, Tel Aviv, Israel. [In Hebrew].

Honig, O., (2014), *Post-graduate art therapy training in Israel: Personal and professional transformation through dynamic artwork-based experiential transformative courses*. Doctoral thesis (Ph.D.), University of Sussex, Available at http://sro.sussex.ac.uk/48310/

Jung, C.G., (1983), *Jung: Selected writings*, Fontana Press, London.

Kubler-Ross, E., (1973), *On death and dying*, Tavistock, London.

Kvale, S., (2009), *Doing interviews: Epistemological issues of interviewing*, Sage Publications Inc., London.

Malchiodi, C.A., (1998), *The Art Therapy Sourcebook*, Lowell House, Illinois, Chicago.

Meitar, D., (2000), 'Thoughts on Kubler Ross's Book', in E. Kubler-ross (ed.), *In Living with Death and Dying*, p. 181 [Hebrew-language edition], Keter, Tel-Aviv.

Naumburg, M., (1987), *Dynamically oriented art therapy: Its principles and practices* (first published in 1966), Revised ed., Magnolia Street Publishers, Chicago.

Regev, O., & Bar-Tur, L., (2015), 'Professional interventions with the family carers of an elderly and sick or impaired parent or spouse', in D. Prilotsky and M. Cohen (eds.), *Practical Gerontology*, Eshel, Jerusalem (vol. 2, pp. 281–319). [In Hebrew]

Reisfeld, S., (2016), 'Who will take care of the caregivers? Most of us will have to care for an aging parent or spouse: What will that do to us?' Available at www.haaretz.co.il/magazine/.premium-1.2984342

Robbins, A. (ed.), (1987), *The artist as therapist*, Human Sciences Press, New York.

Robbins, A., (2000), *The artist as therapist*, Jessica Kingsley Publishers, London.

Rubin, J. A., (2011), *The art of art therapy: What every art therapist needs to know*, Routledge, New York, NY.

Rubinstein, D., (2012), 'Pain, suffering and the issue of transparency in hallucinating patients in the eyes of their professional carers', *Body of Knowledge*, vol. 9, pp. 30–45. [In Hebrew].

Schaverien, J., (2000), 'The Triangular Relationship and Aesthetic Countertransference in Analytical Art Psychotherapy', in A. Gilroy & G. McNeilly (eds.), *The Changing Shape of Art Therapy*, Jessica Kingsley Publishers, London. (Chapter 2, pp. 55–83).

Schulz, R., & Martire, L. M., (2004), 'Family caregiving of persons with dementia: Prevalence, health effects, and support strategies', *American Journal of Geriatric Psychiatry*, vol. 12, no. 3, pp. 240–249.

Shamosh, A., (2015), *Good morning, Alz Heimer*, Massadah, Giv'atayim, Israel. [In Hebrew].

Storr, A. (1991), *The dynamics of creation*, Sifriat Poalim, Tel Aviv. [Hebrew-language edition].

Winnicott, D. W., (1982), *Playing and reality*, Penguin, Harmondsworth, Middlesex, UK.

Winnicott, D. W., (1992), *The child, the family, and the outside world*, Da Capo Press, Cambridge, MA.

Winnicott, D. W., (2011), *Deprivation and delinquency*, Routledge, New York, NY.

Wood, C., (1990), 'The triangular relationship (1): The beginnings and endings of art therapy', *Inscape Journal of Art Therapy*, Winter, pp. 7–13.

# 16 Snapshot of Practice

## Researching the Outcomes of Art Therapy for Caregivers of Patients at End-of-Life

*Girija Kaimal*

## About Me

I am a doctoral research faculty member in the PhD program in Creative Arts Therapies department at Drexel University. I teach research courses, advise doctoral students, write grant proposals for funded research, and manage research teams on my projects. I engage in art therapy clinical practice as part of my professional work as an educator and researcher. My research lab (drexel.edu/cnhp/research/faculty/KaimalGirija/) focuses on a range of studies on health outcomes of visual self-expression. A study we recently completed examined how arts-based approaches might help with physical and psychological well-being of caregivers of patients in home hospice care (end-of-life).

## About the Context in Which I Work

A colleague reached out and asked if I would be interested in collaborating on a proposal to study arts-based approaches at end-of-life. She was a chaplain who used art prints to evoke narratives from patients in hospitals and at end-of-life. I thought about my interest and suggested that we do a combined study where she examines patient experiences and I focus on caregivers. The rationale was that patients perhaps might only be able to engage in receptive experiences (viewing and responding to art) while the caregivers would be more likely to be physically able to create art. We also thought that this would be a way to differentiate between working with an art therapist versus working with a mental health professional who uses art to engage in dialogue.

Much of my work involves mixed methods research designs and so I approached this study with the same intent. Given that we do not have many experimental studies in art therapy, we decided to develop a small pilot intervention study. The study design included two prongs: one group would receive an arts-based intervention (collage) and the other group would receive a narrative-only (interview) intervention. Each participant would meet with the researchers only one time. We had pre and post surveys to assess changes in affect, self-efficacy, spiritual well-being and stress. In addition, we also collected saliva samples to assess changes in the levels of cortisol and oxytocin.

All these elements of the study indicated that we needed funding to implement it. We identified a few potential funders who might provide resources for a pilot study. A foundation in a neighboring state, namely the Foundation for Spirituality and Medicine was identified and we submitted the application. The Foundation responded after two months and asked for a phone meeting to discuss the proposal. They asked us about the art-making conditions and were skeptical that anything would change in a single session. They also asked us why we chose the collage for the art-making session instead of mandalas, for example. We explained that the collage would allow for more self-expression than a mandala. They eventually funded us with a modest sum and we began the study.

## Case Example

Overall the study results indicated that both the narrative-only group and art-based group showed similar improvements in affect and stress. The narrative only group showed greater improvements in spiritual well-being while the art-making group demonstrated trends towards improved self-efficacy and lowered cortisol levels. We were struck by the fact that the narrative group had improved spiritual well-being. It might be that caregivers had such a need to 'talk' that the experience helped them more than art making in a single session format. Perhaps the outcomes might have been different if we had multiple sessions instead of one. The improvement in self-efficacy was only seen more in the art therapy group. This has been fairly consistent in many of our studies (Kaimal, Ray & Muniz, 2016; Kaimal & Ray, 2016; Kaimal et al, 2017). However, given the small samples size (n = 7) in each group, many of the changes seen were not statistically significant.

There were many challenges to implementing this study. Even though we had letters of commitment from three home hospice providers, it was very hard to get referrals for participants. Many social workers and nurses were optimistic about interested participants but given everyone's work schedules and caregiving responsibilities, we waited months for referrals of participants.

The study highlighted the many challenges of recruiting participants. In addition, we had said in the study proposal that we would recruit a diverse sample including from under-represented and socio-economically disadvantaged communities. That made it harder still, because participants who came from more disadvantaged socio-economic backgrounds were even less likely to respond to requests for time to participate in the research study. Even when we were able to identify potential participants for the study, they would at times not respond to phone calls and messages. Caregivers were overwhelmed and unable to spare the hour for the study and were sometimes elderly themselves and unable to complete some of the questionnaires. In addition, patients were often severely incapacitated, which further affected the availability of the caregivers. Thus, although our initial intent was to recruit patient-caregiver dyads, we decided to change that and recruit patients and caregivers independent of each other.

There were also challenges in data collection. Many of the patients were too incapacitated to fill out the pre and post surveys and most could not generate much saliva due to their medications. We also found that those in home hospice care were often extremely ill and neither communicative nor cognitively aware enough to even consent for the study. Elderly caregivers were sometimes not much more able than the patient. A few of them had a hard time reading and understanding the surveys we used in the study. A few others did not produce enough saliva and therefore the samples we collected were not adequate for analysis. One participant in particular had many opinions about the study and did not provide saliva samples or engage in art making. She preferred to talk instead and referred to art making as childish activities that she could not identify with. In the end we were able to recruit about 7 patients who were able to communicate and participate (over 25 were referred but were ineligible for participation due to their physical and mental states). We were also able to recruit 14 caregivers (about 23 were referred but only 14 were able to follow up and schedule a time for participation).

## Advantages of Art Therapy in My Context

Despite all the challenges of recruitment, meeting participants who enrolled in the study was an enriching and transformative experience. The caregivers included parents, spouses, children, and even a neighbor. Caregivers spoke about being 'called' to their roles either because they were the go-to person in the family or that they were perceived as the strongest and most responsive. Many caregivers spoke of feeling a sense of responsibility and duty and giving back to the patient, who had in their own healthy years given much to the person who was now the caregiver. Caregivers also spoke about the many dimensions of care including providing emotional support, helping the patient approach and accept death, taking care of financial or legal issues, providing physical care and company, and protecting the patient by subsuming their own interests and care. Most caregivers appreciated the time to talk about their experiences and the opportunity to create the collage.

## One Idea That Shapes My Work

As an art therapist and researcher, I felt deeply moved by my interactions. I felt honored and privileged to enter the lives of the caregivers. Many had been married for over 60 years and were caring for their spouses in their 80s and 90s. Some were parents who were caring for their children in hospice and struggling with the imminent demise of their child. To me, the time and opportunity to listen to the stories was very impactful. Often on the days when I collected data, I could do little else. I would reflect on what I had heard, make notes, make art, and try to respect and honor the stories of lives around me that I had briefly encountered. Many participants also gave me gifts, which I was ambivalent about accepting: one gave me a large box of cookies (it was the holiday season) and another gave me a book of her artwork. The generosity and kindness might have been somewhat unique to this specific population. The human connection that transcends all demographic barriers was illuminated for me through this study. To listen to each other, to hear the stories of caring and to face the inevitable future that lies ahead for us all: that was the gift I cherished from this study and broadly from all the research that I do.

At present, we are in the process of writing up the results of the study for publication. In addition, we are continuing to study the role of the arts for caregivers of patients with cancer, and continuing to build an evidence base on unique contributions of art therapy for patients and caregivers facing the chronic stressors of a major illness.

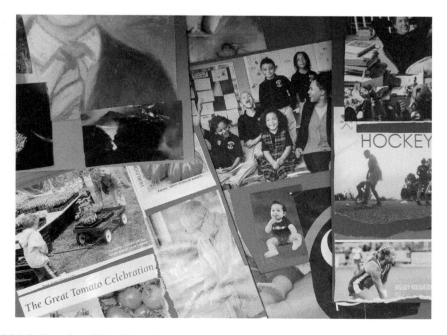

*Figure 16.1* Collage by a Male Caregiver

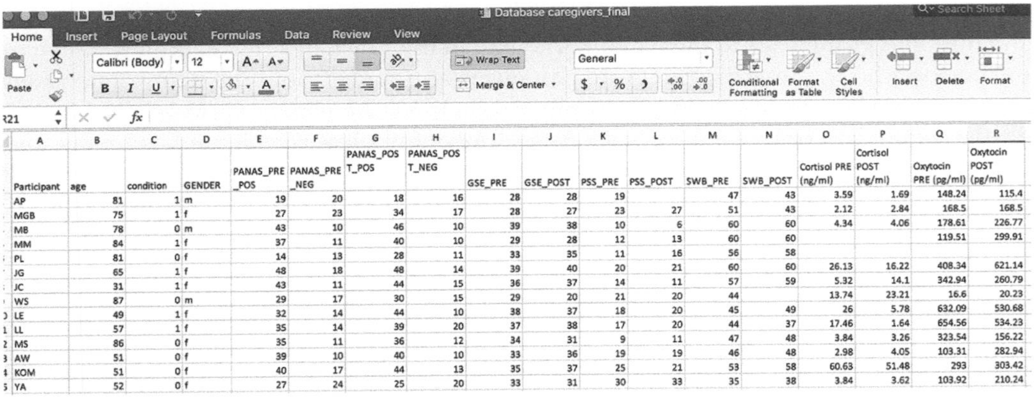

| Participant | age | condition | GENDER | PANAS_PRE_POS | PANAS_PRE_NEG | PANAS_POS T_POS | PANAS_POS T_NEG | GSE_PRE | GSE_POST | PSS_PRE | PSS_POST | SWB_PRE | SWB_POST | Cortisol PRE (ng/ml) | Cortisol POST (ng/ml) | Oxytocin PRE (pg/ml) | Oxytocin POST (pg/ml) |
|---|---|---|---|---|---|---|---|---|---|---|---|---|---|---|---|---|---|
| AP | 81 | 1 | m | 19 | 20 | 18 | 16 | 28 | 28 | 19 |  | 47 | 43 | 3.59 | 1.69 | 148.24 | 115.4 |
| MGB | 75 | 1 | f | 27 | 23 | 34 | 17 | 28 | 27 | 23 | 27 | 51 | 43 | 2.12 | 2.84 | 168.5 | 168.5 |
| MB | 78 | 0 | m | 43 | 10 | 46 | 10 | 39 | 38 | 10 | 6 | 60 | 60 | 4.34 | 4.06 | 178.61 | 226.77 |
| MM | 84 | 1 | f | 37 | 11 | 40 | 10 | 29 | 28 | 12 | 13 | 60 | 60 |  |  | 119.51 | 299.91 |
| PL | 81 | 0 | f | 14 | 13 | 28 | 11 | 33 | 35 | 11 | 16 | 56 | 58 |  |  |  |  |
| JG | 65 | 1 | f | 48 | 18 | 48 | 14 | 39 | 40 | 20 | 21 | 60 | 60 | 26.13 | 16.22 | 408.34 | 621.14 |
| JC | 31 | 1 | f | 43 | 11 | 44 | 15 | 36 | 37 | 14 | 11 | 57 | 59 | 5.32 | 14.1 | 342.94 | 260.79 |
| WS | 87 | 0 | m | 29 | 17 | 30 | 15 | 29 | 20 | 21 | 20 | 44 |  | 13.74 | 23.21 | 16.6 | 20.23 |
| LE | 49 | 1 | f | 32 | 14 | 44 | 10 | 38 | 37 | 18 | 20 | 45 | 49 | 26 | 5.78 | 632.09 | 530.68 |
| LL | 57 | 1 | f | 35 | 14 | 39 | 20 | 37 | 38 | 17 | 20 | 44 | 37 | 17.46 | 1.64 | 654.56 | 534.23 |
| MS | 86 | 0 | f | 35 | 11 | 36 | 12 | 34 | 31 | 9 | 11 | 47 | 48 | 3.84 | 3.26 | 323.54 | 156.22 |
| AW | 51 | 0 | f | 39 | 10 | 40 | 10 | 33 | 36 | 19 | 19 | 46 | 48 | 2.98 | 4.05 | 103.31 | 282.94 |
| KOM | 51 | 0 | f | 40 | 17 | 44 | 13 | 35 | 37 | 25 | 21 | 53 | 58 | 60.63 | 51.48 | 293 | 303.42 |
| YA | 52 | 0 | f | 27 | 24 | 25 | 20 | 33 | 31 | 30 | 33 | 35 | 38 | 3.84 | 3.62 | 103.92 | 210.24 |

*Figure 16.2* Screen Shot of the Quantitative Part of the Study

# References

Kaimal, G., Mensinger, J.L., Drass, J.M., and Dieterich-Hartwell, R. (2017). 'Open studio art therapy versus coloring: Differences in outcomes of affect, stress, creative agency and self—efficacy'. *Canadian Art Therapy Association Journal, 30* (2), pp. 56–68. DOI:10.1080/08322473.2017.1375827

Kaimal, G., and Ray, K. (2016). 'Free art making in an art therapy open studio: Changes in affect and self-efficacy'. *Arts and Health, 9* (2), pp. 154–166. DOI:10.1080/17533015.2016.1217248

Kaimal, G., Ray, K., and Muniz, J.M. (2016). 'Reduction of cortisol levels and participants' responses following artmaking'. *Art Therapy: Journal of the American Art Therapy Association, 33* (2), pp. 74–80. DOI:10.1080/07421656.2016.1166832

# 17 Wading in Knee Deep—The Art Therapist in Different End-of-Life Settings

*Jody Thomson*

In 2015, I interviewed four experienced visual art therapists about their work in cancer and palliative care. The study was inspired and informed by my private art therapy practice over many years with people living with or beyond cancer, and at end-of-life, in hospital out-patient centres and in the community. In that study, themes emerged in relation to the specific challenges, and to the privilege of working with people at end-of-life, expanding on a body of similarly focussed literature by other art therapist-researchers (Bardot, 2008; Bocking, 2005; Connell, 1998; Duesbury, 2005; Furman, 2011; Hardy, 2001, 2005, 2013; Luzzatto, 1998; Schaverien, 2002; Wood, 2005; Wood et al., 2013).[1] To chart my readings of and responses to the interview texts, including the images I asked the therapists to make as part of the interview, I used an art-based method that I called *immersive visual analysis*. This method of analysis showed in visual form how the introduction of art-making into a research interview can radically transform the conversation (Thomson, 2019), so that it becomes more emotionally resonant.

Three years after my initial study, I return to 'peek inside' (Barad, 2007) the stories that stayed with me; that have left a mark on me; that *glow*, or resonate 'in the body as well as the brain' (MacLure, 2013, p. 661),[2] in thinking about how it is to work with the dying and bereaved in different clinical settings. In revisiting these stories, I explore the entangled nature of art-making *as research*, in which the participant(s) and the researcher are open to being affected by the other. Furthermore, these stories call upon me to consider the mutually constitutive relations among art materials, art-making processes, places and objects—and the stories themselves.

I extend my original research by generating further, and qualitatively different, insights by working with Erin Manning's and Brian Massumi's process-focused method of 'thinking in the act' (2014, p. II). This is an emergent process that enabled me to think differently about the ways in which I am *affected* and subtly transformed by the interview texts. Hickey-Moody and Malins described the concept of *affect* as

> that which is felt before it is thought; [that] has a visceral impact on the body before it is given subjective or emotive meaning. Thinking through affect brings the sensory capacity of the body to the fore. . . [and is] very different from emotion: it is an a-subjective bodily response to an encounter. . . [that has] . . . the capacity to disrupt habitual and entrenched ways of thinking.
>
> (2007, p. 8)

By positioning myself not as a 'detached observer, but as entangled witness' (Allegranti & Wyatt, 2014, p. 541), my aim is to offer readers insight into the mutually affective experience of art therapy research, and to generate different understandings that enrich practice knowledge in palliative care.

For readers unfamiliar with the Australian context, the chapter begins by situating art therapy in palliative care within Australian allied health. I then describe a novel, inter-disciplinary art-based approach to inquiry that involves looking, listening and feeling my way back into two of the conversations, to think *with*, rather than alongside, art-making, writing and place. I then apply this method of inquiry to the stories, after introducing the storytellers, Byron and Sarah, using edited excerpts, about how it is to work in end-of-life care. The storytellers' voices are narrated in italics, without parentheses, for in the telling, remembering and thinking, they affectively *become* 'our' stories. After each story, I present my thinking with art-making images (Figures 17.1–17.3), and my experimental writing-thinking in response to my art-making process. I chose an outdoor bush setting for art-making, in which the stories, art materials and the Australian bush where I live became my companions and collaborators, enlarging my artist and researcher palette.

Thinking with writing was done several days later. This space between art-making and writing allowed the affective process time to germinate, and for me to consider the ways in which art-making and the material world are in an iterative relationship with the stories, storytellers and my researching body. The chapter concludes with a discussion of the ways in which distributing the agency (or the ways in which things are made to *matter*) between researcher, storytellers, art, writing and the environment of practice or research contributes to practice knowledge, and what the process allows me to think about.

## Australian Art Therapy in End-Of-Life Care

Australia is a vast urban, rural and often remote landscape and almost a quarter of the population (including many of the Indigenous population) live in isolated communities (AIHW, 2015), suggesting limited access to institutional or multi-disciplinary palliative care. Urban end-of-life facilities or services are located in neonatal units, paediatric services, acute hospitals, general practices, residential and community aged care services and non-profit community-based or charitable organisations. There is also a ground-swell movement towards communities of care and home hospice services supporting the patient, carers and communities for the 70% of the population who would prefer to die at home (Swerissen & Duckett, 2014).

Palliative Care Australia (PCA) is the national peak body[3] for the eight states and territories of Australia, representing the 208 specialist palliative care providers (PCADoS) across the country.[4] The PCA's Service Planning Guide (PCAPG, 2003, p. 28) is endorsed by major Australian stakeholders and promotes the inclusion of allied health personnel in interdisciplinary palliative care teams, as 'an essential component of comprehensive quality palliative care'. Under the heading of allied health, the PCAPG groups together 'music therapy, art therapy, and/or massage, narrative, diversional, complementary therapies etc', noting that 'music and art therapy are professional degree courses [whereas] complementary and other therapists have widely varying levels and types of training'. The PCAGP (2003, p. 29) stated that art therapy can 'significantly increase quality of life and provide normalizing activities' in community-based, acute hospital and hospice-based care.

Art therapy in Australia is a self-regulating allied health profession, represented nationally by the *Australian, New Zealand and Asian Creative Arts Therapies Association* (ANZACATA), which operates as a company limited by guarantee.[5] This association supports differently qualified therapists using a range of theoretical approaches and creative modalities, including visual art therapy. Professional members are bound by a code of ethics and are required to engage in continued professional development and supervision. A membership profile review[6] indicated that while many therapists nominate an interest in palliative care, those who work as specialists form a very small percentage.

The National Arts in Health Framework (NAHF, 2013, pp. 18, 20–21), reported that the arts therapies, 'art therapy (visual, dance, music, drama)' are effective for established disease, tertiary treatment and chronic or clinical management in reducing stress, pain and anxiety, promoting dignity and assisting in 'improved service delivery, supporting staff to deliver patient-centred healthcare'. However, art therapy is marginalised by the Australian Government Health and Welfare Department in their Palliative Care Services in Australia report (AIHW, 2014, p. 3), which noted 'a range of health professionals, other workers, carers and volunteers provide palliative care services. These include . . . other occupations, including personal care assistants, chaplains, pastoral carers, massage therapists and music therapists'.

Australian art therapists are part of a small, emerging profession (Westwood & Linnell, 2011), still negotiating a professional identity (Kelly, 2013; Mallon, 2015), existing at the moment in the margins of allied health. This struggle has several contributing factors:

- 'art therapist' and 'art therapy' are not protected titles in Australia and are inclusive of a variety of modalities
- art therapy is awarded a pay scale in the Department of Health salary awards in only one state (NSW Health, 2010)
- there is an understandable confusion, and a perceived lack of awareness about art therapy in the community (Kelly, 2013) and relatedly
- there are a significant number of artists, arts in health workers, volunteers and students offering services often described as art therapy.[7]

Consequently, art therapy remains marginalised (Kelly, 2013; Mallon, 2015; Westwood, 2010). Within medical settings, employment for art therapists is often tenuous, and obtained through the therapist's entrepreneurial efforts (Westwood, 2010) and years of building relationships with other health professionals. Yet the two storytellers in this chapter (and as researcher and author I am a third storyteller) have worked for over a decade in palliative care, are passionate and committed, and have strong personal identities as art therapists.

## Thinking *With* Art-Making and Writing

> *How do I know what I think until I see what I say.*
>
> —(Forster, 1927, p. 27)

Making images *as research* is not a new concept to art therapists.[8] Those who are artists are always engaged in research at the level of art-making itself (Manning, 2015). Many art therapists engage in *response art* (Fish, 2012) to reflect on practice (for example, Wadeson, 2003; Fish, 2013) and use art-making in supervision (Fish, 2008, 2016). However, the relationship between art-making and words—between the material process of knowledge production through art-making and the words used to discursively analyse, interpret or communicate that process has long been a conundrum in art therapy research and practice.

For Elizabeth St. Pierre 'writing *is* thinking, writing *is* analysis, writing *is* indeed a seductive and tangled *method* of discovery' (Richardson & St. Pierre, 2018, p. 827 original italics). For me, art-making *is* thinking, art-making *is* analysis and art-making *is* seductive and generative in opening a space for the researcher's thinking-writing to develop. My approach, as described in this chapter, uses art-making *and* writing in an interdisciplinary, mutually affective process of inquiry and dissemination.

To help me do this thinking, I draw on the work of poststructuralist and new materialist writers Karen Barad (2003, 2007); Maggie MacLure (2013, 2017); Lisa Mazzei and Alecia Jackson (2012); Bronwyn Davies and Susanne Gannon (2012); and art therapy educators and researchers Patricia Fenner (2017); and Sheridan Linnell and Anita Lever (2017), to explore the notion of *mutual affectivity* across human and non-human bodies in art therapy practice. By this I mean the potential for a non-hierarchical agency, not only between client/research participant(s) and the art therapist/researcher(s), but also between words and images, and the non-human art materials, objects and physical places of therapy or research. This work requires a radical epistemological, ontological and ethical shift that decentres the human being—a startling and yet highly appropriate move for art therapy. In the words of Karen Barad:

> We don't obtain knowledge by standing outside the world; we know because we are of the world . . . The separation of epistemology from ontology . . . assumes an inherent difference between human and nonhuman, subject and object, mind and body, matter and discourse.
>
> (Barad, 2007, p. 185, emphasis added)

My methodology is situated within an onto-epistemological stance of *knowing in being*, 'in which practices of knowing *and* being cannot be isolated from one another but rather are mutually implicated and constitutive' (Mazzei, 2014, p. 745, emphasis added). It uses my affective responses as 'instruments of understanding' (Kofoed & Stenner, 2017, citing Urwin, p. 9) of the ways in which I, as a researcher, am *entangled* within the events I seek to understand.

> [L]istening to the other . . . involves listening not just to oneself and the other, but to the boat, the river, the stars, the changing weather patterns, the waves, and their co-implication in each other. It listens to changing, emergent thought and reflects on it, is integrally co-implicated in it.
>
> (Davies, 2010, p. 57)

If I wade into a pool of water, each movement sends ripples and the reflected view of the landscape, sky and my own reflection changes. The pool is changed—what lies beneath the surface is disturbed, particles of sand, dirt and living matter move through contact with my body. The water's flow, temperature and constitution are also affected. I am similarly changed by this experience—in 'becoming-with' (Banerjee & Blaise, 2013) the river, my feeling-body is changed, affected, as my skin leaves traces in exchange for particles absorbed from the water.

If we art therapists wade knee deep into the waters of another's end-of-life experience, how might we keep our balance when the flow of the current moves around us; or if we wade together into a pool of research—what might germinate in the places where our ripples merge; and what emotional and ecological traces might we exchange in an always-shifting entanglement?

## Byron's Story

Byron is an art therapist, counsellor, playwright and psychodramatist. He has extensive experience in hospital-based palliative care and as a self-employed bereavement and trauma practitioner.

Byron tells me a story about an unrealistic staff culture of death denial in some palliative care settings—*it's really interesting palliative care—no one actually talks about the actual idea of death*. Byron elaborates, *by the idea of death, I mean discussing death as an abstraction from a philosophical perspective, rather than specific deaths—how we feel about it, fear it, how it affects our personal and cultural lives . . . it's all euphemistic . . . and metaphors. It really shocked me one day to hear a [community] nurse say how she dealt with death, she said 'I never drive down that street again, where someone died' . . . but death walks home with her . . . death goes home with you at the end of the day, because you are experiencing whether you want to or not, what is going to happen to you one day.*

Byron's view of art therapy in palliative care is cynical—*the management people liked the look of something like art therapy and music therapy on their brochures . . . so we're window dressing really—we're nice dummies to put in the window . . . the rhetoric of palliative care is holistic and biopsychosocial, but the reality is far more biomedical and the rest is more about image.*

*I've been told not to bother working with people because they are going to die in a couple of weeks . . . I remember exactly being told that about one man—an old builder called Max.* Byron had come across Max enjoying a colouring-in book that a palliative nurse had given him, saying *just fill in your time.* Byron suggested painting, and Max replied *'Oh I couldn't do that, I'm not an artist', I said I'll give you a hand you know.* With a twinkle in his eye and a wry chuckle, Byron continues, *well Max, who was supposed to die in two weeks lived for three months—to the point where they were threatening to chuck him out because he wasn't following the rules and dying . . . you've got to follow the rules if you're in palliative care, if you come in to die that's the contract you've got to fulfil or you get thrown out . . . It's shocking actually—an enormous cause of stress for a lot of people.* Over those months, Max and Byron painted a landscape together, which the hospital exhibited as part of Palliative Care Week. Byron says:

*There's this **big** display and **bang** in the middle of the display is Max's picture—and **bang** in front of the picture is Max in his wheelchair. And he's saying 'I did that, I didn't realize I was an artist ya know'. It was fantastic—it kept him alive for weeks I reckon . . . He had a new view of himself after that . . . that's what I find probably most exciting about palliative care work, you have people who can come to terms with limitations in their life in the last weeks of their life and die in a far more fulfilled state than they would have otherwise done . . . it makes for better death if you're more fulfilled . . . it kind of expanded him in a way. Max was **excited** about where he was at, he died the next week . . . I'll never forget him sitting there in his wheelchair, proud as punch.*

I ask Byron how he has managed to work for such a long time with people at the very end of their lives. He says, *I've been asked that question lots of times and I'm never quite sure. I had a heart attack two years after I started working at the hospice and I'd been through the death of my mum and my dad. All of that helped. When I had my heart attack I had a near death experience—and I lost any fear whatever of death, because I discovered that death is actually really gentle and we shouldn't fear it at all . . . I feel like I seriously have no fear of death, so I see people who are dying and I just feel enormous compassion for their anxiety, their stress and particularly the trauma which is not recognised in palliative care.* Byron's philosophy is that *if you can come to terms with that reality of dying, you are no longer having to hold a defence like everybody else, of immortality, of invulnerability and of denial—of repression really, repression of insecurity, repression of a whole lot of things.*

Byron also talks about loneliness, saying *loneliness is always there with death—in your group of friends, it's very unlikely anyone else is dying,* and says of his own experience, *I've found work as an art therapist to be isolating.*

Waiting at the airport on my way home from meeting with Byron, I receive an email from him. He again takes up the notion of loneliness, saying, in part, *the blank canvas has always been a dangerous place for me . . . because it evokes loneliness, for me, my constant life companion. I wrote this poem a few years ago* [the first few stanzas are included here], *and during our session it came up for me:*

*The danger of writing. . .*
*allow a single word*
*to appear on your blank screen*
*and it will call up its associates,*
*many of which will not be your friends,*
*and like mobsters,*
*may take you on a journey*
*you would rather not be having.*

*The danger of writing. . .*
*especially at certain times,*
*times of vulnerability,*
*when an image,*
*like this image that now confronts my mind,*
*an empty seat facing a river,*
*might evoke a provocative word.*

*I know where this is going. . .*

*Do not allow a single word to appear!*
*Keep staring bleakly*
*at the empty screen.*

*But the word appears*
*on the screen of my mind,*
*impossible to avoid*

*at five o'clock in the afternoon,*
*the winter sun descending,*
*the biting edge of cold dusk*

*settling into my soul.*

*Emptiness. . .*
*life passing relentlessly,*
*second by second,*
*like a river that never stops.*

## Thinking With Byron's Story

Thinking with art-making in response to Byron's stories, I was taken back to the small and windowless meeting room in which we met, experiencing again his kindness and compassion. I remembered feeling that his flashes of anger and frustration were covered by humour; and of how we parted awkwardly outside in the car park—traces of the intimacy of our conversation still hovering, with so much left to say. My image (Figure 17.1) was made three years later, and the thinking with writing that follows it, a week after that, sitting outside on a cold sandstone rock, feeling the winter sun on my back, remembering Byron's warmth.

*A week after making my image, I find that it takes some time to move back into an affective space. The image itself took a long time to make; a long time thinking while I crumbled those sandstone rocks, rubbing one against the other, filling the space, knowing that without glue, it wouldn't stay.*

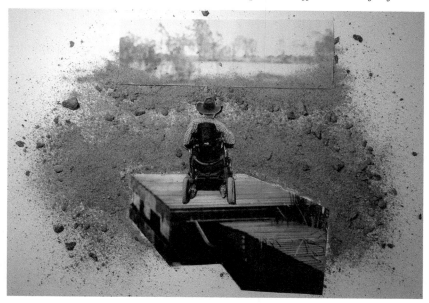

*Figure 17.1* Author's Art Response to Byron's Stories (Mixed Media, 400 × 270 mm)

*The lone figure in the wheelchair is on top of a floating pontoon looking at something in the future. I see the same thing he is looking at, from a different perspective, just behind him. It reminds me of my husband, sitting alone in a wheelchair twenty years ago, facing the reality of death; and of how much of me wanted to go with him. The pontoon is the only thing that is stuck down—a place to arrive and a place to leave. I keep telling myself to stay with the image. I want to walk away. Not speak about it, not think about it . . . to avoid its provocative shadow meanings. Anger and frustration rise and I succumb to an overwhelming urge to brush it all off. Everything not stuck down—the sandstone, view and wheelchair-man, is suddenly gone. All that's left is the pontoon, floating, disconnected from the earth. I need to do something else, take a break from this difficult work, feel the earth and the sun and listen to the birdsong.*

## Sarah's Story

Sarah describes herself as a professional artist and a full-time clinical art therapist in two interdisciplinary home hospice palliative care teams. She also facilitates a community open studio for ambulatory patients, is a trained psychodrama director, and has worked for many years with youth in the community. Sarah makes up to three or four home visits each day as *one specialist, working with a team of other specialists providing care to people in need at home . . . it isn't average to have an art therapist come to your home, talking about either past or current traumas, symptoms, relationships, end of life wishes, legacy needs, where you want to be buried, what you want your funeral to be like.* She provides other staff with *a list of referral indicators that they can use to identify when to offer art therapy*, which might be *to look at how a client uses 'picture words' or metaphor*, adding *we soon identify if the visit is about the spoken word only, I've got colleagues who are best for that—I'm better for the visual and the imaginal domains and sensory needs.* Sarah has worked hard to establish the place of art therapy in the multi-disciplinary teams by making a clear delineation between complementary therapies and art therapy as a specialist profession. . . *so while it is amazing it's still got it's own drawbacks, and part of that is that is the isolation of being specialised.*

Sarah finds that working with families in people's homes requires a great deal of flexibility—*I'm in their home, I'm a guest—I'm traversing all manner of funny role changes, from holding, containment, providing, to when someone comes to the door . . . through to 'here have lunch' . . . so there's a whole range of different skill sets required.*

As we talk together, Sarah takes some paper-based sculpture media and kneads it between her hands, saying *I'm thinking of when I talk to couples particularly, using this media can be about noting the space between their hands . . . there was one gentleman with terrible neuropathic pain—he could no longer be touched or offer touch without pain, and for he and his wife of 50 years plus—it was devastating. They were no longer able to hold hands. The losses in that were taking them down as a couple to such a degree that it was having massive physical effect on him—it also was a subtle yet big point of his wife's carer burden, part of making managing at home together really difficult.*

Sarah shows me the small shell-like object she has made by squeezing the clay between her palms, explaining that it is a *little print of the piece of each other that we don't ever get to materialise or see, because it's a space, the space between the hands we hold . . . it has the other person's half on it, their palm print.*

As part of her private practice, Sarah also provides monthly studio art therapy for up to six palliative clients in the community, where *people can come and go as their energy allows and have that freedom, that sense of being fully living, as if they didn't have anything happening.*

*The lusciousness of it for me is that people who attend studio art therapy commonly use the space to talk about really complex living concerns, decision-making and treatments. They talk about really massive challenges in the changes of relationships across their life and the losses they are facing . . . I can't help but note the 'disguise' and safety offered in the artwork, and the art-making process . . . because it softens the hardness of the words being expressed. It allows people to put their gaze back to the table. It allows people to flick through a book while they are talking about some of their worst life experiences of either being diagnosed or struggling with collapsed veins or being challenged with treatment options, and other such complex decision-making, including where to live and die.*

Sarah uses art journaling for *release and relief* between client visits. I asked her about her other self-care practices—*to look after my self, my container, I have to check what the cracks look like . . . that's with my supervisor . . . you know, the work goes past what you do here or there, you're a person in the world who does many other things. What I am doing in my work, this will have been its own moment, so what impact do I need it to have? And what do I want to think about it, to be able to let it connect in me—so that can be, and is, my work too.* She is also aware of the need to keep her work and personal life in balance—*that can be a walk in nature and feeling connected to the world, it can be reading a great book, it can be art-making or family, just hanging out with the right people that love me back—that sense of connection in my world. So I get that experience of very separate living, of being at work and of being at home.*

## Thinking With Sarah's Story

Engaging with Sarah's story to think with art-making (Figure 17.2), I can hear her voice in my mind. Sarah gave me the little shell-like sculpture that she made in the clasp of her hands at the end of our conversation. It's a little stained now, but clearly shows the print of her palms (the white circle in Figure 17.2). As I hold this precious object in my hand, I feel her enthusiasm, our shared passion as artists and our mutual commitment to art therapy.

*On a quiet, still afternoon, I spend a long time breaking things apart: first in carefully cutting open a difficult landscape, leaving a small, jagged space when I glue it down. Then in breaking*

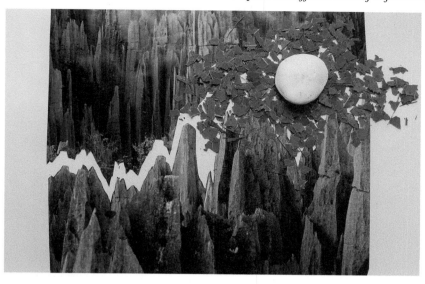

*Figure 17.2* Author's Art Response to Sarah's Stories (Mixed Media, 400 × 270 mm)

*apart gum leaves torn from the tree beside me. I let the pieces fall onto the white spaces. It's soothing and alive, softening the peaks and valleys and some pieces spill off the page. The view is different sitting outside, listening to the quiet sounds of the bush. I place Sarah's sculpture like a sun in the centre of the aromatic leaves. In carefully carrying the artwork inside, a gust of wind changes everything. I stand transfixed, watching the leaf-pieces floating away. An intense feeling of futility rises. When I retrieve the little sculpture, I notice that the strong smell of eucalyptus oil is still on my hands.*

Thinking with art-making and writing in response to Byron's and Sarah's stories together/apart as a third image (Figure 17.3) invited me to think about the multiple ways in which I am a mutually affective, and entangled researching body. This *entanglement* is evident in the questions I chose to ask the therapists in the original interviews; in witnessing their art-making, listening to, transcribing and editing their stories; in holding these stories in the space between the original interviews and this secondary analysis; in being in and of the world of art therapy as a profession, and my practice in end-of-life care; and in the human and non-human spaces of thinking with art-making and writing described in this chapter.

*In the late afternoon under a clear sky, a drawing begins. Layers of tangled half circles painstakingly shaded create a fleshy, churning movement—an entangled maze that's full of dead ends. It bothers me that there is a gaping hole at the bottom, and smaller ones at the side, where 'stuff' can get in and out. I could fix it by continuing to draw, but the light is fading, I have a painful ant-bite and I'm getting cold sitting here outside alone. In semi-darkness I collect a handful of little rocks, all about the same size and colour, and move inside to where it's warm and light. In gluing the almost-circle onto three different papers, I can feel their textures, edges, bumps and lines and where they overlap underneath, like three story-tellers. I then glue the rocks carefully around my drawing, but there are not enough to complete the circle. Again, I am confronted with an open space at the top. This feels like a threshold space-between that is neither inside nor outside, but a vulnerable and mobile space to move between the two.*

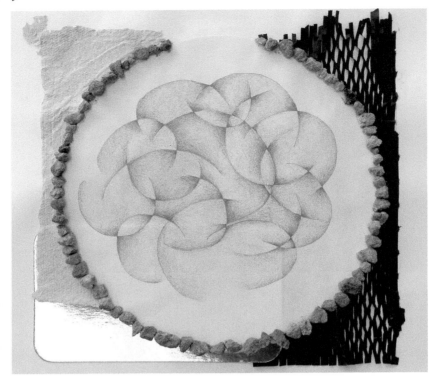

*Figure 17.3* Author's Art Response to Byron's and Sarah's Stories Together (Mixed Media, 300 × 270 mm)

## Discussion and Final Thoughts: What Thinking With Art-Making and Writing Made Possible

During the interviews from which these stories are taken (Thomson, 2019), I asked the art therapists to make an image as part of our conversation. What emerged in my *immersive visual analysis* was a startling qualitative shift in what the art-making process, in the middle of the interview, allowed them to feel and to say. The onto-epistemological process of *knowing in being* (Barad, 2007) by *thinking in the act* (Manning & Massumi, 2014) of visual art-making and writing offered new ways of thinking about how it is to be an art therapist. The method also made it possible for us as therapists and researchers to reflect on, make visible and articulate our experiences of mutual affectivity and entanglement in our work. Re-viewing the same stories through a new materialist theoretical lens, allowed *things to matter* in a way that is equally agentic—the spaces of man-made and natural environments of therapy and research; the material world of art media, art-works and other non-human agents; myself as therapist-researcher; and the therapist-storytellers.

> Being open, and being vulnerable to being affected by the other, is how we accomplish our humanity; it is how the communities, of which we are part, create and re-create themselves. We are not separate from the encounters that make up the community but, rather, emergent *with* them.
>
> (Davies, 2014, p. 10)

By embracing my own vulnerability as an 'entangled witness' (Allegranti & Wyatt, 2014, p. 541) in becoming-with the stories through art-making, I spent time thinking with, and listening to simple things that are normally overlooked, or marginalised in everyday busyness—sandstone rocks, discarded magazine images, the weather, glue sticks, scissors and gum leaves.

In my imag(in)ing of how it is to be Byron, and how it is to be Sarah, I was challenged by my emotional and confronting responses. The process of brushing off everything not glued down in my response to Byron's stories enacted my rage—against the marginalisation of our professional and the personal investment we make as therapists; against our professional isolation; and the marginalisation of palliative care within a medical system that often prioritises cure rather than care. Like so many of the people I have worked with, the gum leaves I used in response to Sarah's story were vibrantly alive until ripped from the tree, torn apart and blown away a moment later. In watching the wind take the leaves so suddenly, I felt *in my body* the fragile and temporary nature of our work, and the sense of frustration and dismay in our struggle to fit into established medical settings. In retrieving Sarah's small sculpture, I was reminded of how incredibly precious, rewarding and unique what we have to offer is.

Adopting a methodology of *thinking in the act* and *thinking with* post-structural and new materialist theories opened a space in which to move beyond a pedestrian thematic analysis of the stories as research 'data', and to consider the mutually affective and entangled relationships that emerge when wading knee deep into the experience of people who are dying, and who work with the dying.

I was startled to recognise the opportunities suggested by the open circle in my final image—ma(r)king the intimate and mutually affective between-space of art-making in therapy and research, and between life and death. It is also an open space of potential and agency for Australian art therapists, made possible through the absence of institutional or governmental regulation. In keeping the art-making process *as research* central to the analysis, what emerged strongly was the affective potential of this form of inquiry on the researcher, and an acknowledgement of the importance of our stories—being told, listened to closely and articulated through images and words, which is our work as art therapists in palliative care.

## Notes

1. All of these studies come from the Northern Hemisphere.
2. These stories are drawn from research (Thomson, 2015) conducted at Western Sydney University Australia for which human ethics approval was granted. The study is reported elsewhere (Thomson, 2017).
3. A 'peak body' is an Australian term for a non-government organisation consisting of smaller organisations with allied interests, whose purpose is to provide a strong and specific community voice for lobbying government and other stakeholders to provide education and share information.
4. At the of time of writing, the majority of these service providers are on the eastern coast of Australia, in NSW, Victoria and Queensland (154), and the remainder (54) are spread across Tasmania, South Australia, Western Australia and the Northern Territory.
5. ANZACATA is supportive of all qualified therapists working with the arts, and inclusive of a broad range of creative modalities including visual art, clay work, dance or movement, music, narrative or storytelling, drama/psychodrama, creative writing, poetry and sandplay therapies. This company was formed in 2018 to amalgamate two previously independent associations, ANZATA (Australian and New Zealand Arts Therapies Association) and ACATA (Australian Creative Arts Therapies Association).
6. The membership review of ANZATA and ACATA (see note v) was conducted in 2017, at which time approximately 2 percent of members indicated a specialisation in palliative, cancer or end-of-life care.

7. See examples ATPC (2017).
8. See for example, Leavy (2015); McNiff (2013, 2014). Also see Fraser & Al Sayah (2011) for a systematic review of arts-based research in health.

# References

AIHW. 2014, 'Australian Government, Australian Institute of Health and Welfare, Palliative Care Services in Australia', viewed 28 July 2017, <www.aihw.gov.au/WorkArea/DownloadAsset. aspx?id=60129548892>

AIHW. 2015, 'Australian Government, Australian Institute of Health and Welfare', viewed 28 July 2017, <www.aihw.gov.au/indigenous-observatory/reports/health-and-welfare-2015/indigenous-population/>

Allegranti, B. & Wyatt, J. 2014, 'Witnessing loss: A feminist material-discursive account', *Qualitative Inquiry*, vol. 20, no. 4, pp. 533–543.

Arts.gov.au. 2013, 'National Arts and Health Framework', Department of Communications and the Arts [online], viewed 1 August 2017, <https://www.arts.gov.au/national-arts-and-health-framework>ATPC. 2017, 'Art Therapy in Palliative and Cancer Care, Online Publications', viewed 3 August 2017, <http://palliativecare.org.au/palliative-matters/tag/art-therapy/; www. smh.com.au/entertainment/art-and-design/sydney-arts/cancer-surivivors-turn-treatment-masks-into-art-at-casula-powerhouse-20160504-gom1qt.html; www.thegroundswellproject.com/new-blog/2015/5/25/meet-flutter-lyon-reflected-legacy-artist; www.mylifehouse.org.au/services/complementary-therapy/arterie/>

Banerjee, B. & Blaise, M. 2013, 'There's something in the air: Becoming-with research practices', *Cultural Studies - Critical Methodologies*, vol. 13, no. 4, pp. 240–245.

Barad, K. 2003, 'Posthumanist performativity: How matter comes to matter', *Journal of Women in Culture and Society*, vol. 28, no. 3, pp. 801–831.

Barad, K. 2007, *Meeting the universe halfway: Quantum physics and the entanglement of matter and meaning*, Duke University Press, Durham, NC.

Bardot, H. 2008, 'Expressing the inexpressible: The resilient healing of client and art therapist', *Art Therapy*, vol. 25, no. 4, pp. 183–186, DOI: 10.1080/07421656.2008.10129547

Bocking, M. 2005, 'A don't know story: Art therapy in an NHS medical oncology department', in Waller, D. & Sibbett, C., *Art therapy in cancer care*, Open University Press, Berkshire, England, pp. 210–222.

Connell, C. 1998, *Something understood: Art therapy in cancer care*, Wrexham Publications, London.

Davies, B. 2010, 'The implications for qualitative research methodology of the struggle between the individualized subject of phenomenology and the emergent multiplicities of the poststructuralist subject: The problem of agency', *Reconceptualizing Educational Research Methodology*, vol. 1, no. 1, pp. 54–68.

Davies, B. 2014, *Listening to children: Being and becoming*, Routledge, London.

Davies, B. & Gannon, S. 2012, 'Collective biography and the entangled enlivening of being', *International Review of Qualitative Research*, vol. 5, no. 4, pp. 357–376.

Duesbury, T. 2005, 'Art therapy in the hospice: Rewards and frustrations', in Waller, D. & Sibbett, C., *Art therapy in cancer care*, Open University Press, Berkshire, England, 199–209.

Fenner, P. 2017, 'Art therapy places, flows, forces, matter and becoming', *ATOL: Art Therapy Online*, vol. 8, no. 1, pp. 1–22.

Fish, B. 2008, 'Formative evaluation research of art-based supervision in art therapy training', *Art Therapy: Journal of the American Art Therapy Association*, vol. 25, no. 2, pp. 70–77.

Fish, B. 2012, 'Response art: The art of the art therapist', *Art Therapy: Journal of the American Art Therapy Association*, vol. 29, no. 3, pp. 138–143.

Fish, B. 2013, 'Painting research: Challenges and opportunities of intimacy and depth', *Journal of Applied Arts & Health*, vol. 4, no. 1, pp. 105–115.

Fish, B. 2016, *Art-based supervision: Cultivating therapeutic insight through imagery*, Routledge, New York, NY.

Forster, E.M. 1927, *Aspects of the novel*, Harcourt, Brace & Company, New York, NY.

Fraser, K.D. & Fatima al Sayah, F. 2011, 'Arts-based methods in health research: A systematic review of the literature', *Arts & Health*, vol. 3, no. 2, pp. 110–145, DOI: 10.1080/17533015.2011.561357

Furman, L.R. 2011, 'Last breath: Art therapy with a lung cancer patient facing imminent death', *Art Therapy*, vol. 28, no. 4, pp. 177–180, DOI: 10.1080/07421656.2011.622690

Hardy, D. 2001, 'Creating through toss: An examination of how art therapists sustain their practice in palliative care', *Inscape*, vol. 6, no. 1, pp. 23–31, DOI: 10.1080/17454830108414026

Hardy, D. 2005, 'Creating through loss: An examination of how art therapists sustain their practice in palliative care', in Waller, D. & Sibbett, C., *Art therapy in cancer care*, Open University Press, Berkshire, England, pp. 185–198.

Hardy, D.C. 2013, 'Working with loss: An examination of how language can be used to address the issue of loss in art therapy', *International Journal of Art Therapy*, vol. 18, no. 1, pp. 29–37, DOI: 10.1080/17454832.2012.707665

Hickey-Moody, A. & Malins, P. 2007, 'Gilles Deleuze and four movements in social thought', in Hickey-Moody, A. & Malins, P., *Deleuzian Encounters: Studies in Contemporary Social Issues*, Pallgrave Macmillan, New York, pp. 1–14.

Kelly, J. 2013, 'Illuminating voices: Perspectives on professional identity', *ANZJAT Australian and New Zealand Journal of Arts Therapy*, vol. 8, no. 1, pp. 5–55.

Kofoed, J. & Stenner, P. 2017, 'Suspended liminality: Vacillating affects in cyberbullying/research', *Theory & Psychology*, vol. 7, no. 2, pp. 167–182.

Leavy, P. 2015, *Method meets art*, Guilford Press, New York, NY.

Linnell, S. & Lever, A. 2017, 'The spaces in-between: The emotional geographies of art therapy and place', *ATOL: Art Therapy Online*, vol. 8 no. 1, pp. 1–18.

Luzzatto, P. 1998, 'From psychiatry to psycho-oncology: Personal reflections on the use of art therapy', in Pratt, M. & Wood, M.J.M., *Art therapy in palliative care*, Routledge, London & New York, pp. 169–175.

MacLure, M. 2013, 'Researching without representation? Language and materiality in post-qualitative methodology', *International Journal of Qualitative Studies in Education*, vol. 26, pp. 658–667, DOI: 10.1080/09518398.2013.788755

MacLure, M. 2017, 'Qualitative methodology and the new materialisms "A little of Dionysus's blood?"', in Denzin, N.K. & Giardina, M.D., *Qualitative Inquiry in Neoliberal Times*, New York, Routledge, pp. 48–58.

Mallon, A.H. 2015, 'How are we able to be here? A creative & narrative inquiry into ANZATA-registered art therapy practitioner personal histories', Ph.D. thesis, Western Sydney University.

Manning, E. 2015, 'Against method', in Vannini, P., *Non-representational methodologies: Re-envisioning research*, New York, Routledge, pp. 52–71.

Manning, E. & Massumi, B. 2014, *Thought in the act*, University of Minnesota Press, London & Minneapolis.

Mazzei, L. 2014, 'Beyond an easy sense: A diffractive analysis', *Qualitative Inquiry*, vol. 20, no. 6, pp. 742–746.

Mazzei, L.A. & Jackson, A.Y. 2012, 'In the threshold: Writing between-the-two', *International Review of Qualitative Research*, vol. 5, no. 4, pp. 449–458.

McNiff, S. (ed.) 2013, *Art as research: Opportunities and challenges*, Intellect, Chicago, IL.

McNiff, S. 2014, 'Art speaking for itself: Evidence that inspires and convinces', *Journal of Applied Arts & Health*, vol. 5 no. 2, pp. 255–262.

NSWH, New South Wales Health. 2010, 'Pay Rates and Conditions', viewed 1 August 2017, <www.health.nsw.gov.au>

PCA, Palliative Care Australia, viewed 30 June 2017, <http://palliativecare.org.au/about-pca/>

PCADoS. nd., Palliative Care Australia, 'Directory of Services', viewed 28 July 2017, <http://palliativecare.org.au/directory-of-services/>

PCAPG. 2003, *Palliative Care Service Provision in Australia: A planning guide* (2nd ed.), viewed 27 July 2017, < http://palliativecare.org.au/wp-content/uploads/2015/07/Palliative-Care-Service-Provision-in-Australia-a-planning-guide.pdf>

Richardson, L. & St. Pierre, E.A. 2018, 'Writing: A method of inquiry', in Denzin, N.K. & Lincoln, Y.S. (5th Ed.), *Sage Handbook of Qualitative Research*, Sage, Thousand Oaks, CA, pp. 818–838.

Schaverien, J. 2002, *The dying patient in psychotherapy: Desire, dreams and individuation*, Palgrave Macmillan, Basingstoke, New York.

Swerissen, H. & Duckett, S. 2014, 'Dying well', *Grattan Institute*, viewed 26 July 2017, <https://grattan.edu.au/wp-content/uploads/2014/09/815-dying-well.pdf>

Thomson, J. 2015, 'From the therapist's brush: Painting a picture of the art therapist's experience in Australian cancer care', Unpublished thesis, Western Sydney University Bankstown, Australia.

Thomson, J. 2019, 'The work of art therapy: An immersive visual analysis', in Westwood, J., Gilroy, A., Linnell, S. & McKenna, T., *Art therapy: Taking a postcolonial, aesthetic turn*, Sense, The Netherlands .

Wadeson, H. 2003, 'Making art for professional processing', *Art Therapy*, vol. 20, no. 4, pp. 208–218, DOI: 10.1080/07421656.2003.10129606

Westwood, J. 2010, 'Hybrid creatures: Mapping the emerging shape of art therapy education in Australia', Ph.D. thesis, University of Western Sydney.

Westwood, J. & Linnell, S. 2011, 'The emergence of Australian art therapies: Colonial legacies and hybrid practices', *Art Therapy Online: ATOL*, vol. 1, no. 3, pp. 1–19.

Wood, M.J.M. 2005, 'Shoreline: The realities of working in cancer and palliative care', in Waller, D. & Sibbett, C., *Art therapy and cancer care*, Open University Press, London, pp. 82–101.

Wood, M.M. Low, Molassiotis, J. & Tookman, A. 2013, 'Art therapy's contribution to the psychological care of adults with cancer: A survey of therapists and service users in the UK', *International Journal of Art Therapy: Inscape*, vol. 18, no. 2, pp. 42–53.

# 18 Coming Up for Air

## Art Therapy With Children Affected by Childhood Cancer

*Claudia Mandler McKnight*

This chapter outlines the development of an art therapy group for children whose families have been living with chronic illness. The art therapy program was developed by a "grass roots" support group for children with cancer and their families. It is held at a public art gallery in Canada and has shown great success. The structure and setting for the group, the criteria for participants, interactions with parents and the use of a spontaneous art therapy approach (rather than group projects or specific directives) are highlighted. Included also are a description of the psychodynamic approach the group has taken on and its benefits, observations of artwork created, common themes that have emerged, the importance of art materials chosen, and the significance of abandoned art pieces. The chapter concludes with a discussion of participants' personal growth as perceived by the parents, the children themselves and the art therapist.

## Health Care in Canada

Health care in Canada is publicly funded and administered on a provincial or territorial basis, with guidelines set by the federal government. Coverage is provided for all Canadian citizens, regardless of age, economic status, or health condition. Canadian Medicare includes preventative care and medical treatments from primary care physicians, as well as access to hospitals, dental surgery and additional medical services (Canadian Healthcare, 2004–2007).

The universal healthcare system in Canada is free in a way, but it is funded largely through taxpayers' money, and there are many who choose to pay monthly or yearly premiums for better health insurance. Public funding only accounts for about 71 percent of Canada's total healthcare spending. Most of the rest is split between private insurers and consumers' out-of-pocket expenses (Canadian Institute for Health Information, 2016).

Many families living with paediatric cancer do not have the medical insurance coverage for out of pocket expenses associated with cancer treatment: transportation, parking, meals, overnight stays, childcare for siblings and counselling. Frequently, parents must take an extended leave of absence from their jobs, so there is also substantial loss of income, creating an additional source of stress for families.

## Childhood Cancer in Canada

Childhood cancer is relatively uncommon: it accounts for less than 1% of all new cancer cases in Canada. However, it remains the most common disease-related cause of death for children. Over 75% of the children will survive, but an estimated two-thirds of childhood cancer survivors will have at least one chronic or long-term side effect from their cancer treatment (Canadian Cancer Society, 2016).

## Candlelighters Simcoe—A Brief History of the Organization

Candlelighters Simcoe was established in the city of Barrie in 1990 by Barbara Johnson, herself the parent of a childhood cancer patient. The name Candlelighters refers to the sage adage "it is better to light a candle than to curse the darkness". Accordingly, Candlelighters Simcoe's mission is to empower families on their childhood cancer journey, lighting the way by providing hope, support and education (Candlelighters Simcoe, 2013).

Barrie is a small, vibrant city of 136,000, situated 100 kilometres north of Toronto, the capital city of the Province of Ontario. Located on the western shores of Lake Simcoe, Barrie is part of the densely populated and industrialized area of Central Ontario. As well, it is part of the scenic Great Lakes area. Summers are hot and humid; winters are cold with much snow. Barrie's population is currently predominantly English speaking and white. But Barrie is the second most rapidly growing city in Canada, and as such is becoming increasingly multi-cultural.

For almost twenty years, I have facilitated the weekly art therapy group which Candlelighters Simcoe hosts in Barrie. Over the years, more than seventy children have participated. Some families travel up to 60 km to take part!

Candlelighters Simcoe began as a small, informal group of parents who met together monthly. It has grown to become a registered not-for-profit organization, serving not only Barrie and area but the entire Simcoe-Muskoka region. Its many social and educational activities are not provincially or nationally funded. Instead, fundraising is done by its enthusiastic Board of Directors, by the members themselves and by community partners. A comprehensive, user-friendly website, www.candlelighterssimcoe.ca, profiles Candlelighters Simcoe's services and events. It also lists the many national and local organizations with which Candlelighters Simcoe interacts, including The Childhood Cancer Foundation, The Ontario Association for Children with Paediatric Cancer (OPACC), The Paediatric Oncology Group of Ontario (POGO) and Gilda's Club of Greater Simcoe and Muskoka.

The major treatment facility for children with cancer in the Barrie area is the Hospital for Sick Children (aka "Sick Kids") in Toronto. Satellite clinics for maintenance and monitoring are in the towns of Newmarket (Southlake Health Centre) and Orillia (Soldiers' Memorial Hospital), each about 40 km away from Barrie. The Candlelighters Simcoe art therapy program is not monitored by these facilities or any associated organizations; it is an independent initiative designed to help local families deal with the stressors of childhood cancer.

## The Stress of Childhood Cancer on the Family

It is increasingly recognized that when a child has cancer, the entire family has cancer. Frequent hospitalizations and lengthy treatment can be overwhelming. Moreover, childhood cancer is for life. Although a child may be cured of the original diagnosis of cancer, impaired vision; difficulties processing language; memory, attention and organizational challenges; and trouble with co-ordination are among the possible long-term effects. Therefore, emotional support for families who struggle through a child's chronic illness is necessary not only during the initial phases of treatment, but on a long-term basis. For those families who sustain the loss of a child through cancer, the pain is devastating, and they too need support in their grief (Nolbris et al, 2010).

The children who are diagnosed suffer both the trauma of being ill and the trauma of invasive and painful treatments. They may encounter surgery, chemotherapy, radiation, scans and pokes and intimidating medical equipment. Hair loss, scarring, significant changes in weight, and/or noticeable disability or injury may occur. Children with cancer may believe the illness is something they did wrong. They are often worried about what other children might think of them. Seeing other sick children, and knowing children who have died, may be frightening. Not knowing what will happen next, intensified by the fear of dying, may result in an attitude of general mistrust and anxiety (Malchiodi, 1999).

The healthy siblings of children with cancer also endure pain. They may think the cancer is somehow their fault. Loss of time with parents and the stress of disrupted family routines create feelings of anxiety. Fear of abandonment by their parents and/or ill sibling is common. Often siblings have been left with family or friends during times of crisis; the younger they are at this time, the greater the abandonment issues seem to be (Malchiodi, 1999).

Siblings may be afraid of becoming sick themselves, dying, or infecting their brother or sister. Complaints of headaches or tummy aches or other minor illnesses, and changes in eating and sleeping habits are common. Clinging to parents or other adults, bed wetting or thumb sucking, being afraid of the dark and reverting to baby talk are other signs of regression due to stress (Huchcroft et al, 1996; McKnight, 2001).

Siblings may show decreased attention span, general irritability or argumentativeness and withdrawal from others. As one mother has observed, "Little disappointments have become A BIG DEAL". At school, siblings may underachieve due to lack of motivation, or overperform in a quest for perfection. Parents often note that in times of crisis, siblings are supportive and undemanding. But when the crisis is past, and the parents are looking forward to a respite, the siblings make their needs known, usually by acting out, refusing to perform routine tasks, or whining and crying in frustration (McKnight, 2001).

Siblings are understandably jealous of the child who is consuming so much of the family's time and attention. Yet they also feel guilty about being mean-minded. A hyper vigilance or compulsion to watch out for potential dangers may develop, with its accompanying feelings of jumpiness and irritability. Withdrawing from others, feeling like an outsider, and/or not wanting to be with friends may be signs of depression. Increasingly, the cancer experience has become linked to the Post Traumatic Stress spectrum of symptoms (Chapman et al, 2001).

## The Candlelighters Simcoe Art Therapy Group

### Structure

Our weekly art therapy program consists of a small group of five or six children. This is a mix of children who have cancer, siblings of children who have cancer and bereaved siblings. Participants range in age from six to eleven. Only one member per family attends the group in a given semester; this ensures confidentiality for the siblings. The program runs concurrent with the school year. There are two semesters of fifteen sessions each; a session is an hour and fifteen minutes in length.

Children are recommended for the group by their parents in consultation with the Candlelighters Simcoe Parent Liaison, a role currently filled by the founder of Candlelighters Simcoe, Barb Johnson. Criteria for participation include the family's ability to make a commitment to bring the participating child to therapy for fifteen consecutive weekly sessions, a willingness on the part of the child to make marks (artistic ability is not a prerequisite!) and the child's readiness to be part of a group. Once the art therapy group is established, it is a closed group to which new members will not be added. After the set of fifteen sessions has been completed, the child may re-register for another semester, pending need and availability of spaces. Often there is a waitlist.

The mix of children with cancer, siblings of children with cancer and bereaved children works well in response to community needs, and in terms of group dynamics. The well siblings are able to experience children outside their own family struggling with chronic illness, and the children diagnosed with cancer can observe and interact with siblings from other families.

Two or three studio assistants, selected in consultation with the parent liaison and the art therapist, provide extra hands for the sessions. Recently, some helpers have been alumni from the program! The assistants are invaluable in providing one-on-one interaction when needed, and creating a friendly, relaxed and attentive atmosphere in the art studio.

Prior to the first session, parents are contacted to confirm arrangements and answer any questions they might have about the program. Halfway through the semester, parents are encouraged to meet with the therapist to confer about their child. Observed strengths and challenges, and support strategies for at home and at school are discussed.

### Aims and Goals for the Art Therapy Group

Our art therapy program aims to increase children's awareness of their feelings and emotions, and to help them express ideas too difficult to talk about. As feelings are identified, anxiety can be relieved, and thereby blockages to emotional expression and growth can be overcome.

### Venue for the Art Therapy Group

Our venue is the beautiful MacLaren Art Centre in downtown Barrie. This award-winning public gallery is a striking hybrid of Victorian architecture (a Carnegie Library) and postmodern additions. The gallery is wheelchair accessible, which is important for children with challenges in mobility.

When the art therapy program first started, parents typically dropped their children off and then left the art gallery to do errands. Over the years, parents have increasingly chosen to stay and chat by the foyer fireplace. This area has become the hearth for family updates, information about treatments and protocols, and parent-to-parent support. Some families have already met through hospital clinics, summer camps for children with cancer, or Candlelighters Simcoe social and educational events. But it is at the art centre that many lasting friendships are formed.

Gallery staff go out of their way to make our Candlelighters families feel welcome. Moreover, for the first three years of our art therapy program, the MacLaren Art Centre was instrumental in securing program funding through special grants and private donations. Since then, the gallery has donated the use of its space, while Candlelighters Simcoe funds the art therapy program.

### The Importance of Snack

When the children enter the art studio, they are invited to partake of a healthy, substantial snack. Tables are organized in a circular formation, so that everyone is at the centre of activity. It is an opportunity for the children to pause, relax and decompress. Some children are quiet and reflective; others are keen to talk. One child recently told me, "I was suspicious about this big room when I first saw it. Then I learned there was SNACK. That made me want to come here! If I could do snack, I could do art!"

### Setting Boundaries

At the start of our first session, while we have snack, I quickly outline a few things we need to remember in order to work well together in the art studio:

- Please enter the art studio when you are invited in (and not before)
- Sit down for hellos and snack first, then start with your art
- Be kind to each other
- Wait until someone else has finished speaking before you speak
- Use your indoor voice
- Walk softly
- Stay in the studio until the session ends; let us know if you need to use the washroom or wash your hands
- Work on someone else's art only if you are invited to do so by that person
- Ask for help if you need it
- Ask one of our teen or adult assistants to man the glue gun for you if you need heavy gluing.
- If an art material came in a box, we really appreciate you putting it back in the box
- when you are finished with it

I also ask the children if perhaps there are some things that I haven't mentioned that could be added. Often the issue of clean-up will be brought forward. I clarify that the teens and adults will do the final tidying and scrubbing, but that it's helpful if markers or crayons can be put back in their boxes. Sometimes a concern for "not copying" emerges, especially from the siblings. In art, I explain, we call it "being inspired" rather than copying.

### Art Therapy Approach Used

The art therapy approach I use is a spontaneous, psychodynamic model. Accordingly, I use few specific directives, verbal prompts or prescribed art tasks. Instead, the children are invited to create what comes to mind, and choose what they would like from the art materials set out. This is important for children who have had to accept many unwelcome events, procedures and interventions. The element of choice empowers them to make their own decisions and to explore, at their own pace, their feelings about themselves and the world. Also, given the wide range of the children's ages and abilities, and differences in the families' situations, it "levels the playing field" of competition and helps create an atmosphere of trust and acceptance. Each child does as he or she is able.

I have found it extremely rare for children in the group to ask what they "ought" to do. But, should a child be uncertain where to begin, I suggest rubbing the hands together and asking the hands which medium they would like to use. Would the hands like to work with something hard and precise, for example, or something soft and flowing? Or maybe something that needs to be squeezed and pushed? This "checking in" and bringing a soft attention to the moment eases the pressure of immediately making a big decision. It also puts the emphasis on exploration and creative play, rather than technical expertise or making a "masterpiece".

Sometimes the children will handle one item and then another, deciding by touch and intuition which material best suits their needs that day. If a child should remain unde-cided, I can provide an open-ended directive, such as, "If you were a creature, what might you look like and where would you be?"

### Art Materials Provided

A wide variety of materials is available for participants to use. Pencils, pencil crayons, fine markers, wide markers, oil pastels, chalk pastels, India ink, watercolours, coloured and textured papers and decorative beads are set out. Plasticine, toothpicks, wooden popsicle sticks, string, ribbon and pipe cleaners are provided for three-dimensional construction. Recycled materials such as boxes, tin cans, egg cartons, bubble wrap and Styrofoam trays are at hand. White glue, glue guns (to be used with the help of a studio assistant), glue sticks, heavy duty masking tape and string ensure that things will really hold together when applied.

Every second week is designated "Goopy Day", with clay and liquid tempera paints added to the array. This encourages the children to give the messier, stickier materi-als a try, because they are not there every session, and are therefore "special". Also, this arrangement provides an element of change in a consistent manner, a helpful experience for children who have become frightened of the unpredictable.

### Seasonal Holidays

Landmark holidays may be especially stressful for families living with childhood cancer. They are similar to anniversaries of diagnoses, treatments, relapses or a child's death. I recall one drawing by a seven-year-old sibling: Santa's reindeer were stuck in the chimney!

### Birthdays

The acknowledgement of a child's special day is particularly important for this popula-tion. It can be hard for parents to plan a festivity at home: it might all have to be cancelled because of a health crisis. A party may be a difficult expense for budgets that are already strained. And some of the children, because they are perceived of as different and/or have poor social skills, are sadly not included in classmates' invitations. Moreover, birth-day celebrations serve as a "reality check" for participants: birthdays are when they are. The children thereby internalize that sometimes they are lucky to be the star, and other times they are in a support role. This helps deconstruct rigid thinking about right and wrong, good and bad.

### Ending the Semester

As we approach the end of semester, we count down the numbers of sessions remain-ing. We want the children to experience a measured, anticipated "good" ending, rather than the abrupt changes and upsets which chronic illness incurs. On the final day, the children's efforts are acknowledged with a celebration of cake, cards, art presents and discussions about work created. The gift of art materials is intended to ensure that after the program is completed, the children have supplies at home to do art independently.

## Common Subjects and Themes I Have Observed in the Art Therapy Group

### Names and Initials

The pleasurable, non-threatening activity of drawing and embellishing letters confirms children's sense of self and marks territory. Elaborate signs for the door of the bedroom, for the school locker or for gift cards are often joyful and exuberant, but sometimes they are dark and edgy and warn intruders to stay out.

### Storms

The force of the weather in drawings and paintings is somewhat contained by the challenge of organizing a scene, yet the amount of chaos mirrors the inner turmoil the child is experiencing.

### Volcanoes

Pictures and sculptures of mountains spewing with lava are particularly favoured by the boys in the group. They are like storms exploding from the ground! The size of the volcano, the amount of lava and the agitation and intensity of the colour reflect the extent of fury in the child.

Zak, a lively nine-year-old in his last year of treatment for leukaemia, was inspired by the rain outside the gallery window. First, he drew a volcano, then clouds and rain, and finally forked lightening and a tornado (Figure 18.1)! Three weeks earlier, he had pounded a slab of clay, stabbed it with plastic knives, and then carved out a disgruntled face with big eyes, a grim mouth, furrowed brow and scratchy hair. Interestingly, the allocation of elements in his "Tornado Alley/Volcano" marker drawing was identical to the configuration of the features in his portrait!

### Aliens

The feeling of being out of place, somehow different, and frustrated with trying to communicate is captured in the children's images of people and creatures not of this world.

Lauren, age eleven, was an older sibling. Shy and reserved, she did not interact much with the other children, but she was content in her art-making, and quietly attuned to what was going on in the room. One afternoon, she drew what she called "The Alien" (Figure 18.2), a polka dot creature that looked simultaneously adorable, needy, irritated and bit menacing. Without going into particulars, Lauren was able to convey the edgy feeling that was consuming her that day.

### Animals and Birds and Fish and Other Creatures

One sibling, six-year-old Freddy, was fascinated by the pop song "What does the fox say?" Inspired by the video, he drew a big fox, standing on guard in a forest of skeletal trees under a dark, cloudy sky. The solitary fox had beady eyes and a long nose, but no

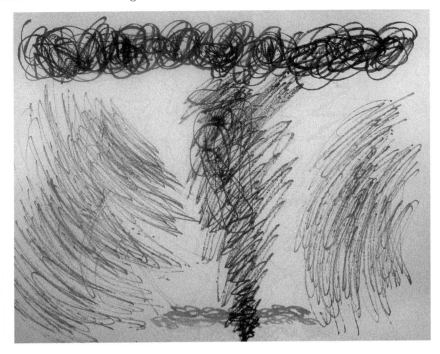

*Figure 18.1* Tornado Alley/Volcano

ears. At school, Freddy had been identified as defiant and oppositional. At home, there was much unrest and arguing. The drawing made it clear that he did not want to hear or could not bear to hear what was being said. After creating this work, Freddy began to talk more about his experiences at school. He was able to discuss the challenging situations in which he found himself, rather than instinctively reacting with outrage to adults' requests.

### Flowers

Especially the girls in our group like to draw, paint and construct flowers, a celebration of beauty. A flower picture may become a kind of family portrait, with each flower representing a member of the family. Often these pictures become a gift for a parent, a favourite teacher, others in the art therapy group, or the art gallery that hosts the program.

### Hearts and Stars and Rainbows

These simple, colourful symbols typically convey love, hope and gratitude, or a wish that may come true. For some children, rainbows have an additional meaning. They may stand for a friend or family member who has passed away.

A bereaved sibling, Cynthia, age six, would occasionally become quiet and reflective, and draw or paint images with rainbows and angels (Figure 18.3). "I really miss Sandy" she would sigh, and we would talk about the qualities she loved about her sibling. She was able to share in images and eventually verbally what she thought heaven was like, and what

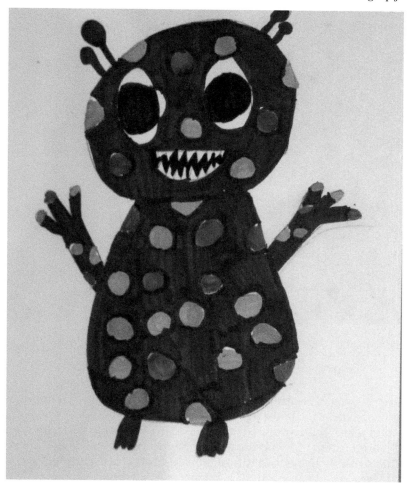

*Figure 18.2* The Alien) (See Plate 2)

she thought her sister was now doing and feeling. At school, Cynthia had been ridiculed for her ideas about heaven and this had been hurtful for her. Cynthia took great comfort in the fact that she could safely mention her deceased sibling with individuals other than her immediate family.

### People

Self-portraits, the family doing something together, characters in stories or movies, or individuals in whom the child is interested figure prominently in the artwork of our group.

Children diagnosed with cancer sometimes create images that express the disappointment of not having the energy to race around and play. Clara, age seven, wanted to portray herself flying a kite. She was very tired and nauseous due to her medication. Her painting showed the kite determinedly soaring through the sky, while Clara herself was lying down and napping. A thin thread connected the figure and the kite. John, age ten,

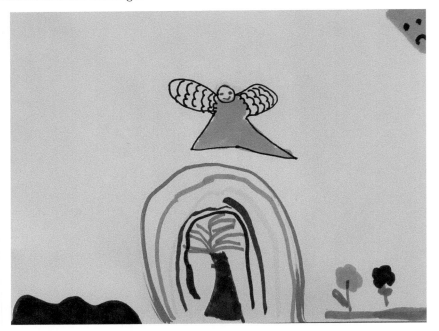

*Figure 18.3* This Small World

made a pencil drawing of recess at his school. All the children were running and jumping and playing ball, except for John, who was seated on the ground. A word bubble asked, "Do you want to play?" John, propped up by the trunk of a big tree, was shown answering, "Not now. I am too tired. . . " The images sparked conversations about the challenge of being grateful for being better, but frustrated at not being entirely well.

Particularly for the siblings, portraits are a way of exploring family relationships. Lucas, age eight, the brother of a child on treatment for leukaemia, painted a picture of his family on vacation. Although he placed himself closest to his mother, he showed himself minuscule in size. Lucas's brother, by way of contrast, was shown as a huge figure, bigger even than Mom. Many raindrops filled the sky. The picture clearly communicated his feelings of insignificance and helplessness in face of his brother's illness.

Bert, age ten, was the bereaved sibling of a child who had died a few months before. Quiet by nature, Bert became even more silent and withdrawn. When his family returned from their customary holiday, Bert drew a picture of his memory of a day at the beach (Figure 18.4). Bert was in the centre of the picture: swimming, just able to keep his head above the tumultuous water. To his left, his mom, exhausted, reclined in a deckchair. To his right, his dad stood upright on a paddleboard. Dad's eyes were on Bert, yet his arms reached up to hold the ballooning parasail. Directly over the sail shone a round yellow sun (son?). Although all were together at the seashore, each family member was facing in a different direction and engaged in a separate activity. The drawing helped Bert convey to himself and his family the heartache of now being the only living child, and the great need to stay connected.

Alice, age seven, employed the art of portraiture to help her understand another sibling in the art therapy group. Alice was shy and thoughtful; Martha, a year older, was

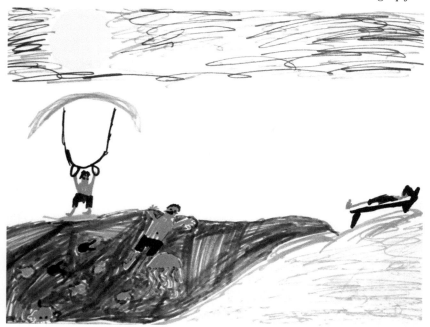

*Figure 18.4* Bert's Family Vacation

energetic, easily distracted and somewhat caustic. Alice not only rendered Martha's physical appearance and mischievous expression, but sought to show Martha's inner thoughts in the plethora of objects and symbols buzzing around her head: cell phones, books, trees, hooks, faces with "real crying and fake crying", hearts (Figure 18.5). The drawing helped create a relationship of respect between the girls. Martha was flattered at being the subject of Alice's sustained attention, and Alice came to know Martha better.

### Boxes

The children in our group are fascinated with boxes. The structure of the containers provides control and safety. Often some kind of treasure is held within: gold sparkles, a loving note. When the lid hides the contents, an element of mystery, secrecy or surprise comes into play. Some boxes are so wrapped in plasticine or twine that they cannot be opened without damaging the box: their secret is not ready to be shared. Frequently the boxes are presents for someone special to the child.

### Buildings

Buildings such as houses, cottages, towers, castles, forts and cathedrals are popular subjects for our group. Some depictions are cosy and inviting; others are imposing or mysterious.

The boys in particular use wooden blocks to build towers of impressive height and majesty, allowing the builders to feel strong and powerful. Often, they will build alongside or with others. The girls usually focus on houses for their pets, or homes for themselves and/or their families. They generally work alongside each other on their own houses, rather

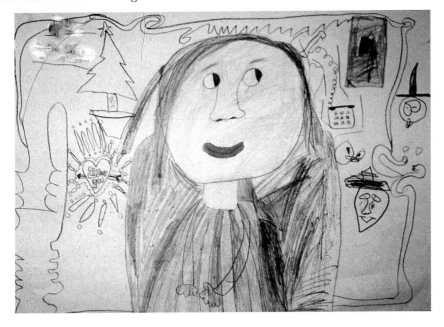

*Figure 18.5* Portrait of Martha

than collaborating. Unlike the boys, who revel in the size and profile of their structures, the girls seem more concerned about the interior comfort and beauty of their buildings. Usually, the bed and a kitchen table are given prime importance. But in one instance, where there had been not only chronic illness but violence in the home, a long narrow space like a shooting gallery was equipped with targets and a helmet and a sword!

### Machines, Instruments and Devices

Packaging materials, tape and glue are regularly repurposed to create new inventions. The children experience the pleasure of transforming "nothing" into something of value. Helmets, tiaras, swords, telescopes and even a "sister trap" (to capture a nosey sibling) have been engineered.

### Vehicles

Cars, trucks, trains and planes are fast and powerful agents of movement and change, and are especially common in the work of boys.

George, age nine, was on treatment for leukaemia. He incessantly drew big black and blue marker pictures of trains, buses, ships and planes. The strong outlines of the vehicles were intertwined with sinister-looking stick figures that hovered inside, outside, above and below. These were robbers, George explained. Over a period of many weeks of robber themes, he began to add law enforcers to his compositions. Eventually, the day came when George drew not only thieves and policemen, but the arrest of the criminals. George was elated! Through his drawings, he had documented his experience of being robbed of a carefree childhood, of receiving help, and finally triumphing.

## Masks

Masks offer the opportunity to temporarily assume another identity. In our group they often show references to animals or superheroes, but they can also signify deeper yearnings for change.

## Nests

Nests in nature are cosy places for eggs or baby birds to flourish and grow. When portrayed in art, the image of the nest reflects a child's perception of home and nurture.

Michael, a nine-year-old child on treatment for leukaemia, enjoyed the tissue paper of birthday and end-of-session gifts more than the art present itself. He tirelessly enacted a scene where he would lie on the ground and cover himself with layers of feather light tissue paper, not only from his own but others' presents. On his request, I would float extra pieces across his face and body. Michael would squeal with delight. Then I would ask wonderingly, "Where's Michael?" A few seconds of silence would ensue. Suddenly, Michael would burst gleefully from his tissue paper nest and cry out, "Here I am!" He would bask in the therapist's apparent wonder and delight to see him appear. The nine-year-old's regression to a much younger age allowed him to experience again and again the relief of being lost and found.

## Landscapes

Some landscapes are green and lush and flowing; others are stark, with skeletal trees, sharp edges and/or snow-capped mountains. They may be painted in broad, thick strokes or meticulously outlined. The outer landscape serves a mirror for the inner world of the child.

Alice, for example, overlapped rich wet brushstrokes of indigo and blue to tell us about her "Everybody hates Alice" day. As the seven-year-old painted, she told us about her horrible feeling of being continually "yelled at" at school. By the time she finished her composition, she had calmed, and proceeded to draw a detailed seating plan of her classroom, so we could visualize exactly who said what and where!

## Food

Renditions of good things to eat show a desire for nurture, and the ability to make things which will feed that hunger. The amount and lushness of the foods often reflects a child's view of how much is available for him or her. One eight-year-old sibling, for example, carefully drew what she called "a banquet". This consisted of a very small banana, one apple and a tiny bunch of grapes on an immense, otherwise empty table.

## Patterns and Dots and Mazes

The artwork of our group often features elaborate pattern-making. In particular, dots are prevalent. The spots or flecks may be playful or jarring, depending on colour and contrast. Often there is a compulsive quality about them. I wonder if the emphasis on blood cells and blood counts in cancer treatment is reflected in this recurring feature in the artwork of our group. Also, chickenpox is feared as a serious complication for those on treatment or newly in recovery, so the dots may echo the dread of this threat.

The dots seem to discharge the restless energy of the child making the dots. They also create a feeling of plenty, and so are soothing to children who have experienced lack. When incorporated into mazes, dots denote tracks to follow and portals to open.

### Split Compositions

Frequently children will create pictures or sculptures divided into two halves. For example, a landscape may show two identical trees, each at a different time of day.

Ginny, age eleven, a survivor of cancer, covered one side of her mask in soft dabs of pale blue, violet and green; the other side was splashed with heavy streaks of silver and gold. She proudly explained that "although [her] illness had created obvious hardships, it also created precious benefits". She chose to embrace these qualities, Ginny said, because it has made her a compassionate loving person.

### Games

Sometimes children will collaborate to create a game. It may feature fortune-telling, sports, a traditional board game format or a popular video game such as Minecraft. The games' combination of luck and skill is a potent reminder of life's up and downs. Satisfaction for the children lies in the fact that at last they have the opportunity to say what counts, which "upgrades" can be contracted, and what the name of the game is. "Maze of Time" and "Haunted House" are not surprising choices of title for a child that has endured repeated MRIs!

## Work Discarded by the Child

Most of the art created in the art therapy group is proudly taken home by the children. Occasionally, a piece is left behind or remains unfinished. These discarded works almost always contain written words. It is my theory that the children, upon reflection, find the words to be too harsh or revealing. They may be afraid of hurting their family's feelings. Also, by parting with these works, the children let go of the pain and heavy weight associated with them.

For example, one day Angela, aged eight, a bereaved sibling, decided to write a story. She chose a quill pen and black ink, painfully scratching each letter into the hard cartridge paper. The sharp metal nib and fluid ink were tricky to handle, and blobs of ink spattered between and across the words. Angela's story was short but eloquent: "*Once a pone uptime there was a girl how was lost and never found her mom and dad, her parintes did not care anymore and one Day she found her Parintes. the End*". When she had finished, Angela read her story out loud to me. I concurred that being lost and unnoticed must have been very difficult for the girl. Slowly the conversation turned to the challenges of having a brother or sister with cancer. At the end of the session, Angela quietly placed her paper into the recycling bin. It appeared she was ready for a new story.

## General Observations About Issues With Which the Children are Struggling

Erikson postulates that the latency years, from ages six to eleven, are a period when children particularly enjoy the satisfaction of being able to do things. Self-esteem develops from being able to master skills and processes (Erikson, 1950). Art therapy meets children's desires to participate and be productive by providing opportunities to engage in activities that are a bit challenging, yet not overwhelming. Thereby, the perfect conditions for "flow", or creative thought, are created (Csikszentmihalyi & Csikzentmihalyi, 1988).

By creating a safe, supportive environment, establishing a strong therapeutic relationship and encouraging the spontaneous creation of artwork, the art therapy process accesses children's inner worlds and so can establish a timely support for the "emotional rollercoaster of experiences" (Shapiro & Brack, 1994).

## Response to the Spontaneous Art Therapy Program

The response to our Candlelighters Simcoe art therapy program has been overwhelmingly positive. Attendance is exemplary, with children missing sessions only when illness, a medical appointment or dangerous weather conditions intervene.

Through personal interviews and brief written surveys, parents and children have shared their thoughts and feelings about the program. Key factors for the program's success are cited as the opportunity for expression through art, the welcoming atmosphere of the art therapy group and the accepting attitude of the art therapist. Observed benefits for participants include increased self-esteem and confidence, decreased anger and anxiety, improved coping strategies, better communication and social skills, greater flexibility and greater ability to focus and stay in the moment. In several instances, a passion for making art was discovered, and the pursuit of Fine Arts in college and university studies was ascribed to children's participation in the art therapy program.

## Support for the Art Therapist

A key factor in supporting my art therapy work has been the ongoing consultation and collaboration with the Candlelighters Simcoe parent liaison, Barb Johnson. As well, I regularly seek out clinical supervision with registered members of the Canadian Art Therapy Association, and engage in the professional development offered by our national and provincial art therapy associations and by the Toronto Art Therapy Institute. A daily practice of mindfulness meditation and hatha yoga helps me cultivate inner calm and optimism, while my studio practice of painting in oil and cold wax allows me to personally benefit from expression through art. Strong roots in the Barrie community and its institutions and organizations create a context of caring and sharing. Swimming, kayaking and hiking at our island cottage on Georgian Bay provide much appreciated restorative time with family and friends.

## Conclusion

In the Candlelighters Simcoe spontaneous art group for children affected by paediatric cancer, participants are provided with the opportunity to take respite from the relentless stress and overwhelming ups and downs created by chronic illness in the family. Children are encouraged to reflect on their own unique situations, and give tangible and visible form to their feelings and ideas. Externalizing and working through the anxiety or pain develops a capacity to sit with uncomfortable feelings; naming the artwork and/or talking about it creates further inner shifts. Sensitivity to not only the art materials but to others grows. By "coming up for air" from their busy days, the children not only experience relief from distressing emotions, but the opportunity to tell their personal stories. A new sense of confidence and well-being emerges.

# References

Canadian Cancer Society. (2016). *Childhood cancer statistics—Canadian Cancer Society.* Available at www.cancer.ca/en/cancer information/cancer 101/childhood cancer statistics/?region=on [accessed 14 September 2016]

Canadian Healthcare. (2004–2007). Available at www.canadian-healthcare.org/page8.html [accessed 14 September 2016]

Canadian Institute for Health Information. (1996–2016). *National Health Expenditure Database metadata,* CIHI. [online] Available at www.cihi.ca/en/spending-and-health-workforce/spending/health-spending-data/national-health-expenditure-database [accessed 14 September 2016].

*Candlelighters Simcoe: Parents of children with cancer.* (2013). Available at www.candlelighterssimcoe.ca [accessed 14 September 2016].

Chapman, L. et al. (2001). "The Effectiveness of Art Therapy Interventions in Reducing Post Traumatic Stress Disorder (PTSD) Symptoms in Pediatric Trauma Patients". *Art Therapy: Journal of the American Art Therapy Association,* 18 (2).

Csikszentmihalyi, M., Csikzentmihalyi, I. (1988). *Optimal experience: Psychological studies of flow in consciousness.* Cambridge: Cambridge University Press.

Erikson, E. (1950). *Childhood and society.* New York: W.W. Norton.

Huchcroft, S., Clarke, A., Mao, Y., Desmeules, M., Dryer, D., Hodges, M., Leclerc, J.-M., McBride, M., Pelletier, W., Yanofsky, R. (1996). *This battle which i must fight: Cancer in Canada's children and teenagers.* Ottawa: Supply and Services Canada.

Malchiodi, C.A. (ed.) (1999). *Medical art therapy with children.* London: Jessica Kingsley.

McKnight, C.M. (2001). *Coming up for Air: Art therapy with children whose family members have or have had cancer.* Unpublished thesis, Toronto Art Therapy Institute.

Nolbris, M., Abrahamsson, J., Hellström, L., Olofsson, L., Enskär, K. (2010). "The Experience of Therapeutic Support Groups by Siblings of Children with Cancer". *Pediatric Nursing,* 36 (6), 298–304.

Shapiro, M., Brack, G. (1994). "Psychosocial Aspects of Siblings' Experiences of Pediatric Cancer". *Elementary School Guidance and Counseling,* 28 (4), 264–274.

# 19 An Art Therapist's Approach to Total Pain

*Sarah Yazdian Rubin*

## Introduction

Palliative care is a natural home for an art therapist. Art therapists and palliative care providers share a common ethos that is rooted in a holistic, relationship-based philosophy in caring for the Whole Person. I am proud to have helped establish the Marilyn E. Baker Creative Arts Therapy Program at the Hertzberg Palliative Care Institute at Mount Sinai Hospital in New York City in 2011. Working as a dually certified Creative Arts Therapist and Child Life Specialist within an exceptional inpatient interdisciplinary team has been a great professional privilege and personal honor. Collectively, our team serves from a place of deep inquiry, witnessing, and advocacy for those we care for.

Dr. Eric Cassell, an early pioneer of the palliative care movement who emphasizes in-depth communication as a hallmark of palliative care once said:

> Similar to scalpels for surgeons, words are the palliative care clinician's greatest tools. Surgeons learn to use their tools with extreme precision, because any error can be devastating. So too should clinicians who rely on words.
>
> (as cited in Wolfe, Hinds, and Sourkes, p. 3, 2011)

But how can palliative care teams serve patients and families when there are no words? When a person loses their ability to speak due to illness or trauma? When people feel silenced, unseen or unheard? Those with *Total Pain*—pain that encompasses physical, social, psychological, and spiritual realms—often require multiple avenues of expressive communication, opening an entry for the creative arts therapist to provide support.

## Total Pain

Pain—the most common and distressing symptom reported by seriously ill patients—is a complex phenomenon that is subjective, complex, and in constant flux (Chai et al, 2014). Founder of the modern hospice and palliative care movement, Dame Cecily Saunders, formulated the concept of Total Pain in 1964—the multifaceted experience of suffering that encompasses physical, psychological, social, and spiritual dimensions of distress. The concept of Total Pain articulates the relationships between dimensions of distress and how this impacts suffering. Total Pain may engulf individuals at various points throughout an illness trajectory, particularly if they are confronting death and dying (Saunders & Baines, 1983). Due to its complexity, Total Pain requires interdisciplinary intervention (Meier & Beresford, 2008) but can be difficult to treat in the acute care hospital, a setting that typically prioritizes medical interventions.

## Art Therapy and Total Pain

From the beginning of time and in every culture, humans have had the need to create to connect, document, and make meaning of their world. One of the reasons art is so powerful in one's experience of loss is that it has the ability to give voice to experience, transcend time, be preserved and shared with generations to come. In the face of loss, and in a web of Total Pain, art therapy provides integrative, facilitative, and creative approaches that hold powerful healing effects.

Figure 19.1 demonstrates how an art therapist may work with patients and families using the framework of Total Pain. While the diagram neatly categorizes four realms that comprise Total Pain, each are interconnected and there is much overlap. Despite universal experiences, people are fundamentally individual in how they experience pain; therefore, each treatment plan, therapeutic relationship and intervention cannot be generalized. This diagram provides a common language for the interdisciplinary team and can serve as a road map to help practitioners facilitate Total Pain relief.

Total Pain cannot solely be treated by an art therapist, or any one team member. However, for the purposes of this chapter, I will illustrate how an art therapist may approach physical, psychological, social, and spiritual domains of Total Pain through case vignettes. The case vignettes highlight specific interventions within a case, rather than the full art therapy trajectory with the patient. Collaboration with team members occurred with all cases presented, although this aspect of care is beyond the scope of this chapter. The cases presented in this chapter will demonstrate how addressing one facet of Total Pain oftentimes leads to other areas of one's pain experience to unfold, emphasizing the interconnections and impact between Total Pain domains.

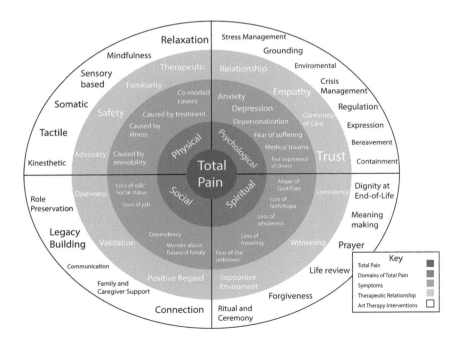

*Figure 19.1* Four Realms of Total Pain

## Physical Pain

Physical pain is a subjective experience with both sensory and emotional components that may be caused by illness, treatment, and various comorbidities. Different types of physical pain—nociceptive, somatic, visceral, neuropathic—can be acute, chronic or terminal, and are managed differently depending on etiology. Etiology of pain is determined through history, assessment of pain, and exams (Chai et al, 2014). For many patients, physical pain cannot be treated with analgesics alone, as emotional pain may manifest physically and exacerbate physical pain. Within the context of end-of-life care, patients experience various parts and systems of the body shutting down (Chai et al, 2014). It is widely accepted that non-pharmacological and cognitive behavioral interventions including complementary and alternative modalities help patients manage and cope with physical pain (Chai et al, 2014). Bolstering one's emotional reserves may impact a person's perception and tolerance of physical pain.

The body is the vehicle through which we think, feel, behave, act, and relate to others. It holds memory in tissue and is the home of one's spirit. The concept of embodied experience acknowledges the body's central place in our personal lives— "the body is not just skin and bones, an assemblage of parts, a medical marvel . . . the body is also, and primarily, the self. We are all embodied" (Synnott, 2001, p. 1). Physical symptoms from illness, treatment, and restriction of physical movement greatly affect the body, and may elicit emotional responses including body dissociation, loss of control, distrust towards and abandonment by one's body.

The creative process is a visceral experience that requires engagement of the body and thus, may emphasize the significance of body in one's experience of illness. The tactile, kinesthetic, and multisensory nature of art materials may be a welcome and pleasurable experience, and support exploration around senses and bodily experiences relating to illness. Art therapy and other mind-body interventions are designed to facilitate the mind's capacity to affect bodily function and symptoms (Nccih.nih.gov). While not all physical symptoms may be appropriate for mind-body interventions, many of these approaches are integrative, non-pharmacological and complement existing medical treatments. The following case demonstrates how one patient used art therapy to cope with physical pain.

### Wilber

Wilber was a bold 36-year-old man who was hospitalized with Crohn's disease for over 200 days. He was bedbound with painful post-surgical fistulas in his groin area and had a history of noncompliance. His refusal of wound care prevented healing and caused physical pain, despite medication. He had developed strained relationships with most of his care team and was labeled a "difficult patient". Wilber was transferred to the palliative care unit for transition planning, goals of care and symptom management. Art therapy was a part of his treatment plan.

Wilber was reluctant to engage initially and tried very hard to reject anyone who displayed an interest in caring for him, including me. Chronic illness and restricted physical movement impacted Wilber's sense of being in the world and was the source of his anger. Most of his early artwork exemplified how he pushed people away. His first piece of art was a sign for his door that read "KNOCK HARDER, AND WAIT FOR AN ANSWER!" Slowly, Wilber began to trust me, and discovered that he could appropriately express his anger using art. Over time he began looking forward to art therapy. He enjoyed being creative and began to demonstrate interest in self-regulation and pain management, especially during wound changes.

I suggested that we make a mask together using art materials and medical materials (gauze and Vaseline). Incorporating gauze and Vaseline in mask making would introduce these materials in a non-medical scenario, and hopefully neutralize his associations to the items associated with wound care. The mask intervention would also require Wilber to tolerate touch, another necessary aspect of wound care, and use a mirror, which Wilber had avoided for many months. Our therapeutic relationship and boundaries created safety that allowed Wilber to tolerate this multifaceted intervention.

When I first applied Vaseline to Wilber's face, he appeared relaxed, but when we began placing strips to create the mask, especially near his mouth, Wilber became anxious about not being able to speak. I introduced deep breathing techniques, and encouraged him to verbally express how he was feeling. He also asked me for an approximate time when the mask would be dry for removal, which helped manage expectations. I brought to Wilber's attention that the strategies he was using to cope with uncomfortable feelings during mask making could also be utilized during dressing changes. This was a breakthrough for Wilber.

Our trusting therapeutic relationship and the intimacy of this specific intervention generated safety that translated towards the rest of the interdisciplinary team. He began allowing wound care and took a more active role in his care, which allowed him to safely be discharged from the hospital. Wilber often requested art therapy to follow dressing changes to self-sooth. During these sessions, we explored metaphorical masks that Wilber wore throughout his hospitalization, and when it was safe, and necessary, to take these masks off. He also created other art pieces with themes of protection, including a shield, that he took with him when he was discharged to a rehab facility. His last art piece was a letter of gratitude that he hand-signed and delivered to each staff person involved in his care.

The relaxation and coping strategies learned during mask making helped Wilber during painful dressing changes. Working with his body in art therapy, specifically skin (the body's boundary), stimulated much symbolic work about boundaries of his body and his world. Active creation, tactile stimulation, the use of a mirror and safe touch enabled Wilber to reconnect to his self and body in a non-injurious way. This was essential in his quest to work through issues of passivity, helplessness, and shame. The mask, representing both self and object, allowed Wilber to simultaneously examine and gain distance from his experience. Our therapeutic alliance, which was strengthened by the mask-making intervention, allowed Wilber to explore the relationship between his wounded physicality and the loss of his sexual and reproductive organs, and how this impacted his identity as a man—all of which was labeled as 'physical pain'. Addressing physical pain was a safe starting point that led Wilber to address other aspects of his Total Pain experience.

## Psychological Pain

People with serious illness and chronic pain commonly experience anxiety, depression, adjustment disorders, and other psychiatric symptoms throughout an illness trajectory. In the palliative care setting, anxiety may affect as many as 25% of patients (Chai et al, 2014, p. 333). For those with advanced or life-limiting illness, 75% of patients experience depression (Chai et al, 2014, p. 325). Untreated anxiety and depression severely impact quality of life, and may be treated with pharmacological and non-pharmacological interventions (Chai et al, 2014).

Several aspects of one's illness experience can contribute to psychological distress. Hospitalization, with its own sensory challenges, complex terminology, and medical culture can render people disoriented and socially isolated, dismantling support systems and interrupting existing coping strategies. Medical trauma, or medical traumatic stress, is the psychological and physiological response to pain, injury, illness, medical procedures, and invasive or frightening treatment experiences (NCTSN.org). People with histories of psychiatric disorders or trauma may be re-traumatized by illness or treatment; a research study on portrait therapy for patients with life-limiting illness revealed that those with childhood trauma expressed the need to heal this trauma when facing end of life (Carr & Hancock, 2017). While social workers and other psychosocial professionals follow patients throughout hospitalization, traditional psychotherapeutic supports in the hospital setting are often limited.

Loss is another aspect of illness that causes psychological pain. Patients who are at the end-of-life face multiple losses including health, functional ability, relationships that give life meaning, independence and control, and sometimes, life itself. People with advanced illness may feel demoralized and appropriately grieve theses losses, referred to as anticipatory grief. When a person with life-limiting illness realizes that life is limited, he or she may experience the 'existential slap' (Coyle, 2004), of which any illusion of security that previously existed is shattered. For palliative care providers, the challenge is to not pathologize grief and responses to loss; equally, providers need not neglect to treat impairing symptoms using medication (Janberidze, 2014). In the setting of serious illness, differentiating between these two experiences can be difficult. The following case demonstrates how one patient used art therapy to cope with psychological pain.

### Alicia

Alicia was a virtuous, soft-spoken 23-year-old woman who was diagnosed with an advanced gastric cancer following a misdiagnosis of pregnancy. Despite high doses of opiates, her pain was largely uncontrolled and the team suspected that anxiety, depression, and existential fears contributed to Total Pain. Alicia was always clutching her Patient Controlled Analgesia (PCA) button, an opiate delivery system and comforting solution to her pain, and pushed it frequently each hour, especially when she felt anxious. She agreed to art therapy to manage psychological symptoms and to support expression around anticipatory grief.

Alicia experimented with several art media though she gravitated towards clay. She responded to the pliability of the material and enjoyed shaping the clay. Comparing the clay to her corporeal form, Alicia poked and prodded the material, perhaps working through the poking and prodding she endured during her treatment. Carving into clay was a powerful nonverbal experience that supported mastery and reversed her passive stance as a patient to an active one. At the end of our first session, Alicia observed that she could take deeper breaths when working with the clay, and stated that the clay, and our conversations, helped her when she felt anxious. She expressed feeling grounded by the clay's "earthy scent" and was able to put her PCA button down while she sculpted. During our sessions, she decreased PCA use to just one push per hour.

Several months later, Alicia was no longer a candidate for chemotherapy and she enrolled in home hospice care. Despite this, her family rarely acknowledged Alicia's dying, which heightened Alicia's anxiety. She felt that she was "leaving her family" and yet, did not know how to begin the process of saying goodbye. At this point in her treatment, art therapy transformed into a safe enclosure for Alicia to explore dying.

Alicia decided to create clay ornaments for her family members, knowing that the upcoming holiday would be her last with them. She also made an ornament for herself, an important statement of her personhood. As she sculpted a heart, an airplane and other meaningful shapes, Alicia shared the symbolism of her choices. I bore witness as Alicia tearfully acknowledged her dying by articulating her hope that her parents would "be okay". In creating ornaments for her family members, Alicia began telling stories and reminiscing, creating space for life review.

Life review is a reminiscing process whereby an individual reviews and makes meaning around life events and relationships, and allows memories to heal and create acceptance (Atkinson, 2002). Importantly, the life review process can help family members, caregivers, and staff to become more aware of the past, present, and future concerns of the dying individual, and thus become more understanding and supportive (Pickrel, 1989). Alicia would oftentimes invite family members to join art therapy sessions, allowing her to share concerns, and allowing family to acknowledge her need to talk about her dying.

When Alicia's ornaments returned from the kiln, she discovered that the two ornaments she created for her parents had cracked. She found this symbolic and explored their feelings of brokenness in losing a child. Alicia decided to repair the ornaments, and in doing so, realized that she played an essential role in her family's healing process, despite her dying.

Of note, I also sculpted a small ornament that I would later give Alicia, to mirror to her own experience of creating and gifting. I was also searching for a way within my professional relationship to express love and gratitude. Sculpting clay alongside her sent a message that I was joining her in her creative efforts and reduced power dynamics that oftentimes mark clinical interactions between patients and staff. This was crucial in supporting Alicia to continue this emotionally challenging project.

During our final art therapy session, Alicia shared her plan to gift her handmade creations when she arrived home. I gifted her the ornament I made for her and expressed my gratitude for her openness to me in times of great pain and vulnerability. Alicia expressed gratitude for our companionship, which "gave her strength". As we said our tearful goodbyes, Alicia realized that our last session served as a rehearsal space for future goodbyes.

Art therapy became a powerful avenue for Alicia to cope with psychological distress, loss, and grief throughout her illness journey. The properties of the clay material—malleable,

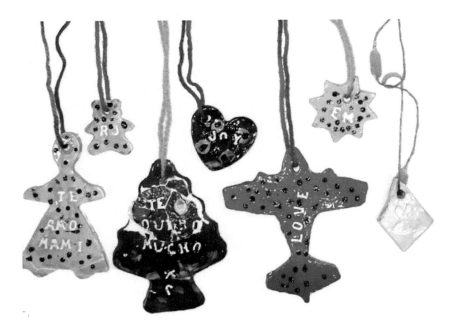

*Figure 19.2* Clay Ornaments (Alicia)

flexible, organic, transformative—served her in nonverbal ways that allowed for deeper processing of her bodily experiences and role within her family unit. Alicia enhanced her connection and awareness with her body, herself and her family through her intentional creations. Her handmade objects supported transparent communication around her dying process and eventually, facilitated the painful yet sacred act of saying goodbye. Art therapy was initially utilized to address psychological symptoms, however it ultimately impacted Alicia from physical, social, and spiritual standpoints.

## Social Pain

Palliative Care practitioners aim to improve quality of life for both patients and their family or caregivers (Chai et al, 2014). Caregiving is known to be a burdensome task, physically, emotionally, and financially. Poor sleep, exhaustion, disrupted activity, sadness, guilt, inadequacy, and resentment are common experiences of caregivers and are associated with increased health problems and mortality (Chai et al, 2014). The concept of reciprocal suffering—the correlation between a patient's suffering and family's suffering—underscores social components of Total Pain. Sherman's (1998) research on reciprocal suffering supports the importance of assessing family dynamics and quality of life intervention for patients' caregivers as an avenue to support patients themselves. Those that provide direct care, and young children, are two groups within a patient's social circle who have unique needs that art therapists are positioned to support.

Patients with young children have unique practical, psychosocial, and existential challenges. In addition to coping with his/her illness experience, parents are tasked with the responsibility to support their children's coping efforts, share information, prepare for life transitions, and, if necessary, engage in permanency planning and legal meetings regarding guardianship.

One of the most common sources of Total Pain for seriously ill patients with young children is the welfare of their children (Greisinger et al, 1997; Cater et al, 2004; Helseath & Ulfsaet, 2005).

There are multiple barriers when identifying and treating the needs of children of hospitalized palliative care patients, including palliative care clinicians not feeling equipped and the lack of training and experience in counseling children and their relatives (Fearnley, 2010; Sutter & Reid, 2012). Children are especially vulnerable to the repercussions of illness due to their cognitive and emotional capacity, developmental immaturity and developing coping capabilities. A child's vulnerability may be compounded by well-intended caretakers, who may be preoccupied with their own grief, and unable to provide adequate support to the child (Krupnick, 1984).

Children's responses may be overlooked, and art therapy presence within an interdisciplinary team brings children's needs to the forefront. Art therapy is often more effective with children compared with traditional verbal-based techniques implemented by other psychosocial team members. Art therapy and child life collaboration fill a much-needed gap on palliative care teams in working with social pain, specifically addressing psychosocial needs of children.

In my experience, patients who request art therapy for their children appear more at ease knowing that their children are receiving additional support during their hospitalization. Likewise, patients who engage in legacy-building activities with or for their children or caregivers report feelings of catharsis and needed release. Legacy-building interventions are experiences and tangible products that support life review, storytelling, and other meaningful connection before or after a death, and throughout a bereavement process. Literature suggests that legacy projects have shown several significant patient benefits, including decreased breathing difficulties, greater social interaction, distraction from pain and negative thoughts, preparation for end of life, increased religious meaning, greater appreciation for self, improved family communication, and decreased caregiver stress (Allen, 2009; Walsh et al, 2004). Legacy projects may be facilitated between patients and loved ones, or created specifically for a loved one by a patient. This portion of the chapter will present a family caregiver case vignette, and a case vignette with young children to show how an art therapist may address social pain.

### Michael's Family

Michael was a vibrant, healthy 19-year-old man who suffered a traumatic brain injury and cardiac arrest after being struck by a vehicle while riding his bicycle. Over five months, Michael suffered several hospital-acquired infections, multiple brain hemorrhages and was ventilator dependent. He was eventually transferred to the palliative care unit for comfort measures, where the family elected for palliative extubation (the removal of the endotracheal tube), expecting him to live only hours to days post extubation. Art therapy was initially considered for short-term legacy work with Michael's family, who were at very high risk for complicated grief, a chronic and heightened state of mourning.

Michael was unresponsive when he arrived to our unit. Our team's main focus was supporting the needs of his family, who presented as emotionally paralyzed and hyper focused on his vitals displayed on the monitors. I introduced a legacy intervention of creating a hand mold in hopes of shifting the family's focus from his respiratory rate and other numbers, to reconnecting with him as a person and his spirit. Laden with symbolism, a commemorative hand mold involves imprinting a casted relief of a hand, filling the mold with plaster, and then peeling away the mold to discover the life-like relief of the person's hand. The process encourages therapeutic touch and gives the family a poignant opportunity to interact with him and sanctify his life. Each of Michael's family members created their own mold of his hand, and told stories of him throughout the process. Michael's mother realized that this art piece would serve as a comforting transitional object, as she expressed "I will be able touch Michael's hand and feel his presence even after his death".

Art therapy took on a new dimension for the family when Michael was in a comatose state for three weeks following extubation. Each morning, the art therapy session itself became a ritual, where the family used art to connect with Michael in various ways. Specifically, creating dream catchers was an impactful art therapy intervention for this family. Historically, Native American dream catchers hang over the bed to protect the sleeper from nightmares, catching harmful thoughts in its web and allowing healing dreams to pass through the center circle. As Michael slept, his family wove intricate webs at his bedside. His mother brought in shells that Michael had collected to hang from the dream catchers, bringing forth specific memories of Michael when he was well. Believing that his body was "merely a shell", Michael's sister Haley explored ways to be in relationship with her brother in his transitional dying process using the dream catchers. Haley shared that the symbolism of dream catchers resonated with her: "Creating dream catchers allowed me to bond with my brother. I would imagine that they were catching all of his bad dreams as he was sleeping. I was able to work through a lot of my emotions when I was weaving and I feel that a piece of him is in each of those dream catchers".

Nurses, doctors, and chaplains joined the family, combing through beads and mosaics for their dream catchers, learning about Michael's life. Several medical staff commented that they felt most helpful to the family when they engaged in art-making with them.

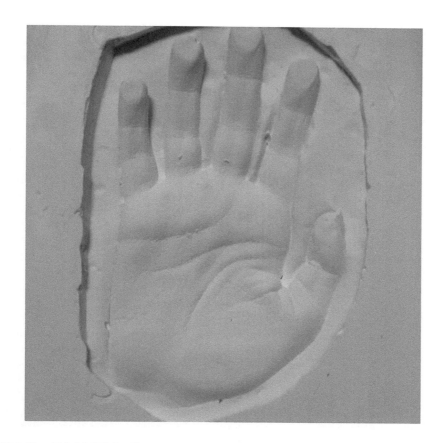

*Figure 19.3* Hand Mold (Michael)

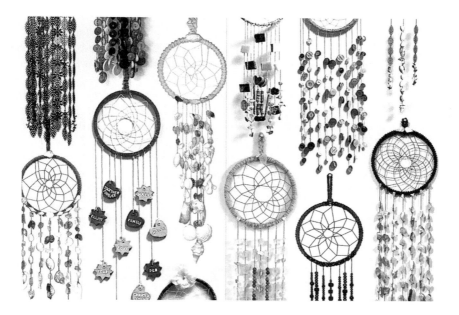

*Figure 19.4* Dream Catchers (Michael)

A special community was created at Michael's bedside as we all draped dream catchers on the walls and windows, wishing to cloak Michael in protection as he slept.

The way in which Michael's family members used art materials revealed their determination to find—and create—moments of hope, connection, and meaning. Michael's family used art therapy to cultivate spaces of spirit, ritual, relationship, and community to cope with the pain of losing their child, sibling, and best friend. Michael's family was held by their art experiences, and reciprocally, their art objects held their multifaceted expressions of life, loss, and love.

After Michael passed away, the family submitted their artwork to our creative arts journal, *The Loom*, which features original work by patients, families, caregivers, and staff. The journal serves as a therapeutic container that allows both families and staff to revisit the creative work of loved ones. Participating in *The Loom* allowed a unique opportunity for Michael's family to memorialize him, safeguard his memory, and perhaps, create another place to visit and remember him. Michael's sister Haley also participated in our art-based memorial service for young people who lost a parent or sibling, a collaboration between art therapy and chaplaincy, which allowed her to share her relationship with her brother with others who were also grieving.

### Julie and Her Children

Julie was a lovely and determined 45-year-old woman and mother of two school-aged children, who was hospitalized and dying of cancer. Throughout her illness, Julie and her husband courageously engaged her children in conversations about her illness, and felt strongly that she would prepare them for her death. The family responded to family art therapy, which became rich experiences for communication and family unity, and preserved their respective roles of mother and children. Julie also requested individual art therapy for her children so they could process their fears within a therapeutic context. The children's anthropomorphic houses and crying rain clouds expressed feelings of sadness that they were not able to verbalize.

As part of preparation for her children and preserving her memory, Julie responded willingly to my suggestions of legacy building. She participated in StoryCorps interview with a close friend, which allowed her to orally record her life story (storycorps.org/legacy). In the interview, Julie directly addressed her children, recounted her experience of their births, and shared life lessons and joyful family moments. Below is an excerpt from the recording:

*I guess I would want them to know that certainly marrying their father was the best thing I ever did. And I feel very confident that he will keep me alive in the same way that my dad kept my mom alive, that he'll tell stories, and he'll make fun of me, and tell them how slow I was at eating, and all the tissues that I used to leave around the apartment. So I know that he will do that for me, and so I feel—I take great comfort in that. I think also my own experience of having lost my parents I know that you can go through great sadness and still be a very happy person. So I'm happy for them that they will have that, but it does make me sad as well to know that I'll be missing big moments in their lives, their weddings. But I know that Craig will find a way to get me there.*

Julie shared that the recording, albeit difficult and emotionally taxing, was cathartic. Knowing that the interview would be available to their children brought comfort to her in her final months of life.

Working with families who have young children, as was the case with Julie, can bring up past experiences that require exploration. The impact of illness summons vulnerability, and may evoke "childlike" feelings and experiences of one's "inner child" that highlights the need for security, protection, and trust from others (Jung, 1993). A patient's own experiences of developmental trauma in childhood also impacts how he or she provides support around dying for their children (Capacchione, 1991). Julie's experiences of losing her parents as a young person, and dying with young children, were the topic of many of our conversations. These conversations affirmed her roles and identity of both daughter and mother.

During Julie's final hospitalization, she and her husband planned for each of their children to have time alone with Julie to say goodbye. Julie asked for art materials for these final moments. I supplied the clay and tools, and then excused myself, respecting the family's need for privacy. I remained available to the children and to Julie in the days that followed, and kept the objects safe until Julie's husband felt ready to return to the hospital to collect the artwork, a month following her death. Julie's husband shared that art therapy created many special experiences for the family that they would cherish in years to come.

## Spiritual Pain

Understanding the spiritual dimension of a patient's life is an integral part of healthcare. Spirituality can be difficult to clearly define because it means different things to different people. Generally speaking, spirituality is the aspect of humanity that refers to the way individuals seek and express meaning and purpose. Likewise, it refers to the way people experience connection to the moment, to self, to others, to nature and to the significant or sacred (Puchalski et al, 2009).

Illness can cause spiritual distress, which is associated with anxiety, depression, increased mortality (Puchalski et al, 2009), and renders people demoralized and less whole. Doka (2014) writes that in finding meaning in life, spiritual, and existential needs are often accentuated as clients face death (p. 219). Providing spiritual care involves responding to needs of the human spirit and supporting individuals as they reconstitute their global meaning of life.

Art-making specifically is permeated with transcendent, ephemeral, and non-materialistic qualities of experience that support patients to explore spirituality. Symbolic language may enable transformation, "revealed truth" and existential questions to surface, bringing into awareness what is subconscious or hidden. The interpretative nature of looking at a piece of art further facilitates personal meaning making and spirituality (Bell, 2011). Art therapists working in palliative care have described art therapy as a form of "spiritual medicine" (McNiff, 2004) to "awaken spiritual realities" (Bell, 2011), "cast the spirit" (Rutenberg, 2008), "create sanctuary", "leave traces", and "find one's way home" (Fenton, 2008). Finding meaning through illness and at the end of life is no small endeavor; it takes courage, commitment, and conviction to reflect upon and take ownership of one's existence.

Creative processes and spiritual expression have many similarities and can become intertwined in a clinical setting. Music, art, prayer, meditation, community, and ritual are just some of the shared practices and resources of this blended domain. The role of ritual in particular is significant to consider in palliative care. Rutenberg cites a quote by Seftel (2006) that "rituals provide a focal point of awareness that we are moving through an obstacle, transitioning to a new sense of self, or letting go of something lost" (Rutenberg, 2008, p. 109). In the hospital setting, daily or weekly art therapy sessions may morph into rituals themselves (as was the case with Michael's family), creating space within an environment that so often neglects the person living with disease.

This portion of the chapter aims to exemplify how spiritual needs may be met in art therapy, and specifically, how the creative process can enable a patient to transcend discomfort to experience the self that is whole, intact, growing, and living. The following case demonstrates how art therapy bolstered one patient's faith and supported spiritual healing.

### Kyla

Kyla, a thoughtful and resilient 31-year-old woman, was diagnosed with osteosarcoma after a pathologic femur fracture. I met her a month into her hospitalization as she was beginning chemotherapy before limb-salvaging surgery. At this time, Kyla was bedbound, with a cast that spanned from her hip to her ankle. Her physical mobility was severely limited. She enjoyed art and agreed to art therapy as a part of her treatment plan.

Her first oil pastel drawing was of a sea with a super moon above. She worked silently but shared with me that she did not know what she was making. All she could think about was a deep sea. We spoke more about her sea—its vastness, depth, and unknown elements. Kyla began to cry. Her art, a version of an "underworld", had brought subconscious feelings to the surface, giving voice to her fear. With one wave, her body could be consumed, disfigured, broken. Together we identified metaphorical buoys for rest and recovery—her family and friends, and her faith. Spending days and weeks away from her home, we also

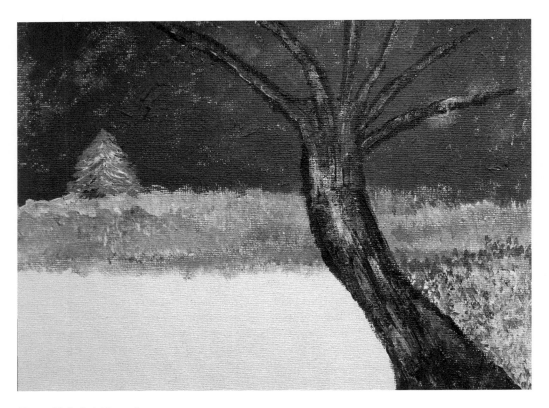

*Figure 19.5* Oak Trees 1

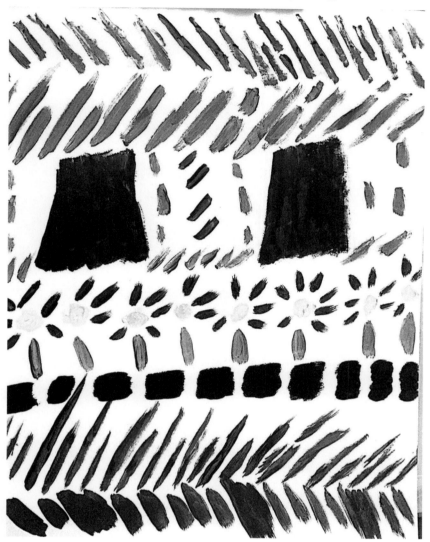

*Figure 19.6* Oak Trees 2

explored the power of place—physical places and ones created in our hearts, minds, and through prayer.

Nature emerged as a recurring theme in Kyla's artwork. Confined to her bed as she spoke about her illness-related losses (her job, her home, her ability to walk, her appetite, her independence), Kyla's artwork transported her to faraway places that were safe and vibrant. She began creating "scapes" in her artwork that grounded her in nature, her faith, and her values. She gravitated towards collage and reflected on how collaging related to her lived experience of wholeness: "collage became a deep reminder that I could make something beautiful out of broken fragments. I start out with pieces, but through creativity and faith, they always come together in the end", Kyla shared.

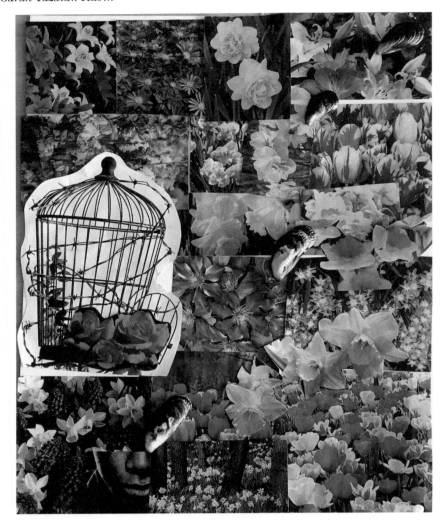

*Figure 19.7* Oak Trees 3

Oak trees became a prominent symbol that represented strength and growth. She identified with these trees—how they swayed instead of snapped in extreme weather conditions, how their extensive root systems grew as deep as the tree's height and as wide as its branches. In her paintings and in collages, an oak tree would almost always appear, reminding her of her own "rooting". We even co-created an oak tree that spanned her leg cast, which concealed her body's "trunk". Humming as she worked, Kyla drew a hole in the tree trunk over the site of her tumor, and asked family and friends to write their signatures on the bottom to form the roots of her oak. As we worked on her cast, she spoke of her faith in things unseen, and prayed that healing was happening underneath the cast— "like roots, you trust that they are there, anchoring".

Kyla's images and conversations oftentimes brought light to the paradoxical nature of existence—life and death, hope and despair, relation and isolation, absence, and presence. Art-making helped Kyla mark the liminal and threshold states (Turner, 1995) as well as the rites of passage (Van Gennep, 1960) that marked her cancer experience.

Undergoing chemotherapy but holding the possibility of leg amputation, Kyla was betwixt and between two worlds, and used art to ground her in the present moment. Despite the pain and suffering, Kyla searched and found lessons from her diagnosis. She reflected on familial relationships that healed because of cancer, her "angels on earth", and her experience of giving and receiving support. Most of all, she reflected on the necessity to "embrace brokenness" in her journey towards wholeness.

Kyla tapped into an inner resource of creativity that allowed for spiritual healing and post-traumatic growth. Art therapy became sacred space, Kyla's metaphor became a vehicle for healing, and her art became prayer. A faithful individual, cancer shook Kyla's belief system to its core. Through her identity as an artist, Kyla discovered personal agency to make meaning of her cancer experience. Her psychospiritual achievement of integrating cancer into her life transcended disease or a cure.

## A Note on Staff Pain

An African proverb states: "If you want to travel quickly, go alone. But if you want to travel far, you must go together". The delivery of palliative care is complex and therefore always involves a team approach to care. The interdisciplinary team represents a unified model of care, and in many ways, reflects the Whole Person. Each team member has unique skills they bring to patient care and to the team itself (Spruyt, 2011). Palliative care teams take care of patients, but they also must take care of each other.

Staff Pain, another aspect of Total Pain, is the suffering clinicians feel from continuous loss. While not on the diagram, it is important to note because the wellbeing of staff affects work with patients. In our program, various psychosocial professionals assist with staff pain. Though not discussed in this chapter, currently, I facilitate art-based self-care groups as needed for staff, fellows, and medical students rotating with our team to sustain and support my team members. Providing and receiving support from the team helps to keep the team and our patients as safe and supported as possible.

## Conclusion

Our palliative care unit is a place of transitions and extremes—immense strength and raw vulnerability, frightful isolation and exquisite human connection. As the concept of Total Pain highlights, illness can affect all domains of life, threatening the intactness of a person (Cassell, 1982). By acknowledging the Whole Person and Whole Experience, and considering the framework of Total Pain, we as clinicians can help people see themselves holistically to support reintegration of self.

Concurrent with medical care, art therapy is one of the few parts of treatment where a patient may choose to participate and direct its course. Noninvasive and inherently productive, creation that occurs in art therapy mitigates loss and provides symbolic planes for intentional connection. Active engagement also challenges the tight grip of illness and the victimization of time. Palliative care patients utilize art therapy for a multitude of needs—to regain control, find resolution, say goodbye, or to find peace, even for a moment in time.

When the power of words can go no further, art may pick up where words fall short. Wilber, Alicia, Michael's family, Julie and her children, and Kyla were all relatively young when illness or injury entered their lives, propelling them into a premature sense of recognizing their death. At critical junctures of their illness journeys, their lives were destabilized and sometimes, dismantled. Using art therapy and creative experience, each cultivated a path to take control over how to live and die. These individuals and families found ways to start conversations, cultivate awareness, and move through illness (and sometimes, towards death) with dignity. Their art products carried something that words could not.

The stories in this chapter illuminate how art therapy can help people traverse liminal, painful and indescribable spaces of loss, and transform them into tangible, soulful and resilient expressions of hope, connection and love, with the most raw and creative material of all: the Whole Self. I am deeply grateful for those who bared their souls during seemingly impossible circumstances, teaching that we all have the creative resources to grow, renew, and become until the moment that our bodies die. It is my hope that their stories inspire people and palliative care programs to discover the wellspring of art therapy in dying and in living.

## Acknowledgements

I would like to thank my colleagues at Mount Sinai for support of the art therapy program. Joining you all in the meaningful quest to relieve suffering has been a sacred, transformative experience and has revealed a new way of seeing. Thank you to Christina Grosso and Suzy Goldhirsch for their time and mentorship in helping to develop this chapter.

## References

Allen, R.S. (2009). The legacy project intervention to enhance meaningful family interactions: Case examples. *Clinical Gerontology*, 32(2):164–176.

Atkinson, R. (2002). The Life Review Interview. In *Handbook of Interview Research Context & Method* (J. F. Gubrium & J. A. Holstien, Eds.). London: Sage Publications.

Bell, S. (2011). Art therapy and spirituality. *Journal for the Study of Spirituality*, 1(2):215–230, DOI: 10.1558/jss.v1i2.215

Capacchione, L. (1991). *Recovery of Your Inner Child*. New York, NY: Simon & Schuster/Fireside.

Carr, S., & Hancock, S. (2017). Healing the inner child through portrait therapy: Illness, identity and childhood trauma. *International Journal of Art Therapy*, 22(1):8–21, DOI: 10.1080/17454832.2016.1245767

Carter, H., MacLeod, R., Brander, P., McPherson, K., Carter, H., & MacLeod, R. (2004). Living with a terminal illness: Patients' priorities. *Journal of Advanced Nursing*, 45:611–620.

Cassell, E.J. (1982). The nature of suffering and the goals of medicine. *New England Journal of Medicine*, 307(12):758–760.

Chai, E., Meier, D., Morris, J., & Goldhirsch, S. (2014). *Geriatric Palliative Care: A Practical Guide for Clinicians*. Oxford: Oxford University Press.

Coyle, N. (2004). The existential slap- a crisis of disclosure. *International Journal of Palliative Nursing*, 10(11):520.

Doka, K. (2014). *Living with Life-Threatening Illness: An Adolescent Perspective*. Washington, DC: Hospice Foundation of America.

Fearnley, R. (2010). Death of a parent and the children's experience: Don't ignore the elephant in the room. *Journal of Interprofessional Care*, 24:450–459.

Fenton, J.F. (2008). "Finding one's way home": Reflections on art therapy in palliative care art therapy. *Journal of the American Art Therapy Association*, 25(3):137–140.

Greisinger, A.J., Lorimar, R.J., Aday, L.A., Winn, R.J., Baile, W.F., & Greisinger, A.J. (1997). Terminally ill cancer patients: Their most important concerns. *Cancer Practice*, 5:147–154.

Helseth, S., & Ulfsaet, N. (2005). Parenting experiences during cancer. *Journal of Advanced Nursing*, 52:38–46.

Janberidze, E., Hjermstad, M., Haugen, D., Sigurdardottir, K., Løhre, E., Lie, H., Loge, J., Kaasa, S., Knudsen, A., Brearley, S., Caraceni, A., Cohen, J., De Groote, Z., Deliens, L., Francke, A., Harding, R., Higginson, I., Linden, K., Miccinesi, G., Onwuteaka-Philipsen, B., Pardon, K., Pasman,

R., Pautex, S., Payne, S., & Van den Block, L. (2014). *Journal of Pain and Symptom Management*, 48(4):678–698.

Jung, C.G. (1993). *The Practice of Psychotherapy* (2nd ed.). East Sussex: Routledge.

Krupnick, J.L. (1984). Chapter 5: Bereavement During Childhood and Adolescence. In *Bereavement: Reactions, Consequences, Care* (M. Osterveis, F. Solomon & M. Green (Eds.), (pp. 99–145). Washington, DC: National Academies Press.

McNiff, S. (2004). *Art as Medicine*. Boston, MA: Shambala Press.

Meier, D., & Beresford, L. (2008). The palliative care team. *Journal of Palliative Medicine*, 11(5):617–681.

Pickrel, J. (1989). Tell me your story: Using life review in counseling for the terminally ill. *Death Studies*, 13(2):127–135.

Puchalski, C., Ferrell, B., Virani, R., Otis-Green, S., Baird, P., Bull, J., Chochinov, H., Handzo, G., Nelson-Becker, H., Prince-Paul, M., Pugliese, K., & Sulmasy, D. (2009). Improving the quality of spiritual care as a dimension of palliative care: The report of the consensus conference. *Journal of Palliative Medicine*, 12(10):885–904.

Rutenberg, M. (2008). Casting the spirit: A handmade legacy art therapy. *Journal of the American Art Therapy Association*, 25(3):108–114.

Saunders, C., & Baines, M. (1983). *Living with Dying: The Management of Terminal Disease*. Oxford: Oxford University Press.

Sherman, D.W. (1998). Reciprocal suffering: The need to improve family caregiver's quality of life through palliative care. *Journal of Palliative Medicine*, 1(4):357–366.

Spruyt, O. (2011). Team networking in palliative care. *Indian Journal of Palliative Care*:S17—S19.

Sutter, C., & Reid, T. (2012). How do we talk to the children? Child life consultation to support the children of seriously ill inpatients. *Journal of Palliative Medicine*, 15(12):1–7.

Synnott, A. (2001). *The Body Social: Symbolism, Self and Society*. London: Routledge.

Turner, B.S. (1996). *The Body and Society*. London: Sage.

Van Gennep, A. (1960). *The Rites of Passage*. London: Routledge & Kegan Paul.

Walsh, S.M., Martin, S.C., & Schmidt, L.A. (2004). Testing the efficacy of a creative-arts intervention with family caregivers of patients with cancer. *Journal Nursing Scholarship*, 36(3):214–219.

Wolfe, J., Hinds, P., & Sourkes, B. (2011). *Textbook of Interdisciplinary Pediatric Palliative Care*. Philadelphia: Elsevier Saunders.

# Plate section

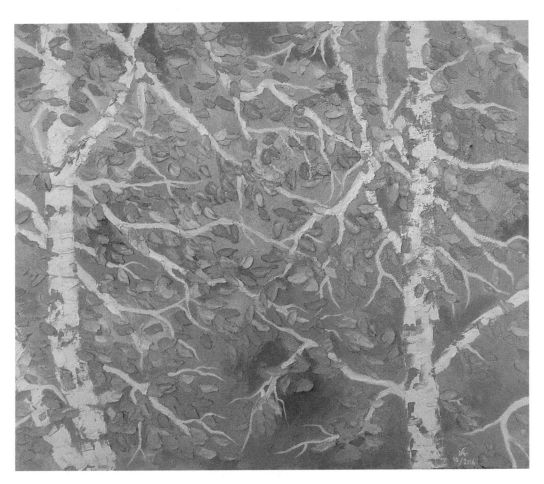

*Plate 1*

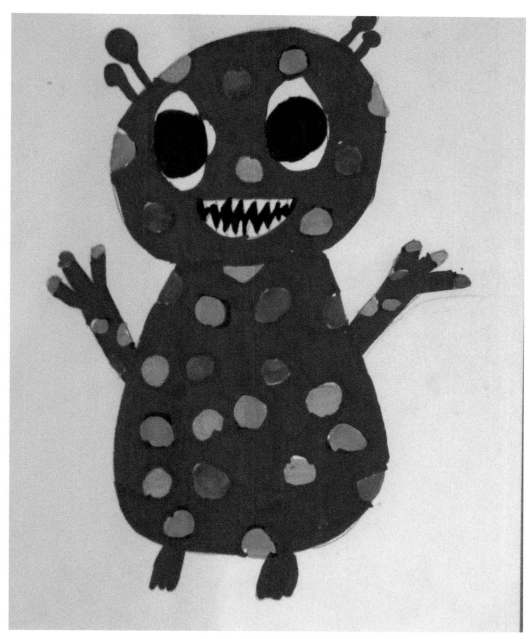

*Plate 2*

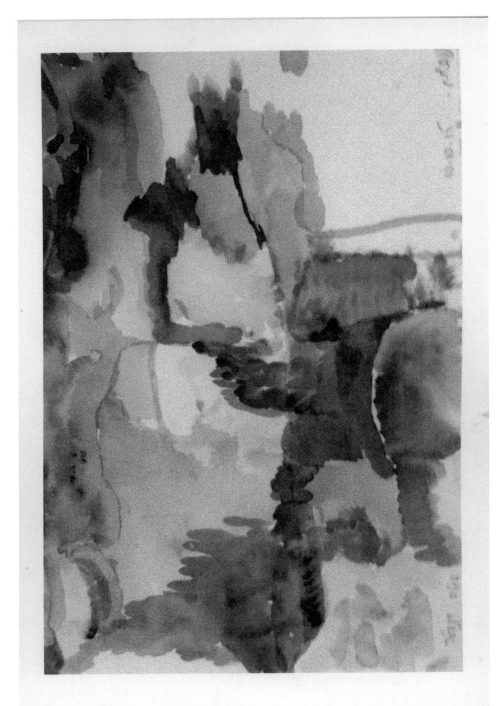

Plate 3

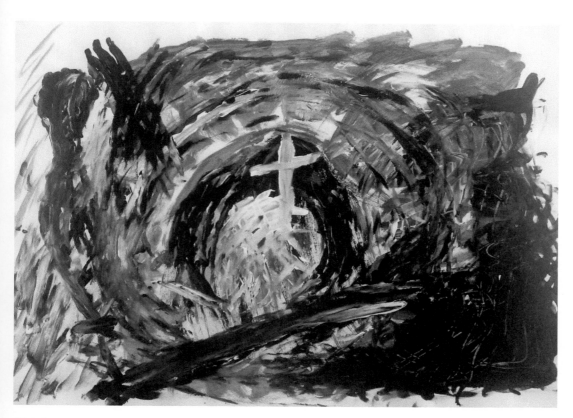

Plate 4

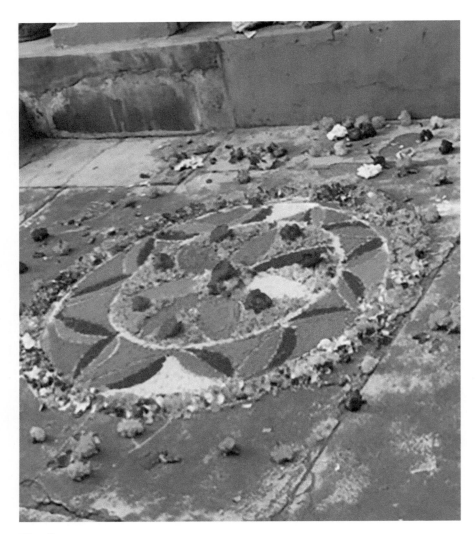

*Plate 5*

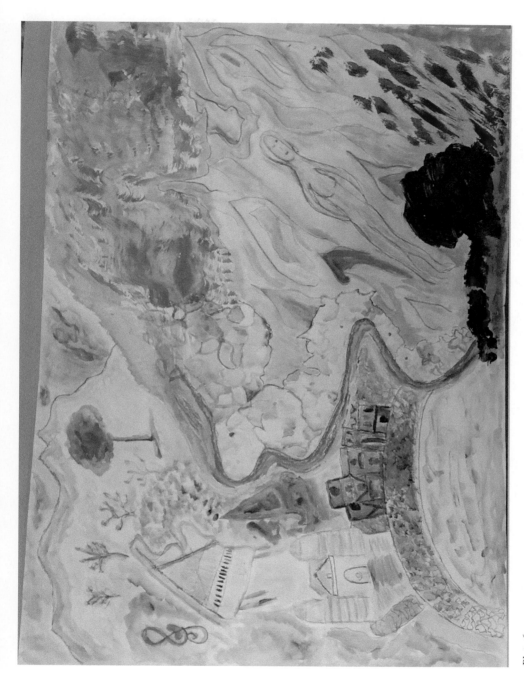

Plate 6

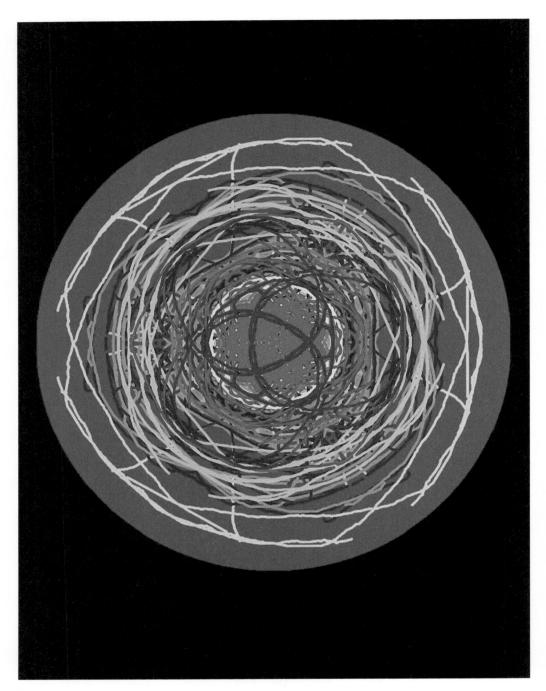

*Plate 7*

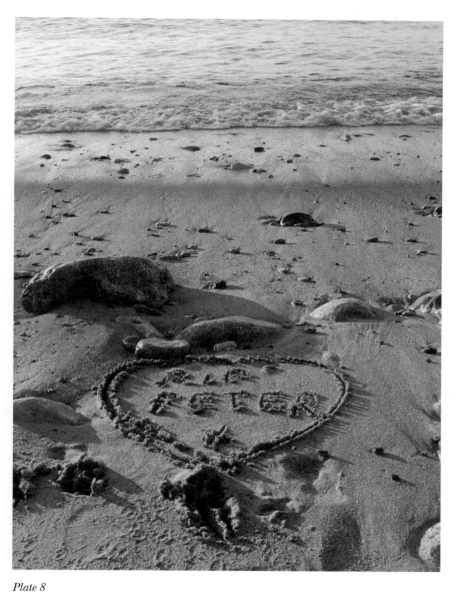

*Plate 8*

# 20 The Power of Creative Expression and Ritual

## Integrating Art Therapy Into a Bereavement Camp

*Heidi Bardot and Jean McCaw*

The death of a loved one is often a life changing experience. When children or adolescents are dealing with the loss of a family member their lives can be filled with challenges that make enjoyment, happiness, and understanding difficult to achieve. Feelings of sadness, fear, isolation, separation, anger and guilt can be overwhelming and difficult to navigate for any child or teen.

In 1996 a large hospice in Northern Virginia responded to this need and expanded their outreach and support in the community by creating an annual weekend bereavement program called Point of Hope Camp to support children who were grieving the death of a loved one. After two years it became clear that adolescents and adults were also in need of a program that could provide this same comprehensive bereavement support. As a result, in 1998, Point of Hope Camp expanded to include three programs that were held simultaneously at the same campsite—programs for children ages 6–12, adolescents ages 13–17, and adults ages 18 and older. This camp provided a caring environment with therapeutic and recreational activities to assist each participant in coping with their loss.

Point of Hope camp offered a special combination of therapeutic activities, educational and supportive discussions, and fun recreational activities to help participants, build trust, learn coping skills, and enhance their sense of self through connecting with the staff, the adult volunteers, and their peers. This camp was provided free of charge for up to 35 children, 15 teens and 25 adults. The three programs were designed to be separate, focused on each specific age group with minimal interaction during the weekend.

The adult camp was focused on rest and rejuvenation, understanding that grieving can be taxing physically as well as emotionally. Massage, yoga, and art therapy were offered as a means of reducing stress and allowing for quiet reflection, introspection, and personal understanding and growth, along with opportunities for group discussion and connection with peers. The focus of this chapter will be on the programs for children and adolescents, covering the therapeutic elements of the weekend, structure of the camp, importance of volunteer support and concluding thoughts.

Programs for both the children and teens were art therapy focused, combining many opportunities to have fun, laugh, and play together with more reflective moments for contemplation, expression, and quiet conversation.

Although each camp varied in approach and activities, the goals were primarily the same; to provide different avenues through which the children and teens could address their feelings and memories, learn ways to cope with their grief, and become more aware of their strengths and unique, special qualities. The children and teens participated throughout the weekend in a variety of large and small group activities. Art therapy and grief education were a primary component of each program which provided a safe and non-threatening method for participants to express feelings and to memorialize their loved ones.

A significant aspect of this weekend program was the pairing of each child and teen with a trained adult volunteer called either a "Big Buddy" or "Teen Buddy." The Buddy provided support to the child/teen camper and participated in every activity with the child or teen, providing companionship, someone to talk with and confide in, and a partner in all of the therapeutic and recreational activities. A crucial role of the Buddy was being witness to the child or teen's grief process and supporting their inherent resilience.

Throughout the weekend the children and teens were given the opportunity to talk openly about the events leading up to the death of their loved one as well as the funeral or memorial service and what life was like for them and their families after the death. They understood the purpose of this camp and realized there was a common bond with the other participants as they were all invited to share their stories and grief experiences. With the foundation of a supportive environment in place, the children and teens learned that this was a safe setting in which feelings were respected, valued, and validated not only by the staff and big buddies but also by other children or teens participating in Point of Hope Camp.

## Therapeutic Elements of the Weekend

**Art Therapy**: Creating art provides an effective and meaningful way to express feelings. It promotes healing and can facilitate the process for a child or teen to address what they are thinking, feeling, and remembering. Many memories or feelings can be challenging and sometimes frightening or overwhelming. Addressing these thoughts and images through the art process often provides a more gentle and manageable way to address that which is most difficult (Bardot, 2008, 2013; McCaw, 2013). Therefore, art therapy directives and rituals were woven into the fabric of this weekend camp, providing deeper meaning through these modes of expression. Each of the art therapy themes and projects built upon the one before and once combined became an important part of the final ritual.

**Healing Circles**: The Healing Circles occurred four times during the weekend, providing the children and teens with grief education focused on the different aspects of the grieving process: telling their story, identifying and discussing feelings related to grief, remembering and memorializing their loved one, looking at their personal strengths as well as their wishes and dreams for their future. Art therapists led the Healing Circles and campers were grouped together by age. In the Healing Circles, children/teens were given an opportunity to talk about their experiences related to the death of their loved one. One key element was telling their story, an essential process in the healing of loss (Neimeyer, 2012). Children and teens listened to the experiences and feelings of others, which was helpful as they began to understand that they were not alone. So often grieving creates a feeling of isolation in children and adolescents as they often sense they are alone in dealing with their loss. In addition, the Healing Circles provided opportunities to learn about the many other aspects of grief as well as to normalize and validate the children/teens personal responses.

**Rituals**: Rituals became an integral aspect of this camp, providing opportunities for expression and connection to other participants as well as to those who have died. Art therapy enhanced the experience of ritual by providing a creative framework within which the participant could express feelings and gain understanding of their experiences.

> Ritual or ceremony can provide meaning to those who have been affected by the death and unite a group of people who are grieving. In this way rituals can touch us personally and collectively, acting as a uniting force. Often words cannot touch the depth of our grief, but ritual and the symbols used in ritual can touch those places and help us to express feelings that are beyond words.
>
> (McCaw, 2013, p. 21)

This process provided increased personal meaning and connection during the rituals, which helped to connect past experiences with present life as well as offered comfort and support making it easier to look toward the future with hope (Doka, 2000; Zulli, 1998).

**Music:** At the beginning of the Healing Circles, music was played as a quiet reminder that the group was gathering and preparing to start. Each song was carefully chosen for the words it expressed and the tone of the song. It provided a gentle and quiet way to enter into the sacred aspects of the Healing Circle. Music was also integral in the final ritual on Sunday, providing reverence and meaning to this closing ceremony.

**Other Meaningful and Recreational Activities:** Yoga provided relaxation and focused on calming the body through movement and breathing. Other modalities of expression included journaling, drumming circles, storytelling, poetry therapy, music therapy and therapeutic pets. Participants journaled in memory books that were often worked on beside their Buddies or shared with them afterwards. During these private moments more personal information or concerns were often raised and shared. Recreational activities included the parachute, swimming, group games, hiking, volleyball, and basketball.

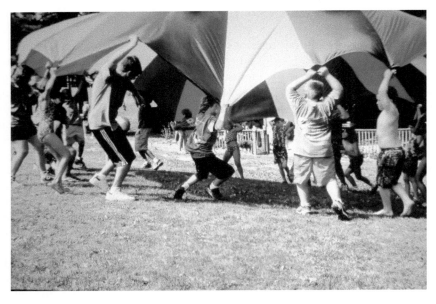

*Figure 20.1* Recreational Activities Offered Were Games, Drumming, Storytelling, Yoga, Hiking, and Swimming

## The Structure of Camp

An important aspect of the camp was helping the children and teens get settled in, feel welcomed, and manage separating from parents. This was achieved by Big/Teen Buddies immediately connecting with their Little/Teen Buddy, getting their camp t-shirt, making wooden nametags, and collecting donated items (i.e., handmade blankets, stuffed animals, water bottles, journals, ponchos in case of rain). For some children, these were items they had never owned before.

*Friday Evening Healing Circle:* After dinner, the groups gathered for the first Healing Circle. The structure and purpose of the weekend was discussed and each child or teen was given an opportunity to share their story of loss. Neimeyer (2012) discusses how this is a core element in the healing process—being able to tell your story to others and to be really heard. Often people are not allowed to tell their story due to society's discomfort with death and for a child/teen the need to revisit and retell their story is important (Bardot, 2013). Additionally, it provided that moment to connect, as stories were being told and the feelings of loss were experienced, which allowed the group to come together in their common grief (McCaw, 2013). The first Healing Circle then closed with the first of many rituals.

*Friday Evening Ritual:* To honor the importance of their shared stories and to set the stage for the entire weekend, the first ritual was dedicated to the loved one who had died. The ceremony began in silence and then each family member's name was read and a bell was rung. As the name was read, each child and/or teen in that family was presented with a silk Memory Flag with their loved one's name written in calligraphy on the flag. The solemnity of the ritual and the sense of the loss and grief were evident in the children and teen's serious and attentive approach to this ceremony. Once every name was read and every participant acknowledged, the Memory Flags were strung together across the main gathering area as a way to honor their loss and as a reminder of the purpose and importance of this weekend. At the end of this three-day camp the flags became part of the final ritual and were taken home.

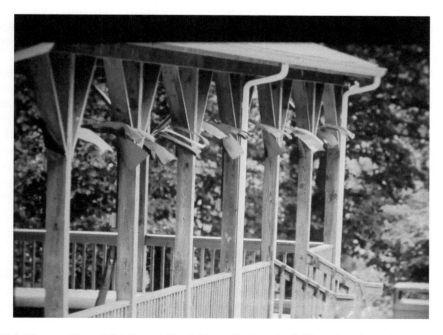

*Figure 20.2* Memory Flags, With Loved One's Name Written in Calligraphy, Fluttering in the Breeze Throughout the Weekend

*Saturday Morning Healing Circle:* The morning Healing Circle began by acknowledging again why we were all gathered at camp and then exploring all the feelings the children and teens were experiencing related to their grief. It was important to name all the feelings and to accept and validate them, as grief is not limited to just sadness, but often includes: fear, anger, guilt, loneliness, shock, shame, peace, relief, and even happiness. Oftentimes, children feel alone and isolated when grieving, so hearing peers share similar feelings and experiences was important. Children and teens often felt guilty that they did not spend enough time with their family member or they argued with them before they died. They sometimes felt anger at the doctors for not "fixing" the person or angry with the deceased for leaving them. Very often they felt relieved that their loved one was no longer in pain or suffering but then felt guilty for that sense of relief and were reluctant to share that emotion. Therefore, it becomes essential to validate and normalize all emotions that are experienced (Bardot, 2013; McCaw, 2013). Additionally, we explored the importance for each child to express feelings rather than internalize them and discussed productive and non-productive ways to express emotion and techniques to help them manage all that they were feeling. Each child and teen was then asked to choose three feelings related to their loss and write them on small slips of paper, kept in a small coin envelope, as part of a larger art therapy project.

### Art Therapy Activity: Hope Books (Page One)

The Hope Books were introduced as a visual, hands-on method of exploring and processing grief. The goal was to have the participants focus on different aspects of their grief experience and then bring these together in one tangible space. They worked in dyads with their Big Buddy who provided assistance and facilitated discussion on the topic. In this session they created the first of three pages for their Hope Book. The morning Healing Circle was focused on feelings; therefore, this theme was continued in their art work. Some children addressed one emotion while others included numerous feelings. Participants were provided with oil and chalk pastels, markers, glue, scissors, collage word sheets, and a feelings chart with a list of emotions and animated faces depicting the corresponding expression (Feelings Poster, 1994).

*Saturday Afternoon Healing Circle:* The Saturday afternoon Healing Circle focused on memories and the past. The children and teens were given the opportunity to reminisce and tell the group their favorite memories as well as the difficult memories surrounding the death of their loved one. In this circle children/teens often spoke about the circumstances related to the death, which were stories they often had been told not to talk about by their family, friends, or even school personnel. Other topics of discussion included why memories are important, worrying about forgetting details about their loved one, and how in talking and reminiscing about their family member they kept them more present. Each child/teen was then asked to write down three memories related to their loss and put them in their envelope.

### Art Therapy Activity: Hope Books (Page Two)

Following the afternoon topic, the Big and Little Buddies created the second page of their Hope Book, which focused on their memories. Art supplies included oil and chalk pastels and markers; as it seemed these media encouraged greater expression due to the nature of the materials. Big/Teen Buddies encouraged the child/teen to talk about their experiences as it was often easier for them to talk one on one than sharing in the larger group and feelings and concerns could be explored more deeply.

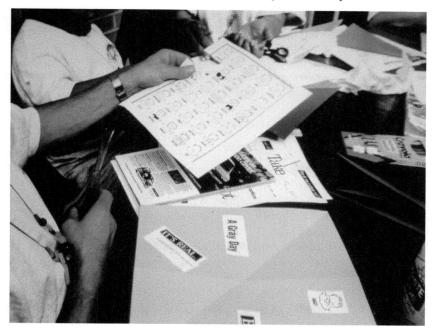

*Figure 20.3* Page One of the Hope Books Focused on Expression of Feelings Related to Grief

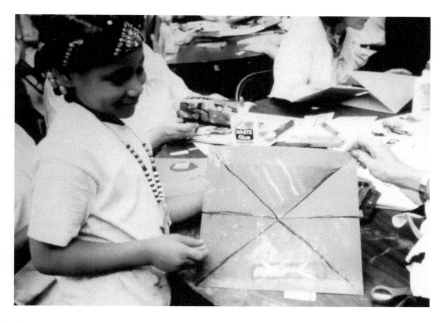

*Figure 20.4* Page Two of the Hope Books Focused on a Memory Related to the Death of Their Loved One

***Sunday Morning Final Healing Circle***: The final Healing Circle focused on wishes, dreams, and the future. Because children grieve in a different manner than adults, often fluctuating between periods of sadness, anger, happiness, and fun, this session not only focused on moving forward into a future without the person who died, but also discussed the importance of fun and laughter, and in essence gave them "permission" to experience these feelings in their lives. They were able to acknowledge what wishes and dreams had been lost because of the death and then they thought about and shared three wishes focused on moving forward: a wish they had for themselves and their own future, a wish they had for their family, and a wish the deceased may have had for them. These three wishes were then written down and put into their envelope.

### Art Therapy Activity: Hope Books (Page Three)

The group then worked on the final page of the Hope Book alongside their Big/Teen Buddies, who helped them explore what their wishes might be, how the future would be different, and what it would be like when they returned home from camp that afternoon. In addition to the previous materials, tissue collage supplies were offered as a way to expand their means of expression.

*Assembling the 3D Hope Book for the Ritual* (*descriptions and visuals for the origami fold for each page, how to assemble the book, and how to create the star are included at the end of this chapter*).

With all three pages of the Hope Book completed, the pages were glued together to create a book and the small envelope, containing the slips of paper with the child/teen's feelings, memories, and wishes, was glued to the outside back page. The book was hole-punched, strung with twine or ribbon, and hung from a stick to create a 3D star. The Memory Flag was also attached to the stick and became part of the final ritual.

*Sunday Ritual:* The ritual began with a silent procession, led by the beat of a single drum. Buddies walked beside the children and teens as they carried their Hope Books and Memory Flags aloft above their heads and processed down to the camp fire where they gathered quietly in a large circle. Readings were provided by staff and volunteers and words of reflection and blessings were given by a chaplain. The children and teens were then invited to take out the papers on which they had written their feelings, memories, and wishes and to release any pieces they wanted to into the camp fire. Children were assisted by their Big Buddies when needed and music was played during this process. This was a time of silence, contemplation, and tears and even the youngest and most active children were drawn to the seriousness of this ceremony and the enormity of their loss. Each participant was then given a river stone, which they dropped one at a time into a pitcher of water. As the stones were collected together the whole of the camp and those that died were represented and honored in that moment. Every participant was then given the opportunity to pour water or to throw a handful of sand onto the fire to extinguish the flames. Once the water was emptied from the pitcher and the fire was out, each child and teen was invited to take a river stone from the pitcher as a symbol of remembrance. As the fire was extinguished the group stood in silence for a final moment as a poem was read to close this important and meaningful ceremony.

*The Final Farewell:* As the weekend was coming to a close a final activity provided a way for all participants to say goodbye to each other. Polaroid pictures were taken of Big and Little Buddies and Teens and Teen Buddies and they were attached to blank note cards. All participants wrote goodbye notes to each other as well as words of encouragement and hope. This created a formal and fun way for the children, teens, volunteers, and staff to say goodbye and end on a joyful note.

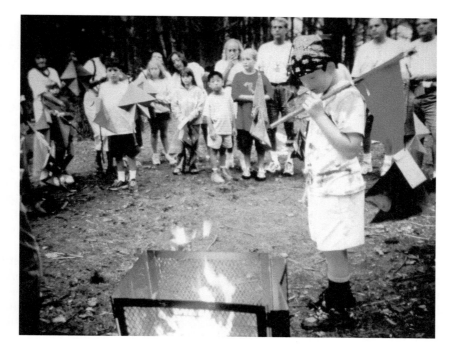

*Figure 20.5* The Final Ritual: Letting Go of Difficult Feelings or Memories or Future Wishes

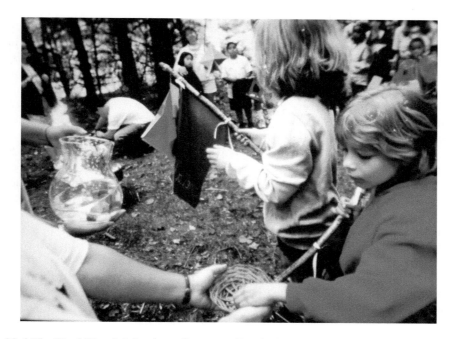

*Figure 20.6* The Final Ritual: Selecting a Stone as a Reminder

## The Importance of Support for the Volunteers

*Training:* A mandatory volunteer training was important for many reasons. This type of camp experience was not only physically and emotionally taxing, but often triggered feelings, memories, and responses from the volunteers' own grief experiences. Therefore, training was provided to help prepare the volunteers for the demands of this weekend program including ways in which to help manage their personal responses to what they would hear and experience during the three-day weekend. This training emphasized how volunteers could find support during the weekend and when it was important to ask for help. During this day-long training volunteers learned specifics about child and adolescent grief, setting limits, creating healthy boundaries, ways in which to provide support to their Little Buddy, as well as someone else's Little Buddy and to fellow Buddies. They were encouraged to ask questions at any point in time, report concerns and ask for support. This training also provided a chance for new volunteers to meet the staff and returning volunteers prior to camp, and for returning volunteers to reconnect.

*Friday Volunteer Gathering and Ritual:* Once volunteers and staff arrived and settled in and before the children and teens arrived, everyone gathered together. There were a few moments dedicated to introductions and what the volunteers were looking forward to. They voiced their hopes and concerns, and most importantly, they each set their intention for the weekend. As a result of this initial ritual, the volunteers felt connected and supported when the children and teens arrived, and they set a positive and welcoming tone for the weekend. They began this challenging and rewarding weekend with a sense of connection, confidence, and positivity, and they understood they were supported throughout this experience.

*Evening Debriefings:* Each evening, once the children and teens were in bed and were supervised by designated volunteers, all the adult volunteers and staff gathered to debrief about the day. Questions and concerns were addressed, problems raised, and information shared. Successes and poignant moments were also shared as Big/Teen Buddies processed their experiences. The role of Big/Teen Buddy could be quite intimate, intense, and challenging when campers shared details of their stories, their thoughts, feelings, and grief. Staff became more aware of where additional support was needed for the next day and Buddies were provided with added support if their Little Buddy or Teen Buddy had limitations or specific challenges. Oftentimes a tag-team approach was put in place when two Little or Teen Buddies had connected, which provided Buddies support for each other and an opportunity to take breaks, if needed.

*Sunday Final Meeting and Debriefing:* Once all of the campers had departed on Sunday and before the cleaning and packing began, the volunteers and staff gathered one last time to debrief about the weekend as a whole and reflect on the challenges and successes. A great deal was shared during the weekend by the children and teens, and it was often emotionally challenging for the volunteers to hold all that they had witnessed. It was imperative that there be an opportunity to give voice to that which was most challenging as well as that which was enjoyable and most meaningful. Gathering the volunteers together also provided a formal way for them to say goodbye to each other and the staff, as meaningful connections were often made within this dedicated group. In this way, camp was then concluded the same way it had begun, with the team gathered together to reflect on the intentions that were set at the very beginning and then to reflect on all that had taken place during this very important and emotional three days. Each volunteer and staff member had dedicated the weekend to these children and teens in support and in the hope that they would grieve, connect, and begin to move forward.

## Concluding Thoughts

Coming together for this weekend camp proved to be a valuable experience for all three age groups. Although the programs were separate and did not interact, the goals were the same for each participant regardless of their age. Each child and teen was provided an opportunity to address, process, and express their grief through many different therapies and activities, which included art therapy, journaling, discussion, and other expressive therapies and a variety of recreational activities. Through the use of art in their grief process, the children and teens were given a means through which they could express the inexpressible—emotions, thoughts, concerns, or hopes that they could not otherwise describe (Bardot, 2008). The Hope Books provided a tangible means by which to validate their feelings, honor their memories, and explore their wishes and dreams. Because of the non-threatening aspects of art, their thoughts, feelings, and concerns were expressed and the process in and of itself was healing. The images and expressions were explored more deeply through discussion with their Big Buddy or Teen Buddy or within their group. Each camper had the opportunity to tell their story, talk about what was hard, their favorite and challenging memories, and the many feelings they were experiencing. With the support of their Big Buddies, Teen Buddies, adult volunteers, staff, and peers, a safe and supportive therapeutic environment was created. The children and teens were able to share a great deal of their experience with each other as well as have fun together which provided connection, release, relief, and a chance to build new friendships in a safe and understanding community. One of our regular volunteers was quoted as saying, "Volunteering as a Big Buddy for several years of these camps was a truly rewarding and meaningful experience for me. I came to see how art, healing circles, and other forms of openly expressing feelings of grief could provide comfort to a child."

Though the work proved beneficial and far reaching, due to budgetary cuts, the art therapy program at this hospice was discontinued after being in existence for twelve years. Therefore, other clinical staff took responsibility for implementing the Point of Hope camp, but the programs were greatly changed without the continuity, community, and expression that the art therapy focus provided. In addition, because the funding sources that had supported the camp were not actively pursued, it became increasingly difficult to deliver such a comprehensive program and the camp closed after two years. The discontinuation of the Point of Hope camp and the hospice art therapy program was a significant loss to the community.

The basic idea for Point of Hope camp was shared with us by another organization in the southeast. This model was then enhanced with the art therapy, adapted to the needs of the children and families we served, and fine-tuned through years of experience. Point of Hope camp then became a model which was shared with other organizations on the east coast providing much needed grief support to families.

## The Creation of the Hope Books

**The Fold:** The star books are created with a simple origami fold. If used with an older child, he/she can be taught the technique for the fold; if used with a younger child, the pages should be pre-folded so that the child can move immediately into creating the art. The size of the paper used is 12" × 12"; however, this can vary. The paper must be square and large enough for drawing and collage. Scrapbooking paper, which is found in many arts and crafts supply stores, works well because it can be found in a heavier weight like card stock, and provides a large surface on which to work. This origami fold is called the

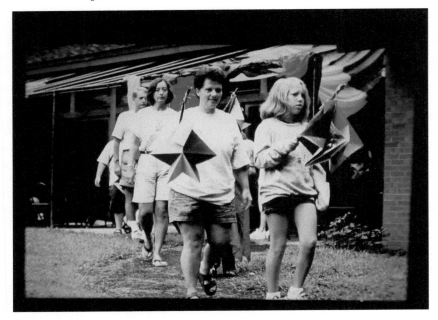

*Figure 20.7* Close Up of the Assembled Hope Books Attached to Sticks

Water Bomb Base (www.origami-instructions.com). The page can be opened up in order to work on it and view and easily folds back into a triangle.

**Making a Book:** Fold three sheets of paper using the Water Bomb Base fold. Each page can be a different color if desired. Once the pages have been folded, stack the pages on top of each other to create a three-page book and glue the layers together. When each page is opened it becomes a square but resumes the fold easily when closed. Using card stock or heavier paper will hold this fold very well and creates a durable book.

**Creating the Star:** Once the pages are glued together it is possible to create a star. Hold the book so that all three pages open up, and bring the first page and last page together so they are back to back. Hold the pages by one corner, and it creates a three-dimensional star. A hole punch can be used to make a hole in the front and back sheets and ribbon, twine or yarn can be tied in the hole so that the book can be hung as a star or the twine or ribbon can be wrapped around the book and to secure it when closed. This was originally designed so that the books could be hung from a stick or dowel and used as part of a bereavement ritual, but this can also provide a method of displaying the book.

## References

Bardot, H. (2008). Expressing the inexpressible: The resilient healing of client and art therapist. *Art Therapy*, 25(4), 183–186.

Bardot, H. (2013). The universality of grief and loss. In P. Howie, S. Prasad & J. Kristel (Eds.) *Using art therapy with diverse populations: Crossing cultures and abilities*. London: Jessica Kingsley Publishers.

Doka, K.J. (Ed.) (2000). *Children, adolescents and loss*. Washington, DC: Hospice Foundation of America.

*Feelings Poster*. (1994). *Feelings Poster*. Cincinnati, OH: Creative Therapies Associates, Inc. Retrieved from www.ctherapy.com

McCaw, J. (2013). *Touching grief: Frequently asked questions about child and adolescent grief*. Fairfax, VA: Walker's Cove Publishing.

Neimeyer, R. (2012). *Techniques of grief therapy: Creative practices for counseling the bereaved*. New York, NY: Routledge.

Zulli, A.P. (1998). Healing rituals: Powerful and empowering. In K.J. Doka & J.D. Davidson (Eds.) *Living with grief: Who we are, how we grieve*. Philadelphia, PA: Bunner/Mazel.

# 21 Saying Goodbye
## Grieving Families

*Kayleigh Orr*

The focus of this chapter is on how art therapy is used when working with family members in a child and adult hospice based in England. As an art therapist working across children and adult services, I have found that there is a constant need to adapt to meet the needs of patients and their families during their journey through the hospice. This chapter will explore my perspective on the experience and knowledge that is required when working with families within palliative care; the UK's healthcare system; and how hospice care relates to this and differs when working with adults, children and families during various stages of pre-bereavement, end of life care and post-bereavement. Three case studies will illustrate the breadth of work I undertake which includes working with an adult patient during end of life care, a sibling's experience of their brother dying, and an example of revisiting a death ten years later.

## Palliative Care Within the UK

In England, the primary healthcare provision is the National Health Service (NHS); a publicly funded healthcare system for all legal residents of the United Kingdom. Its main source of funding is from the taxation system; therefore, the majority of services are free. The NHS is overseen by the Department of Health, a ministerial department of the UK Government that develops guidance and policy for improving patient care and expectations.

According to National demographics, approximately half a million people die each year in England and this is expected to rise by 17% by 2030. Out of these deaths approximately three quarters were expected, suggesting that specialist care in the final year of life is required. This specialist care is most commonly known as palliative care. The National Institute of Health and Care Excellence, which provides the national guidelines for clinical care in the NHS define palliative care as,

> The active holistic care of patients with advanced progressive illness. Management of pain and other symptoms and provision of psychological, social and spiritual support is paramount. The goal of palliative care is achievement of the best quality of life for patients and their families. Many aspects of palliative care are also applicable earlier in the course of the illness in conjunction with other treatments.
>
> (NICE: 2016)

At present in the UK, up to 170,000 adults receive specialist palliative care each year (NHS England: 2014). It is estimated that at least 49,000 children and young people in the UK have life limiting or life-threatening illness that may require palliative care services (Together for Short Lives: 2011). In response to these numbers, the NHS endeavours to meet individual preferences around death and dying but also follows NICE guidelines. Furthermore, coalitions such as 'Dying Matters', which consists of the NHS, voluntary and independent sectors, aim to meet the Department of Health's Strategy for End of

Life Care (2012) by encouraging people to talk openly about death and dying. The NHS also partially funds hospices, which provide specialist holistic palliation services to people within hospitals, care homes or within their own homes.

## Keech Hospice Care and Its Provision

Keech Hospice Care currently provides care for people in three counties across the East of England (Hertfordshire, Bedfordshire and Milton Keynes). It was instigated by a retired GP; Dr Wink White in 1986 who felt that a provision was required for terminally ill adults in South Bedfordshire. After five years of fundraising and planning the adult hospice became operational in 1991. After a charity appeal in 1997, a second hospice for children with life limiting illnesses from a further two counties was established on the same site. Keech Hospice Care's statement of purpose (2014) explains how, like other English hospices and palliative services, partial funding is provided by the NHS and the rest from charitable funds (Keech's figures state approximately 30% NHS and 60% from fundraising and donations.) Keech Hospice Care is run by a board of trustees who have ultimate responsibility for the hospice, its assets and activities. The Hospice Service is regulated by the Care Quality Commission who is responsible for regulating and inspecting voluntary and private healthcare organisations in the UK.

The adult service provides palliative care to individuals aged over 18 years who have a life limiting condition and are in the palliative stage of their illness. Keech Hospice Care has an 8-bed inpatient service which is purpose built with specialised medical and nursing care. It provides care for patients whose symptoms and complex needs are not readily relieved in the home or care setting and the primary focus is on symptom control, psychological support and end of life care. The staff use the Burford Model of Care (Johns, 1991) which is a tailored and holistic approach. In addition to the inpatient services, a palliative care centre provides additional holistic support to patients and families whilst they remain under the support of their general practitioner and Community Nursing Team. Individualised programmes are developed to help the patients achieve their goals. Keech Hospice Care also has a care co-ordination team that provides a single point of access for coordinating care packages for adults in the local area with palliative care needs.

The children's service provides specialist palliative care for children and young people up to their 19th birthday who have a life limiting illness. Services provided include the use of a 5-bed inpatient unit for symptom management, respite care in urgent situations and end of life care. The children's unit also offers specialised play and educational activities, treatment and therapy sessions. In addition, the hospice has a palliative community service for hospice care within various community settings such as the home, school or hospital. This community team will offer support in partnership with other agencies such as the NHS or social care.

## Supportive Care Team and Art Therapy

As an art therapist at Keech Hospice Care, I am part of 'The Supportive Care Team' which provides a service to both the adult and children's hospice. Clinicians on the team include family support workers, complementary therapist's, music and art therapists, chaplains and a hospice-at-home co-ordinator (volunteers provide practical and emotional support in the home). Social workers, a physiotherapist and occupational therapist also regularly link into the team to provide a holistic approach to care. These clinicians can work with a family at any stage during the patient's illness.

The art therapy service is open to the patient or any family member or friends who are affected by the palliative condition. Interventions provided include 1:1 or group sessions using a directive or non-directive approach.

The criteria to access the art therapy service include the following:

1. A recent or significant event—end of life care, changes within treatment, bereavement etc.
2. A willingness to engage with art materials and would benefit from accessing a visual media.
3. Currently not accessing any other psychological services.

I also provide clinical supervision sessions for staff at the hospice.

## Differences in Children and Adult Services

Working across both adult and children's services, I have observed noticeable differences between these areas which can impact practice. In both services, the approach to palliative care is holistic in nature and focussed upon the quality of life for the adult or child patient. Again in both cases, support can be provided to family members including spouses, siblings, parents and other extended family members and friends.

For children and young people accessing palliative care services, the range of conditions are varied, some of which are rare. It is also accepted that children with cancers with a positive prognosis such as acute lymphatic lymphoma (ALL) will also be accepted for hospice support. Medical interventions can be a combination of palliative and curative. It is not uncommon for children with a palliative diagnosis to survive into adulthood. Therefore, hospice care is provided over a longer period of time as the service is offered from diagnosis to end of life care. Keech Hospice Care offers emergency respite care, a day care service for children and young people unable to access education, symptom management and end of life care. Another factor which must be taken into consideration is that children and young people continue to develop physically, emotionally and cognitively throughout the course of their illness, whereas adults generally deteriorate. There are additional practicalities of providing a service to children such as capacity and consent depending upon the child's age, involving the primary carer as well as additional health or educational services and ensuring that confidentiality is maintained across all of these. Finally, psychological support for the whole family is integral to ensuring positive well-being during this life changing journey.

Typically, for the adult service, the hospice usually only becomes involved as the disease progresses. General practitioners (GP's) are normally involved with the overall care of an adult patient and links are readily made with local hospitals and district nurses (nurses who provide community care). The hospice, from a medical perspective, provides symptom management and end of life care; therefore, medical interventions are palliative in nature. The majority of deaths follow a period of chronic illnesses such as heart disease, cancer, strokes, neurological illnesses or dementia. However, it is also worth noting that many young people with palliative conditions such as cystic fibrosis are living into early adulthood and therefore require transition into adult services. Following the holistic approach as adopted by children's palliative care, support for adults encompasses family members; however often this tends to be spouses and the patient's own children. At times, the patient and their partner may require support together to consider the impact of illness and future plans.

Although differences are noted between the two services, it has become apparent that clinicians require a set of skills to implement psychological support which requires sensitivity and flexibility on the part of the therapist. Although not an extensive list, the following are areas in which I feel that a clinician working within this field needs to have an understanding:

1. **Knowledge and understanding of palliative conditions**

   - Knowing the trajectory of the illness.
   - Identifying the family's knowledge and understanding of the illness.
   - Answering questions or clarifying terminology, treatment options, etc.
   - Being able to use age appropriate medical language.
   - Signposting families to other clinicians.

2. **Awareness of the dying and grieving process**

   - Knowledge and understanding of the dying process and being able to witness this experience alongside a family.
   - Recognising the normality of the grieving process and when grief becomes complex.
   - Awareness of funerals/ceremonies held by different cultures after death.
   - Knowing when the therapist is unable to continue to provide support and referrals to other agencies are required.

3. **The family**

   - Considering the impact of illness on each of the family members as individuals and as a whole.
   - Acknowledge each individual member's own experiences and assumptions about illness.
   - Recognising whether the individual or family are ready and able to accept psychological support.
   - Honouring the patient (child or adult's) wishes around care or treatment when these may differ from their family.
   - Being able to maintain confidentiality and boundaries between family members.

4. **The role of the art work in art therapy**

   - Allows unconscious thoughts and feelings to be expressed.
   - An opportunity to reflect upon past experiences, behaviours or feelings.
   - Primarily a non-verbal intervention.
   - Provides a sense of mastery and control.
   - Enables legacies or memories to be created for loved ones.

The following case studies show a range of work that I have undertaken at Keech Hospice Care. They demonstrate some of the skills and knowledge highlighted above as well as the flexibility and sensitivity required to work with a holistic approach in a hospice setting.

## Joining the Journey

I met with James, an intelligent 8-year-old sibling who suffered with Asperger's syndrome and Attention Deficit Hyperactive Disorder (ADHD), for an art therapy assessment. His brother Kevin, aged 10 years old, had a number of conditions including cerebral palsy, autism, epilepsy and ADHD as a result of oxygen deprivation to the brain shortly after birth (perinatal hypoxia leading to ischaemic encephalopathy). The family were becoming increasingly aware that James was struggling to verbalise his feelings about his brother's diagnosis especially in light of learning that his condition was palliative and it was felt that art therapy may be beneficial. James became easily frustrated towards himself and others, which resulted in challenging behaviours. James's youngest sibling, aged 5 years, was also referred for additional support and began music therapy sessions at the same time.

James accessed art therapy sessions during and after his brother's death. Kevin died at the hospice after he developed complications with pneumonia approximately seven months after James began art therapy.

Due to James's Asperger's syndrome he struggled to use art making as a way to express himself as he found understanding his emotions confusing. However, James' intelligence, directness and black and white thinking enabled the use of psycho-educational components and semi directive tasks, which invited him to channel his thinking about his brother's condition and his own emotions. It took time to develop a method which worked effectively for James; this included using body mapping, 'worksheets' and inviting James to ask questions.

Over time, James began to trust me and developed his own method of using the sessions, which primarily involved talking, playing games, writing lists and occasionally drawing. I found that I often had to enter into James's world, whether this would involve listening to descriptions of Star Wars characters, playing battles with weapons that protected/

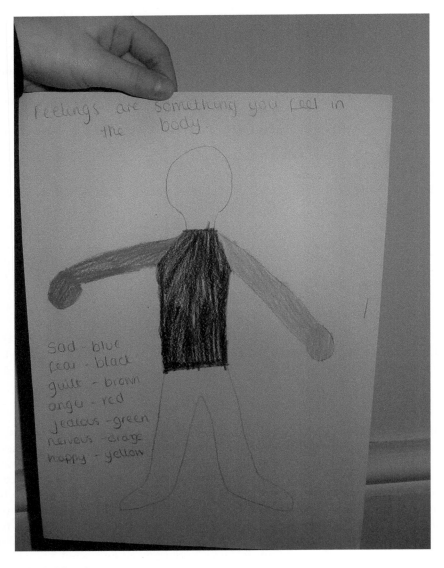

*Figure 21.1* Body Mapping

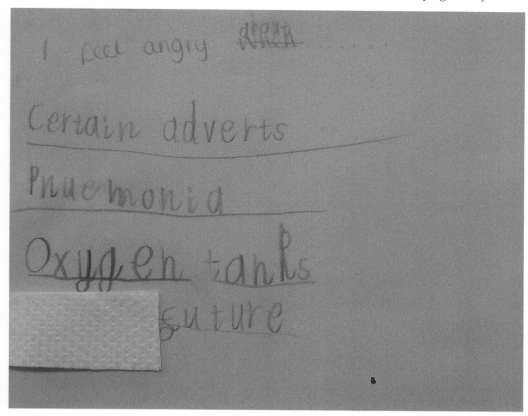

*Figure 21.2* I Feel Angry

attacked or playing board games such as 'Operation.' Although not a typical art therapy approach, the content of the sessions inevitably linked to James' emotions even though these were rarely verbalised.

James often needed to know information in advance, allowing him to process his thoughts. Therefore, his parents informed me of changes in his brother's condition and James often came with questions. This led to in-depth conversations about terminology used to describe death and grieving ('Why pass on?! Where do people pass to?), the medical and practical aspects of dying ('So the body shuts down and is no longer needed? . . . like when a car breaks down and needs to go to the scrap yard?') and religious beliefs ('I'm not sure I can be a Christian anymore, I'm too angry at God for allowing Kevin to get ill'). These conversations allowed James to make sense of his brother's death.

James showed me that he had normalised Kevin's death: 'Kayleigh! Guess what? Kevin has died,' and requested that we went to say good morning to him, therefore beginning the session alongside Kevin's body. James had decided that for his art therapy session he would like to take photos of his deceased brother on his iPad. When this was explored, James explained that his family were upset because they could not 'see' Kevin after the funeral and therefore he wished to create images which could go on the fridge so that Kevin could be 'seen' every day. In light of James's condition and with the support of his parents this was facilitated as it allowed James to create memories for himself and his family.

James sessions were expanded further to include a family music/art therapy session about the forthcoming funeral and a large family painting was created in memory of

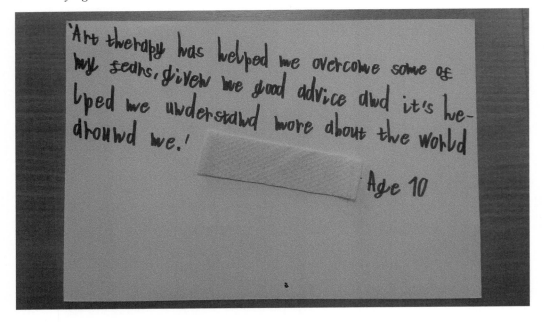

'Art therapy has helped me overcome some of my fears, given me good advice and it's helped me understand more about the world around me.'

Age 10

*Figure 21.3* James's Words

Kevin. James painted an image of Kevin's spirit going to heaven and his diseased body remaining on earth in his grave. James was invited into a dialogue with his family about the funeral, which allowed him to express his fears of crying and there being large volumes of people attending. This process showed James's knowledge and understanding of the funeral process, his religious beliefs and allowed him to express his fear. The music element of the session invited James and his brother to show the family how they felt and other family members were invited to 'meet' the boys in their playing.

Although not typical of everyday practice, with the music therapist I attended Kevin's funeral. It was felt that attending allowed the journey to continue for James and his brother without them having to verbalise their feelings. I was then able to refer to Kevin's death and funeral experience in future sessions. James continued to attend art therapy for several months after Kevin's death, allowing James to process the experience and express his own worries about being the eldest child, other family members dying and the effect the death had on individual family members. In his final session James was invited to create an image which reflected his experience of art therapy.

## Revisiting Death: 10 Years Later

Sally, a 16-year-old twin requested psychological support from Keech Hospice Care due to anger issues towards family members. Sally's father had died at the hospice from cancer when Sally was 6 years old. At the time, she had accessed group bereavement support. Sally vehemently denied that her anger issues related to the bereavement of her father and categorically stated that she did not wish to discuss this. Initially Sally accessed six 1:1 sessions with a male family support worker; however, she withdrew from these sessions due to feeling as though they were not 'helping.' It was suggested a referral to art therapy may be beneficial and she agreed.

To begin, I encouraged Sally to use the art work to think about how she responds to situations. She identified that other people angered her and when she felt in a pressurised situation she would verbally and physically lash out at her mother and brother. She identified that she did not wish to share her problems for fear of upsetting others, therefore leading her emotions to overspill. Sally also identified the need to be busy all the time, therefore undertaking many additional hours of school work and extra curriculum activities. Sally spoke about the demands and pressures of being a teenager, such as feeling self-conscious about her body image, peer relationships and sexual exploration.

Sally showed many avoidant behaviours during art therapy. During art making, she would re-create images from her school art and design projects. She questioned me repeatedly about my background and became angered when I informed her that this information could not be provided to ensure the therapeutic boundaries were maintained. It was also noted that Sally would attempt to provoke and analyse my comments or gestures. I felt that through the transference process, I had come to represent her family members, specifically the mother and therefore it was important to tolerate Sally's frustrations.

After ten sessions and without prompting, Sally suddenly spoke about her father's bereavement, stating that the art room overlooked the bedroom in which her father had died. She discussed the practical aspects of his death, the surprise of being able to discuss this openly, her experiences of bereavement groups and her own feelings about death and the afterlife. Although Sally had begun to talk about her father, it still felt that she was unable to connect emotions. However, from this point on Sally was able to tolerate reflections that I made, occasionally returning to wanting to control me. She identified that 'feeling out of controlled to aggression' and the need to suppress her emotions for fear of upsetting others. She was able to link these feelings to starting around the time her father had died. Sally's art work during this phase of therapy was of a mask which could be seen to represent her need to be controlled and brave in front of others but also reminded me of a death mask.

Another period of transition in Sally's therapy occurred when Sally's grandfather (on her father's side) was diagnosed with cancer. Sally continued to mask her true feelings, stating 'that everyone dies so there is no point in being upset about it.' However, her art work allowed her true feelings to be expressed. Sally used water and salt to create an image reminiscent of tears.

As Sally became more open about her feelings through her art work, it was mutually agreed that an end to her therapy should be set. This coincided with finishing an academic year for school and allowed a further eight sessions to consider the impact of ending and what this would mean.

When discussing the ending, Sally requested to dispose of her art work, specifically through burning it. Sally's reasoning behind this was that through burning, no parts of the art work would be left as the ash would disperse, whereas shredding or cutting could allow for parts to be seen. Although it was not verbalised, I was mindful that burning was reminiscent of cremating and contained ritualistic elements. It was not surprising to find out that both Sally's father and grandfather were cremated. I undertook a risk assessment and was able to provide Sally with an outdoor space, fire proof container and fire safety equipment. Sally was allowed to undertake the burning ritual she had in mind, whilst I observed quietly by her side. She burnt all of her art work in the garden, an area between the art room and the room in which her father had died. Afterwards, Sally requested that I dispose of the 'remains.'

## Loss of Art Work, Time and Boundaries

I was requested to work with a female inpatient, Alice, aged 40 years old, who had entered the hospice for symptom management for cancer of the stomach and tissue. However, Alice's deteriorating health meant that she was unable to return home and end of life care was required. Alice's husband and three teenage children were regular visitors to the hospice.

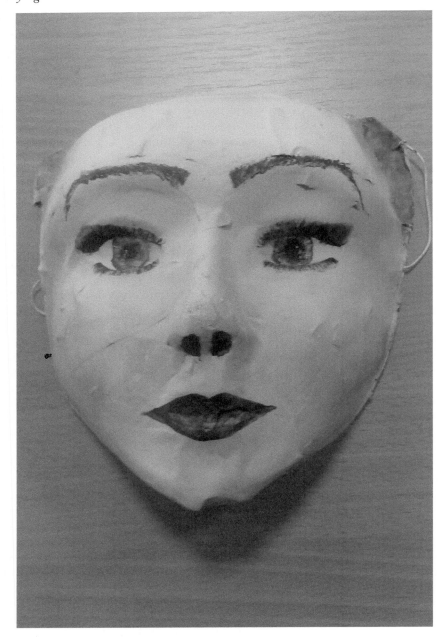

*Figure 21.4* Mask

During Alice's admission, staff were struggling to manage her pain and this was caus-ing frustration for Alice, who was concerned that her death would be painful. Alice had experienced a difficult childhood and had challenging relationships with her extended family members. Her husband had been her carer leading up to Alice's admission but this had been a difficult period for them both. It was identified by the nursing team that psychological support was required for staff and it was agreed that an external clinical psy-chologist would support the nursing team whilst I would offer art therapy sessions to Alice.

*Figure 21.5* Tears

Alice was clear that she did not wish to talk about her past relationships with family members, that they had come back into her life, but she felt there was not enough time to resolve these 'traumas' before she died. However, Alice was receptive to having weekly art therapy sessions at her bedside and it was agreed that the therapy would focus on the 'here and now.'

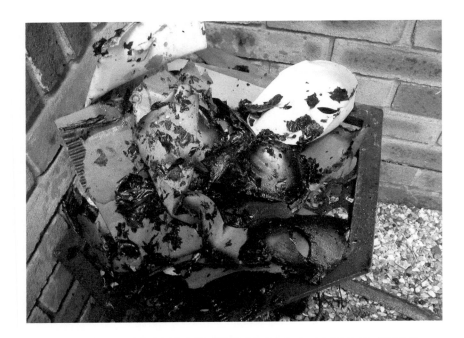

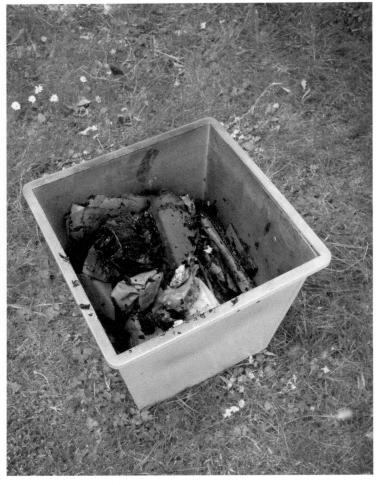

*Figure 21.6* and *21.7* Burn

Due to Alice's physical weakness it was suggested she used model magic, a soft modelling material which could be easily manipulated. To begin, Alice's sessions focussed on creating 'gifts' for her children. She recalled memories from their childhood and spoke about how proud she felt of her 'boys.' Alice also spent time creating a delicate drawing of a flower whilst discussing her pain, medications, care provided by the hospice and other palliative services. Alice was also able to speak concretely about her impending death and the fears she had of dying in pain. Alice's children and husband were always at the forefront of her mind and she spent sessions highlighting concerns about their ability to cope with her death and beyond. Although Alice's sessions continued on a regular basis, I offered to meet each of the family members and assess whether they wished to have any additional support. Using model magic once more, each family member was given the opportunity to discuss their own fears and uncertainties about the future. This alleviated Alice's concerns and also introduced her extended family to art therapy.

During Alice's therapy, I received news that one of my family members with a palliative diagnosis had moved into end of life care. I felt extremely conflicted in whether I should withdraw from the sessions because of the uncertainty about my availability for Alice and being able to use the transference and counter-transference effectively. I decided that rather than withdrawing from sessions I would inform Alice of my situation and would outline the impact it may have on future sessions, being mindful that it may have a negative impact upon the relationship. However, before this could happen, Alice asked me to tell her what was happening in my personal life, sensing that I was struggling with my own emotions. It was felt that Alice had invited me to share my own experiences of my family members illness and impending death. This appeared to be a positive experience for Alice and changed the way in which she used the sessions. She said, 'Nobody tells me how they feel. They are scared it will upset me. You've shared your pain with me and it makes me feel real.' Alice then went on to speak on an emotional level about her impending death and how it impacts upon others, how she felt ready to say goodbye and had come to terms with it but witnessing my pain had made her realise the importance of her family continuing to live fulfilling lives. Together, we cried about the losses we were both experiencing. It was felt that Alice's thinking had shifted from the present situation to facing no future.

As end of life approached, Alice would request for me to stay with her as she drifted in and out of consciousness. I would make art work alongside Alice and shared this with her when able to. Alice took particular interest in a piece which she titled 'straw hat.' This evoked memories for Alice as she touched briefly upon her childhood and the enjoyment she had experienced from nature. Alice saw pleasure in the art work whilst I saw a cancerous tumour and the lack of colour felt symbolic of further loss.

As Alice's body deteriorated the sessions with her became shorter and more fluid. Multiple losses were present including the art work, length of sessions and conversations. I witnessed each of these changes quietly at Alice's bedside until she died.

## Final Thoughts

Reflecting upon the cases above, it has become apparent that being faced with death and dying on a regular basis provides challenges. There is difficulty entering into a therapeutic relationship in palliative care without entering into the world of the client and therefore being led on a potentially painful, yet rewarding, journey. I found the need to relax the rigid boundaries learned in my formal training. By focussing less on the art making or keeping a therapeutic distance I was more able to be authentic in my responses to Alice. This made me query whether there was any 'art' or 'therapy' occurring and required confidence to advocate the significance of my practice to colleagues.

Furthermore, working within a hospice setting can expose clinicians to their own vulnerabilities and therefore there is an increased risk of burnout. Preventative measures

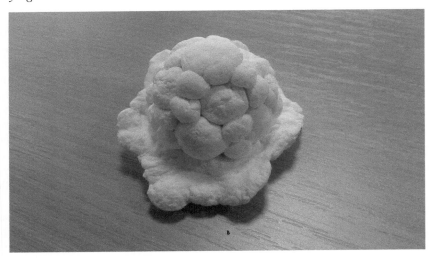

*Figure 21.8* Straw Hat

can include discussing cases within supervision, sharing pertinent information with other team members, reflecting upon case work, ensuring personal well-being is maintained and recognising when to step out of the work.

To ensure that the therapy has a positive impact, the art therapist has to be willing to expose themselves and adapt their practice to meet the needs of the individuals. As shown in the cases of Alice, James and Sarah this may mean tears may be shared at a bedside, photographs of deceased children may be taken and funerals may be attended.

**Confidentiality:** To maintain confidentiality of the families who have accessed support at Keech Hospice Care, permission to use details of art therapy sessions has been agreed and names have been changed.

## References

Department of Health. (2012) *End of Life Care Strategy.* [online] Available at: www.gov.uk/government/uploads/system/uploads/attachment_data/file/136486/End-of-Life-Care-Strategy-Fourth-Annual-report-web-version-v2.pdf [Accessed 14th April 2016]

Factsheet: How many children and young people are affected by a life limiting or life threatening condition? (2011) *Together for Short Lives.* Available at: www.togetherforshortlives.org.uk/wp-content/uploads/2018/01/ProRes-How-Many-Children-Young-People-Affected-By-A-Life-Limiting-or-Life-Threatening-Condition-Factsheet.pdf [Accessed 14th March 2016]

Johns, C. (1991) 'The Burford Nursing Development Unit Holistic Model of Nursing Practice'. *Journal of Advanced Nursing,* 16, pp. 1090–1098.

NHS England. (2014) *Actions for End of Life Care: 2014–2016.* [online] Available at: www.england.nhs.uk/wp-content/uploads/2014/11/actions-eolc.pdf [Accessed 17th April 2016]

Statement of Purpose. (2014) *Full Text.* [online] Keech Hospice Care. Available at: www.keech.org.uk/assets/000/000/213/STATE'Tof_PURP'_2014_FINAL_low_originalpdf [Accessed 29th April 2016]

Care Quality Commission
www.cqc.org.uk/
Keech Hospice Care
www.keech.org.uk
Together for Short Lives
www.togetherforshortlives.org.uk/professionals/resources
(National Charity for children and young people with a palliative condition)

# 22 'Time to Unwind'

## Meitheal at the Crossroads—An Open Art Therapy and Music Therapy Group on the Specialist Palliative Care Inpatient Unit

*Jennifer Newson McMahon, Neasa Whelan, Karen Kelly, and Meghan Treacy*

### Introduction

Milford Care Centre is a voluntary, non-profit organisation and a registered charity; it comprises a Specialist Palliative Care Inpatient unit, Specialist Palliative Care Day unit, Specialist Palliative Care Hospice-at-Home Community service, Older Persons' Day Care and a Nursing Home. The mission statement comprises core values from 'The Little Company of Mary' (the founders of Milford Care Centre) of Justice, Compassion, Respect, Communication and Accountability and the aim is to provide the highest quality care both in the area of palliative care and of the older person. Milford Care Centre, integrated within Ireland's Healthcare system, provides palliative care for the Mid-west region of Ireland encompassing the City of Limerick and County Limerick, County Clare and North Tipperary.

In this chapter, we will illustrate the value of a collaboration between art and music therapies in providing a therapeutic space for patients, families, friends and staff in the thirty-one bedded Specialist Palliative Care Inpatient Unit (hereafter referred to as the Inpatient Unit). We will document our journey through project planning, running an initial pilot group, the challenges, benefits and feedback that shaped the onward development of the group to the present where we run an established group. We have recently obtained ethical approval enabling us to collect data for more formal research on the benefits of this group.

### In the Beginning

Over the past ten years, in Milford Care Centre, the art and music therapists have collaborated with each other and with other members of the multi-disciplinary team. These collaborations included various projects such as creative reminiscence therapy or similar closed groups in the Nursing Home, Older Persons' Day Care and the Specialist Palliative Care Day Unit.

Our rationale in starting 'Time to Unwind' was to set up a therapeutic space for an open art therapy and music therapy group in the Inpatient Unit for patients, families and friends. We felt it was important to give them a space or 'time out' to leave the medical environment behind for a while and additionally give them a chance to experience pleasure or express themselves through art and music.

We held information sessions with the multi-disciplinary team and discussed with our nursing colleagues which area might be a suitable venue on the Inpatient Unit where we could hold the sessions. We chose the foyer / reception area as it is a large, comfortably furnished open area near the patients' rooms giving ease of access for participants to leave and join as they wished. It also gave an opportunity for people who were passing by to join in. Our plan was to run a pilot of six sessions that we could evaluate informally through verbal feedback given by the participants. The art and music therapists would meet after each session to discuss any observed benefits or interactions together with any issues that needed to be addressed. Evaluations would then determine whether this open group was a viable and worthwhile project to be incorporated as a regular part of our service.

As with previous collaborations, we were conscious that there were differing elements coming together that required discussion, including our different theoretical influences (Waller, 1993; Yalom, 1995; Schaverien, 1999; Kitwood, 1997; O'Kelly and Koffman, 2007). The result was an integrative approach, which we felt would provide an effective framework for this client group. We also discussed the format for the sessions and how the space would be set up. It was agreed that the piano/keyboard would be playing as participants arrived and they would be welcomed by the therapists. There was a selection of photographs, songbooks, objects and art materials displayed on the tables with an informal art gallery of images positioned on the wall behind one of the sofas. Busch (2001, p. 120) reflects on the use of photography as giving "the opportunity to experience a healing connection uniting the past with the present, weaving together inner and outer landscapes of memory and time."

Weiser (1999, p. 347) speaks of photographs as "effective keys that unlock doors to previously hidden information, feelings and memories." We also feel that this extends to the objects, art materials and songs or music used throughout the group.

In addition, a selection of instruments would be available for use by participants, such as a guitar and percussion. We aimed to provide opportunities through partaking or listening to live instrumental music, choosing a song/piece of music, using photographs, objects and art materials in order to reminisce, relax or reflect with other participants and the therapists.

When we discussed what name we should give this group, we wanted to incorporate both the intended relaxed nature of the group, giving participants "Time to Unwind", plus the Irish ethos of 'Meitheal'. Meitheal is the Irish tradition whereby neighbours came together socially, for example, sharing songs, stories, poems, dancing at the crossroads or assisting with various important life tasks such as gathering the hay or turf.

The group location being at a crossroads on the unit made this both relevant and meaningful. Figures 22.1 and 22.2 show the foyer area on the specialist palliative care unit.

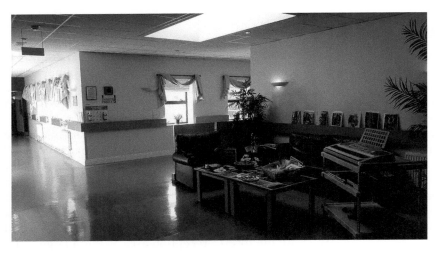

*Figure 22.1* The Foyer at the 'Crossroads' on the Unit (Angle 1)

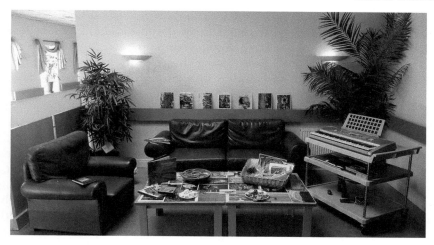

*Figure 22.2* Photo Gallery With Art and Music Materials

## Time to Unwind—Running the Pilot Project

The six sessions in this pilot project took place once a week for an hour and a half in the afternoon. The hour and a half time slot allowed for consultation with the staff, time setting up, collection of patients and running the group. We discovered that the afternoon was more suitable as the morning was busy with ward rounds and various appointments. We liaised with our nursing colleagues for an update on patients' conditions and then met available patients and their families on the unit during the morning, inviting them to the afternoon sessions. We displayed a 'Time to Unwind' poster in the foyer giving information about the afternoon art therapy and music therapy group.

## Running the Open Group

The fostering of creativity and self-expression within these therapeutic conditions began not on entering the "Time to Unwind" space but the moment the therapist arrived to introduce themselves to the patient; this was most commonly at their bedside. Either the art therapist or the music therapist approached the patient to invite them to attend. The introduction was short and succinct, emphasised attendance as voluntary and not mandatory. The element of choice is of the utmost importance for patients as they may have but a few choices left in their lives.

Not only was the challenge to introduce the patient to the premise of 'Time to Unwind' in a short period but it was important to describe briefly the space they would be entering, who would possibly attend, the facilitators and their respective disciplines of art and music therapy. We also discussed any particular needs they may have had in order to attend the session.

After setting up the space, we, along with our nursing and multi-disciplinary team colleagues, assisted in bringing participants to the group. Participants included those who were ambulant or in wheelchairs, and staff occasionally brought a patient in their bed. While participants were gathering, the music therapist played the piano/keyboard, letting the music float down the corridors, which in itself became a musical invitation. Weinstein Kaplan (2014) highlights the efficacy of gentle music playing in open clinical spaces as a way of engaging people and by providing a welcome distraction.

The introductory music played provided a warm relaxing atmosphere. The live music during the session, selected by participants or by the music therapist, included some Irish melodies, ballads and songs as well as some contemporary popular pieces. Participants had opportunities to request music/song choice or to sing or play an instrument throughout the session. Often the chosen music or songs have particular meaning for the individual. O' Callaghan and Magill (2016, p. 112) outline the importance of song/music choice as it enables individuals "to choose music that reflects feelings or thoughts they may have and for which they desire to gain support, or connect with special memories."

Art materials on display included a variety of images such as flowers, seascapes, landscapes, occupations, animals and olden day Irish photographs. There were also art, poetry and photography books available along with fabrics and tactile objects including shells and buttons. Some participants would select an image, material or object themselves and reflect on the reasons for their choice. At other times the art therapist invited them to select something if they so wished, as having a photograph or object in hand enables an easier avenue for reflection and or discussion. This approach is also supported by Case and Dalley (1992).

During the session, participants had the opportunity to move between the art and music elements with natural links occurring, for example, between an image, poem and a song. With participants being positively engaged with the art and music it gave relief from other issues. The value of the creative process is also described by Trauger-Querry and Haghighi (1999).

As you can see in Figures 22.2 and 22.3, the main area of activity for the group centred around the piano/keyboard and gallery in the brown sofa area, leaving a quieter space for others on the smaller sofa opposite.

Five minutes before ending the group, we gave clear notice that the session was drawing to a close and offered final song/music choices. We thanked participants for attending and participating, advising them we would be there the following week. In addition, we informed them we were available for individual art therapy or music therapy sessions in the interim if they so wished.

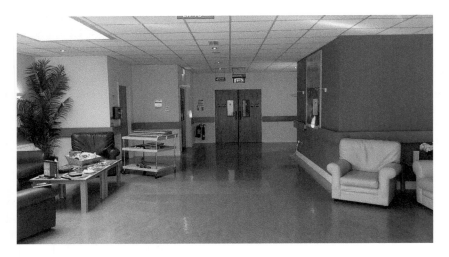

*Figure 22.3* The Foyer at the 'Crossroads' on the Unit (Angle 2)

## Evaluation and Reflection From the Pilot Project

Spontaneously during the group, participants would make verbal comments, or we asked for feedback after the group. There were three ways we collected feedback; firstly, from our own observations during the group sessions. Here we learnt the value of having two therapists as there was greater awareness and quicker responses to participants' reactions and needs in the group. From our observations, we noticed that onlookers, who were initially standing nearby, gradually moved nearer and sat down sometimes spontaneously or by invitation from one of the therapists.

Secondly, from participants as to how they found the group and what aspects were most useful for themselves. We also gave them the opportunity to say which elements they did not like and any changes they would prefer for the group format, and we asked whether they would wish to attend again. Thirdly, from staff observations.

The feedback received from participants during this pilot was extremely positive with many repeated comments on it being enjoyable, relaxing, uplifting, and calming. Additional comments were that it gave patients and families a break from their rooms, offered an opportunity to exchange coping strategies, being with their families in a positive way and that they enjoyed meeting other patients and families. Our observations confirmed their feedback and is echoed by Ward (1999), in observing art therapy with families. Aldridge (1999, p. 18), describes it as being, "an experience of time that is qualitatively rich."

We noted that staff, on passing the session, reacted positively to the music playing—smiling, moving to the music, giving music/song requests, clapping and responding to patients and families. This increased our awareness of the value sessions held for staff, but also how it served to change their perception of their patients' capabilities when they saw them communicating creatively through art and or music. This shift in focus is also observed by Obrian (2001, p. 164), who states "patients work may also help to create a focus for change in identity shifting the emphasis from 'terminally ill' to an individual actively engaged in pursuing and constructing meaning."

Informal evaluation of this pilot project highlighted the value of having an art and music therapy open group with patients and their families or friends in the Specialist Palliative Care Inpatient Unit. Consequently, we decided to incorporate it as part of our regular service and now describe in further detail the onward planning, the therapeutic space, and session themes before discussing both challenges and benefits.

## Our Current Weekly Art Therapy and Music Therapy Open Group

Encouraged by our findings from the pilot project we kept in mind the institutional factors important when deciding to run this weekly group. Group attendance is influenced by its allocated time schedule and its synchronicity with meal times, patient personal care, Mass times, routine staff checks, family meetings and medical updates. Even with all these factors taken into account, there may be very few patients available due to their current level of health, having visitors or having no interest participating in the group.

Just as the therapists' intuition within the session is integral to the group's success, it is also important that this apply when deciding to run the group. As discussed previously in relation to the pilot project, it is important to be considerate and respectful of what is happening on the unit. At times we decided to cancel the group session for different reasons such as recently bereaved relatives using the foyer area or one of the therapists being unavailable.

This consideration begins early in the morning of a group by attending meetings regarding medical updates, planned discharges, discussions in relation to patient care and availability of staff. A good relationship with consultants, doctors, nursing staff, carers and other multi-disciplinary team members is essential. They can relay a broad overview of patient care in the previous twenty-four hours prior to the group and may influence the materials chosen.

It is important to have a good understanding and insight into the needs of the patients; their interests, history, and present mood. Even with all this information and preparation circumstances can change quickly and affect group attendance.

## The Therapeutic Space

O' Kelly and Koffman (2007), state the importance of collaborative work in creating an easily accessible public therapeutic space. Inviting patients, families and friends to step into a neutral space, temporarily transformed into a creative one, takes them away from the purely medical landscape that they inhabit at that particular time. Waller (2002) also describes the importance of the surrounding environment with families and staff for patients with progressive illnesses.

The presence of two qualified and experienced therapists ensured a safe space; they were mindful of maintaining boundaries, and understanding of group dynamics and the changing needs of the participants. This was essential as it provided an environment where all could contribute as they wished; integrate, support each other and share both emotionally and creatively. Rogers states that his "experience in psychotherapy leads me to believe that by setting up conditions of psychological safety and freedom, we maximise the likelihood of an emergence of constructive creativity" (Rogers, 1967, pp. 356–357). Both art and music therapists, Schaverien (1999) and Salmon (2001), agree on the importance of the therapeutic space with its potential for transformation. This space, which is one of three elements, together with the therapeutic relationship and the art/music materials, enable participants to engage in the session safely. Sometimes family members or friends need a quiet break from the intensity of their loved one's bedside, to be distracted or soothed by an image or a melodic interlude, simply to just be within a space with no expectations required of them.

Figure 22.3 illustrates that in this 'crossroads' venue one sofa provides a central focal point, while the other, a space away from the immediate music and imagery for people who wish only to observe.

## Session Themes and Events

Sessions can occur where all attendees are unfamiliar to each other and the space, or it may be that they have attended or met before. The latter may experience a sense of belonging and begin looking forward to sharing their chosen song or awaiting new images they will encounter. Some participants will experience the group only once whereas others may have multiple sessions. According to Wood (2005), there is evidence that even a single session can be of value.

Soft relaxing melodies played at the beginning of the session help to set the tone of the group in creating a warm, welcoming atmosphere. During the group we invited participants to select a personal song or piece of music or they may create musical links with images or objects they are handling. The aim is to give ownership and autonomy to individuals in the group

The content of the conversations occurs, either spontaneously or through the use of art materials or via a song/melody. The conversations may include experiences of being in a hospice environment, treatment experiences, support from someone in a similar situation, family members and friends getting support from each other. Other frequent themes are: places they have travelled/holidays, nature, how times have changed, reminiscing through art and music. We have found that some of these themes arise stimulated by art and music.

The two media allow for the use of symbolism and metaphor in their communication which as we have previously stated can make it easier to express how they feel in their current situation. Examples include, through the use of imagery; participants describing themselves as a lighthouse being battered by storms, of being upside down in a bed because their world has been turned upside down or musically through chosen songs echoing how a participant feels. A client has shared his feelings on awaiting death by comparing it to being at a horse racing event, knowing the race has started but not knowing when the horses will reach where he is standing. What he does know is that when they do get to him they will be gone in a flash.

The use of the image or art objects not only stimulates conversation but also connects people physically through sharing and passing to each other within a common experience. Additional examples in how group participants connect with each other include one making a nest out of clay and others making eggs and filling her nest; one participant or the whole group singing a significant song for another participant either for a special event or on request. Individuals' music choices can at times mirror their moods or be a conscious decision to take them in a different direction at the "crossroads." Both serve to bring up memories or create new realities. Other authors such as Falk (2002); Simon (1997); and Birtchnell (1984), also speak of the importance of symbolic images as holding memories.

During sessions, participants have celebrated events such as birthdays and anniversaries. They have also participated by performing a song or playing an instrument or by reading a poem of their own composition. Through our own observations, we have found like O' Callaghan (2013), that there can be private family moments within the hospice setting.

## Challenges

Some of the initial challenges from the pilot project continue to be pertinent in our regular group such as the changing composition of the group.

There are a number of factors here such as not knowing in advance how many participants there will be or what proportion will be patients, family members or friends. Numbers of participants have varied from one person to twenty people. There was a need to not only observe how the main group was progressing but to be cognisant of those sitting or standing on the periphery.

Keeping the cohesiveness of a large group, with all wishing to participate, occupying both sofas and additional seating presented a definite challenge. It required great attention and skill to ensure that each was offered an opportunity to handle materials, have a song /music choice and share with those nearest them. Any connections arising would be highlighted by one of the therapists if another participant was too far away from the speaker and it was appropriate to make the connection. Again having two therapists managing the group enabled one to move around the group. We endeavoured to allow participants to be part of a group but still unique in themselves and their reflections, memories and comments were valued. Naturally there were differences of opinions at times and that needed to be acknowledged and the reality of people having opposing viewpoints. This highlights the strength of having therapists used to group dynamics.

A common issue is managing participants joining or leaving during the session which can be for a variety of reasons such as fatigue, an appointment or a visitor arriving unexpectedly. We do advise participants of this probability when we conduct the initial meeting with them. Departures from the group session can take two forms, either a quiet one or one where other participants voice their positive feelings about being with the person who had to leave. This is where having two therapists is necessary, as there is always one therapist to work with the group whilst the second copes with the changes. Our challenge is being ready to facilitate either event.

Being open about the interruptions and apologising when appropriate, has met with general understanding by participants. There are influences outside our control such as visitors asking for directions, traffic to and from the lift, new patients arriving on the unit or staff trolleys moving through the space. We also needed to manage this area by ensuring that the main walkways through the Inpatient Unit were kept clear in line with health and safety requirements. Practical issues also included putting in boundaries around the taking of photographs by participants to ensure the maintenance of confidentiality of others in the group.

Working together lessened the challenge in providing a balance in the 'Time to Unwind' sessions between supporting serious issues with lighter ones and found that fun and laughter often happened spontaneously within the group.

## Learning Points: Benefits for Patients, Family, Friends and Staff

- We found that the co-facilitation of two therapists offered participants greater choice with whom they would like to interact during the session.
- We observed that the inclusion of objects, art, poetry and music offered patients alternative avenues through which to communicate a range of feelings and memories.
- The relaxed nature of the group encouraged participants to engage at their own pace.
- The open group sessions form a temporary community 'Meitheal', for participants with time to express, be acknowledged, have fun, pass on advice or receive support whilst they are away from their usual communities.
- The regular nature of our current group now means that participants can look forward to other sessions or on their next admission to the unit.
- Some participants who may have found connections to each other, or formed friendships or renewed past acquaintances during sessions can continue to provide support for each other.
- Staff become accustomed to the regular group day and time and so keep people in mind who may like or benefit from attending.
- Members of the multi-disciplinary team are also aware and drop in to join a patient or the group in general.
- Staff see patients participating in a meaningful manner and perhaps showing abilities or life skills not previously known about.

## Learning Points: Benefits for Therapists

- The advantage of having two therapists was apparent to us from the beginning, as it allowed both general and more personal interactions to occur, for example, some participants could be listening to music played by the music therapist whilst the art therapist could be holding an in-depth conversation with another.
- We found support in having another therapist working in tandem to address the changing needs of the group.

- By co-facilitating the group, the therapists instinctively supported and learnt from each other, which made for effective and empathic management of the group.
- Afforded the two therapists an opportunity to try different materials and assess their suitability, for example, the introduction of soft white modelling dough that proved to be successful with patients choosing to leave their pieces or take them back to their rooms.
- The longer the two therapists work together the more it became second nature in knowing who was to take the lead and when that needs to change.
- The trust and surety in each other's therapy built and gave greater understanding of how best to 'marry' the two therapies in sessions.
- These ongoing sessions increased the therapists' knowledge about the use of art therapy and music therapy in palliative care.
- Working alongside a supportive colleague decreased the pressure that can arise from holding stressful issues, provided natural peer support.

## Conclusion

This 'Time to Unwind' project has developed from an initial successful pilot project to an evaluated study, and has led onto more formal research. Based on feedback from patients, families, friends and staff, and from our own observations and evaluations, this project is a worthwhile and valuable resource. It enhances and extends conventional ways of working to a wide range of participants with differing needs. The group provides a therapeutic space with an atmosphere that encourages creativity and interconnectivity, whilst supporting participants in their unfolding of their life experiences. Meitheals can meet their need to be with family, friends or fellow patients, taking the time to literally 'unwind' in a creative way.

Our project concurs with research on the benefit of effective interdisciplinary team work by Edwards et al (2006), who conducted the first collaborative art and music therapies research study in Ireland. We would encourage other Creative Arts Therapists' to collaborate and develop their own "Meitheals" in palliative care both at home and abroad.

## References

Aldridge, D. (1999) 'Music Therapy and the Creative Act' in Ed. Aldridge, D. *Music Therapy in Palliative Care: New Voices.* London and Philadelphia: Jessica Kingsley Publishers, p. 18.

Birtchnell, J. (1984) *Art Therapy as a Form of Psychotherapy in Art as Therapy.* Ed. Dalley, T. London and New York: Routledge, p. 39.

Busch, C. (2001) *Pilgrimage Revisited: Celtic Spirituality in Spirituality and Art Therapy: Living the Connection.* Ed. Mimi F.-H. London and Pennsylvania: Jessica Kingsley Publishers, p. 120.

Case, C., Dalley, D. (1992) 'Introduction' in *The Handbook of Art Therapy.* New York: Routledge, pp. 1–18.

Edwards, J., Ledger, A., Loane, R., Newson McMahon, J., Wale, S., Hiscock, R. (2006) 'An evaluation of the effects of combining music therapy and art therapy to reduce challenging behaviour in people with dementia on a specialist care ward', *National Institute of Health Sciences Research Health Bulletin,* 3(3), 51–55.

Falk, B. (2002) 'Arts Therapies and Progressive Illness: Nameless Dread' in Ed. Waller, D. *A Narrowed Sense of Space: An Art Therapy Group with Young Alzheimer's Suffers.* Hove, East Sussex: Brunner-Routl edge Publishers, pp. 107–121.

Kitwood, T. (1997) *Dementia Reconsidered: The person comes first.* Buckingham: University Press, p. 8.

Obrian, J. (2001) 'Providing scope for creative growth in palliative care', *European Journal of Palliative Care,* 164.

O' Callaghan, C. (2013) 'Music therapy preloss care through legacy creation', *Progress in Palliative Care,* 21(2), 78–82.

O' Callaghan, C., Magill, L. (2016) 'Music Therapy with Adults Diagnosed with Cancer and Their Families' in Ed. Edwards, J. *The Oxford Handbook of Music Therapy*. Oxford: Oxford University Press, p. 112.

O' Kelly, J., Koffman, J. (2007) 'Multidisciplinary perspectives of music therapy in adult palliative care', *Palliative Medicine*, 21, 235.

Rogers, C.R. (1967) *A Therapist's View of Psychotherapy on Becoming a Person*. London: Publications Constable and Company Ltd., pp. 356–357.

Salmon, D. (2001) 'Music therapy as psychospiritual process in palliative care', *Journal of Palliative Care*, 17(3), 142–146.

Schaverien, J. (1999) 'The Picture Within the Frame', in *The Revealing Image: Analytical Art Psychotherapy in Theory and Practice*. London and Philadelphia: Jessica Kingsley Publishers, pp. 62–78.

Simon, R.M. (1997) 'The Circle in the Square' in *Symbolic Images in Art as Therapy*. London and New York: Routledge, pp. 4–14.

Trauger-Querry, B., Ryan Haghighi, K. (1999) 'Balancing the focus: Art and music therapy for pain control and symptom management in hospice care', *The Hospice Journal*, 4(1), 28.

Waller, D. (1993) *Group Interactive Art Therapy: Its Use in Training and Treatment*. New York: Routledge.

Waller, D. (2002) *Arts Therapies and Progressive Illness: Nameless Dread*. East Sussex and New York: Brunner-Routledge.

Ward, C. (1999) 'Shaping Connections—Hands on Art Therapy' in Ed. Cattanach, A. *Process in the Arts Therapies*. London and Philadelphia: Jessica Kingsley Publishers, pp. 103–131.

Weinstein Kaplan, B. (2014) 'The healing arts program at Montefiore: A collaboration that heals patients and nurses', *Oncology Nurse Advisor*, 5(3), 46–47.

Weiser, J. (1999) 'Using Photo Therapy to Promote Healing and Personal Growth' in *Phototherapy Techniques: Exploring the Secrets of Personal Snapshots and Family Albums*. Vancouver, Canada: Photo Therapy Centre, p. 347.

Wood, M.J.M. (2005) 'The Contribution of Art Therapy to Palliative Medicine' in Eds. Doyle, D., Hanks, G., Cherny, N. and Calman, K. *Oxford Textbook of Palliative Medicine*. Oxford: Oxford University Press, pp. 1063–1067.

Yalom, I.D. (1995) The Theory and Practice of Group Psychotherapy. New York: Basic Books.

## Acknowledgements

We wish to thank our Milford Care Centre colleagues for their support, assistance and professional advice.

# 23 Group Art Therapy Using Telemedicine Technology for Patients Undergoing Chemotherapy

*Gudrun Jones, Rachel Rahman, and Martine Robson*

*I switched the video screen off at the end of the session. I didn't understand what the problem was. In the silence I thought: I cannot carry on with this project. I am an art therapist not an I.T. specialist!*

The experience of running a group therapy session using video conferencing was my biggest challenge yet. Telemedicine looks very similar to a Skype connection, both sides able to view and hear the other on a television screen. But in this session, the fragile connections that held me and three patients together kept breaking, as we repeatedly lost visual and audio links.

As an art therapist in a Welsh rural hospital, working within the Oncology and Palliative care team, my role has traditionally involved providing a two-core approach, psychodynamic art therapy as well as 'First Aid' Cognitive Behavioural Therapy (CBT), working to level 2 of the National Institute and Clinical Excellence (NICE, 2004) Guidelines using CBT techniques in cancer care. Art therapy aims to provide a safe, supportive, and consistent place where patients can discuss their issues and experiences of living with a cancer diagnosis. The creation of artwork offers an additional vehicle for communicating and sharing meaningful experiences through symbol and metaphor. I have always seen the meaningful personal connections that are made with individuals in a small rural community as an important component of my therapeutic role, which includes visiting clients at home as well as in hospital.

The official name of the Welsh National Health Service is Gwasanaeth Iechyd Gwladol Cymru (GIG Cymru), and it is divided into seven health boards that are publicly funded and are the responsibility of the devolved Welsh Government. The health board I work for covers rural Mid Wales and palliative care is part of the community services. Our service is supported by a 'Hospice at Home' service run by a local charity. We don't have a hospice in our county. Clients will often have to spend an hour-long journey to visit the local hospital, which can be a significant burden for both patients and their families. The alternative is that I spend time travelling between clients and so manage to see fewer in a day. An opportunity arose to be part of a PhD research project with the Aberystwyth University Psychology Department. The title of the thesis was "The feasibility and acceptability of telehealth to support palliative care in Mid Wales: Exploring professional perceptions and patient experiences" (Keenan, 2018). This offered a way of exploring an innovative service working with a full-time postgraduate researcher to support the technology, which I would not have had the knowledge or confidence to do alone.

The PhD project involved a one-to-one connection, using laptops and videoconferencing software, from clients' homes. The technology worked well and clients reported significant benefits to accessing the service from the privacy of their own homes. The telehealth connection afforded them the relief of engaging in their care without the pressure of the associated travel. They experienced an improved sense of autonomy, as their day was now theirs to plan as they wished, rather than being dominated by healthcare appointments. Most encouraging to me was that the distance created by the technology did not seem to impact the closeness of the therapeutic relationship. Clients reported feeling well supported and spoke of the understanding and beneficial relationship that developed between us. In sum, the benefits exceeded our expectations and led to us to develop a second, more ambitious piece of research. In this latest project, we decided to form two eight-week virtual therapy groups, using the telemedicine technology to connect two to three individuals from their own homes to me as the art therapist in the local hospital. In this chapter, I outline the therapeutic approach that was adopted to deliver this virtual group therapy, and reflect on the challenges and successes of the service, with a particular focus on the ability to maintain psychologically meaningful connections via telehealth technology in a remote environment.

## The Research Set Up

The researchers (Rachel Rahman and Martine Robson), both psychologists, worked with me to consider unmet needs within our service that could benefit from the technology that had worked so well in the first project. We identified a lack of psychosocial support for patients undergoing chemotherapy in a rural area. The benefits of peer support were well documented in many different contexts (Dale et al., 2012; Thompson et al., 2007; Ussher et al., 2006). However, the immunosuppression faced by chemotherapy clients clearly limited our ability to deliver face-to-face group sessions, even without the added burden of travel. Chemotherapy patients already regularly travel significant distances to receive their treatment, and also often suffer nausea and fatigue. A systematic review had suggested positive outcomes for online group peer support (Hoey et al., 2007), and so it seemed an ideal opportunity to trial videoconferencing. After the project received ethical approval, clients on the chemotherapy ward were approached by the oncologist and chemotherapy nurses and offered the opportunity to participate.

The first challenge was that recruitment was slow, but this arose more from the reluctance of the team to broach the subject with clients than from clients declining to take part. The staff all appeared supportive of the project, but were also concerned about increasing burdens and stress for their vulnerable patients. It was interesting to see healthcare staff use their own preconceptions to decide who would and would not be open to using technology in their care. I couldn't blame them—this was something that I had struggled with in the first project. Surprisingly, age, gender, and stage of illness had no bearing on how acceptable technology would be to someone, and I had learnt through that experience that there really was no way of telling in advance.

In the end, we ran two small groups. The first included two women, aged between 45 and 55 living close to the local hospital. The second included a man, Ashley, aged 69, and two women, Kate, in her 60s, and, Gemma, in her late 30s. These participants lived in more remote locations, between half an hour and an hour away from the hospital. The research team interviewed participants before, during, and after the art therapy groups to gather their expectations, concerns, and experiences whilst I delivered eight weekly sessions of art therapy to each group.

## The Therapeutic Approach

An art pack was delivered to each participant: an A4 spiral bound journal, chalks, pastels paint, brushes, glue, and a variety of coloured papers. The journal was theirs to keep, and the participants were encouraged to use the journal between sessions for writing or creating further images.

Each of the eight sessions lasted an hour and half, and followed a regular pattern, beginning with a sharing round, then approximately 20 minutes of making pictures and/ or writing, based on a weekly theme. Participants then shared their work and each session ended with a five-minute relaxation exercise.

I have run art therapy groups in different ways over the years depending on the needs of the client group, including brief or longer term, slow, open groups (Jones, G. 2000, 2007). I have used a directive approach, providing clients with themes, visual exercises, and with groups who have worked together on joint images, as well as a more traditional non-directive, psychodynamic art therapy approach, which allows clients' own ideas and themes to emerge in the moment. In this relatively short-term therapy group, I suggested a theme at the first session, and subsequently offered participants the option of choosing their own topic. However, participants of the two cohort virtual therapy groups chose to take up my suggestion each time. For the first session, I chose the metaphor of a boat as a vehicle for describing where clients felt they were on that day, which enabled discussions about personal journeys, their own resources, isolation, sources of support and difficulties, and internal and external worlds. They interpreted the theme in their own way with any of the materials available. I subsequently used the previous session's discussions as a starting point for each week's theme.

Although I was initially surprised that clients preferred my choice of themes/topics over their own, on reflection, I think this format helped focus the work in the session, which was especially valuable in view of the limited number of sessions. Freed from the pressure of having to choose or design their own theme, my suggestions provided a container for clients' feelings and structured and enabled discussion in this different environment.

As a therapist from a psychodynamic background, I am always conscious of the therapist's influence on the work of the group. In thinking about how this therapy group developed over the eight weeks I considered how the structure might influence the end result. Bion (1961), in his theory on group development, identifies 'dependency' as an emotional stage in the life of a group, where the 'basic assumption' is that the therapist will take on the responsibility for the themes. Was this group more dependent on the therapist because of the intervention of the technology and physical distance of the virtual therapy room? I thought the distance created by telecommunication might impact the time available for everyone to share their story, which together with the potential for delay in the flow of audio communication would influence how the group would bond together. Another consideration is the impact of the illness and treatment on patients' physical condition, energy, and concentration.

## Running the Two Virtual Therapy Groups

From my point of view, the first few sessions of both cohorts were technologically disastrous. In the initial eight-session group, one of the participants connected online with ease, and we were full of optimism. However, the second participant faced a major stumbling block in linking in to the NHS conferencing software from her workplace because of firewalls, which are used by large companies and now home users, to protect against potential hackers and offensive websites. It took several weeks of trials with expert technical support from the University to help us. By week three, both participants were linking in with ease, even when one had to relocate in order to undergo surgery. Without a research team and their technical support, I doubt we would have been able to continue.

We had assured ourselves that the second eight-session group with its new participants would be far less problematic, given that everyone was linking from home, with no dreaded firewalls to overcome! Ashley, the first participant, linked in with ease and

Kate joined second. However, once the third patient, Gemma, joined, it became apparent that the broadband struggled to support the visual link between all four of us. Imagine a face-to-face group, where participants run in and out of the room, where you cannot keep people together in one place for any length of time. This is how I experienced the poor network links, where people dropped in and out of vision and sound and sometimes disappeared altogether. One participant was unable to join at all, so I phoned her, and relayed the other participants' conversations and described their artwork to her, and hers to them throughout that first session. For me, this was my 'session from hell'.

It was a session where all of the core principles of the 'right way' to run an art therapy group had been challenged. It left me questioning whether the therapy course was going to make people feel worse, and I felt that I could not put the clients through another session like it. It had been almost unbearable for me, so I could only imagine how people felt who were unwell after chemotherapy. Surely, they would not be able to bond as a group with us connecting in this unreliable manner? At the end, I had to ask whether they want to carry on. To my amazement, they all said yes. They had clearly connected with each other and benefited from that tenuous contact. But my heart sank, as I was not sure I could cope with the continual risk of connectivity failure. I was very conscious that the situation echoed the fragility and uncertainty that their illness, treatments, and test results can cause, and I was having a direct experience of this through the difficulties with the technology. However, at their request, we persevered with two participants successfully linking in and the third joining the sessions by phone via a conference call, so that at least the other clients could hear her voice.

The format for a typical art therapy session in my setting is to begin with a discussion of topics; these can cover the whole range of emotions and experiences that accompany a cancer diagnosis, day-to-day concerns, and thoughts about the future. Then follows a period of image making based on a chosen theme, after which group members share their artwork and experiences before the session comes to an end.

Art therapy groups in my experience offer a place to express thoughts and feelings that are not voiced elsewhere. They provide a welcome safe space where negative or angry feelings can be expressed without overburdening families or friends. The candid discussions and sharing that followed the making of images via telehealth technology indicated that the group had developed into a safe space to share their experiences and artwork. Despite being inexperienced in making art, clients showed ingenuity and confidence in interpreting themes and describing their experiences. This in turn gave me confidence to pursue this way of working, with technology as a partner in therapy.

Over the weeks I began to feel more confident that the virtual group had engaged with creative processes, and that the making of visual images and poems added a valuable layer of connection and meaning over and above the verbal communication. The sharing of thoughts and ideas around the work gave an insight into each person's thinking and approach to their illness and experience. The images became a shared language for the group, a way of reviewing progress or describing each other's position, often being referred to in subsequent sessions. For example, a sailing boat with a torn and tattered topsail in a rough sea is later seen in tranquil surroundings, with a mended sail, perhaps implying a change in the state of mind of the maker. I was pleased and excited to find that the image making came into its own and provided a rich layer of sharing in the group, despite the technological difficulties we encountered.

In art therapy, the therapist is traditionally the caretaker of the visual work until such time as the therapy comes to an end. At this point, clients can choose to take the artwork away, or leave it with the therapist to be destroyed confidentially in due course. It struck me when I first began working via telemedicine, how much I had invested in that caretaker role, and how much I missed reflecting on the artworks as I tidied them away after sessions. The length of time the artwork was on screen was short, and we were dependent on the maker to give a verbal description. I did miss the tactile experience of observing work being made, and was surprised to learn from participant interviews that this was not so for participants, who valued the privacy the technology offered. Many discussed how they enjoyed the 20 minutes when the others were 'there' on screen, but not intruding into their space whilst they created, reflected on, and considered their art. Not being observed by others meant that they felt more relaxed and confident about their artwork and some talked about taking inspiration from their own surroundings that held personal meaning for them. Telemedicine thus provided generative experiences that would not have been possible in a village hall or hospital setting.

However, I still questioned whether the same supportive interpersonal relationships would develop between members of the group when we were all so remote from one another. My question was clearly answered in the session I describe below.

## The Island Session

I have chosen extracts from one group session to explore how the artwork enabled a discussion about their sense of the gathering as a group. This followed the 'session from hell' that had been disrupted by technological connection difficulties.

In this session there are three members: Ashley, Kate, and Gemma.

Gemma had connected briefly by conference phone before the session began to tell us she was going back to bed, because she felt so ill after her chemotherapy treatment.

I proposed the theme of 'The Island' and suggested that if they wanted more space for their artwork, they could open out the journal as a double page spread. This extended space would be a topic of conversation later. I asked the group to make a picture of an island of their own, but also to think about their island in relation to each other. I wanted to give them the opportunity to share their experiences of the connections between the group members. I was very curious, as well as anxious, to understand what made them want to carry on with this project.

The two participants in this session, Ashley and Kate, worked on their images for around 20 minutes as usual. Ashley then shared his island picture with us saying, 'this is my green island with a tree on it', a reflection on his rural and remote location and the importance of the wild uncontrolled nature and landscape that he valued. He then said to Kate, 'I've given you a gold shiny island, it's nice and bright'. Kate was delighted, and she playfully named it 'treasure island'.

Despite being absent that day, Gemma was still present in our minds, and on paper—Ashley said,

> 'I have given Gemma a purple island and the sea around her is a bit rougher, a bit up and down (and her island) a bit rocky, because I feel perhaps she is in a rougher place than we are.'

Despite only meeting Gemma once, briefly on screen, Ashley's picture encapsulated her physical and emotional situation, and his insight and empathy for her.

The closeness I observed between them was the common experience of each having been through chemotherapy and knowing what those bad days were about. Two of the participants were receiving palliative chemotherapy. The group hoped that Gemma, who was only at the beginning of her treatment, would survive and get to the point where Ashley, who had completed his treatment, and Kate who was mid treatment, were. Ashley's islands seemed to reflect these different stages—his own smooth, peaceful, green island, Kate's shiny golden island reflecting her very positive and hopeful view in her art work and through her poems, and Gemma's more troubled and difficult space. There was also a common hope that their treatment would work and give them all a future.

Kate had used one side of A4 paper to draw her archipelago of islands. She had included an island for Martine, the research assistant 'trying to make sure the connections do work', and for me 'the host keeping the group in contact with each other'. She then reflected on the limitations of her one ferry boat that she had drawn, which she realised could only go to one island at a time. She said,

> 'There is no permanence about that, it only connects two at a time, whereas, I think there must be a way to bring everyone together, maybe put a central island and everyone can go by ferry and go to the central island and then we'll all be together.'

Ashley responded by describing his island; he had also given each island a boat.

> 'There is the little boat here with lines going to each island (as you might see on a map to depict a pathway) this is Gudrun's little boat keeping us all in communication.'

After seeing Kate's image, Ashley was concerned that since he had used the double page spread it had made the islands look far apart, which did not accurately describe his experience of the group.
He said,

> 'I think if I'd made smaller islands and kept them together as a group, that would show that we are a group you know, that we are connected rather than spread out.'

He added another dimension to their connectedness, one that was not limited to their technological, once a week contact, but affirmed that they were present in each other's thoughts and reflections throughout the week. He asserted that, 'we're not only a group on a Tuesday morning, because we are a group all week, we are there all the time, so we are still connected to the group, we still have the connection which is important and not only on a Tuesday morning'.

A description of the session and the images was emailed to Gemma after the group session, and who then made her own drawings of islands in her journal.

Can drawing islands and sharing thoughts, explain anything about the quality of the cohesiveness? I believe that by engaging imaginatively, creatively, and visually, a rich and multi-level connectedness had been established between them, despite the technological barriers; and this was only their third session.

Whilst I had been anxious and distressed by the technical connectivity problems experienced by Gemma in particular, I was surprised that this did not figure in any of the participants' images nor was it identified by Gemma as a problem. I perhaps held the anxiety for the group about the tenuous nature of the connectivity, while the group itself achieved a sense of oneness.

I was also struck that without any discussion group members had both given Martine (researcher) and I an island each with very definite roles. I did wonder about our roles as facilitators in group therapy, often referred to as parental figures. Martine could be seen as representing the father, as she was involved in the practical technical connections in each of their homes. I represented the mother as the one who managed the emotional world of the group. I was also reminded of Winnicott's (1971) phrase 'good enough mother' and continuity of care in the therapeutic relationship. The technology was responsible for a loss of continuity in a very concrete way in the previous session. I had to accept that neither of us could solve the connectivity problem and compromises had to be made with Gemma on a phone conference call. But the connectedness was evidently 'good enough' for all the clients to be content to continue in this way.

Interestingly, what I experienced and reflected on in this session was echoed in the interview data later. The researchers had conducted participant interviews before, at the midpoint, and at the end of the eight weeks. They had been equally fascinated about how the technological challenges would influence group dynamics. Participants said that they felt well connected to the others in the group, holding each other in their minds and reflecting on the themes and each other's art work and writing in between sessions. There was some discussion about the group sizes and one limitation of the technology was that it could in reality only support small numbers of people in the group at one time.

However, my role in the group was discussed and raises some interesting reflections. At times I had seen the groups getting along so well that I had questioned myself about my role in this—was I actually needed once the group got to know one another? To my relief, the interview data indicated a clear yes. Participants discussed the important role of having someone to direct the session and of feeling that there was someone with overall responsibility, emotionally, and practically. It made them feel more at ease that their participation was to benefit their own well-being without the pressure of worrying about managing the emotions of other people, something that many had experienced in their communication with family and friends. Some discussed how the questions posed by the therapist encouraged more insightful consideration of their own thoughts and feelings and, to me, showed that the sessions were serving their purpose.

However, I was also discussed as being 'an equal'. I always aim to provide a space that is comfortable for participants and view myself as group facilitator. In this context, participants said that although I was facilitating the session, I was not seen as being 'in charge'. It seems that the distance afforded by the technology created equality, not just with me, but also with all members of the group. With video conferencing technology, if more than one person speaks at a time, it becomes very difficult to understand two voices speaking at once. Participants need to allow the other person to finish talking before they respond. Both virtual groups were very good at this; I had to work hard not to respond with my automatic "hmm" response I realised I was partial to. This meant that each person had time to talk meaningfully without fear of interruptions, whilst others were forced to actively listen as opposed to jumping in with their own interpretations and experiences. Any dominant oppressive voices were not as apparent in this forum. Similarly, despite the fact that, in reality, we all varied in physical size from a petite 5'6" to 6' tall (five foot six to six foot), one participant noted that they took comfort in the fact that the head and shoulder view afforded by the technology meant that there were no physical size differences apparent between us, removing any perceived physical intimidation or power differences. It may be that in a virtual therapy group context there is greater equality experienced in the relationship between healthcare professional and client.

I was surprised to hear that almost all members indicated that they would not have participated in a group support session had it been in person. It seemed that the technology had facilitated access to services that would not have been taken up otherwise. Participants felt comfortable connecting to others knowing that this connection could be discontinued easily if they wanted to. This could imply a lack of engagement with the group; however, this is not what I experienced. Participants were engaged for the eight sessions, and they were clear in the interview data that they had gained meaningfully from the experience. Again, it seems as though the technology offered new possibilities for control and self-management of their therapy and communication.

## Conclusion

The 'session from hell' taught me a great deal about what makes meaningful connections. I started the project with many assumptions about offering therapy through technology. What I have learnt from initial interview transcripts has given me hope that, with a solid technical infrastructure in place to support this type of therapy service, it has something to offer clients living in a rural location, particularly where chemotherapy can prove to be psychologically and socially isolating for those still undergoing treatment. These two telehealth art therapy groups have shown that technologically mediated communication can be meaningful, close, caring, supportive, humorous, cheeky, fun, and at the same time allow for serious discussion about fear, loss, depression, and anxiety as a result of diagnosis and treatment side effects.

It is also clear that group sessions through technology reached an audience that would otherwise have been unlikely to engage, not just because of their immunosuppression, but because of the pressure of face to face group dynamics and their fears of being made to feel worse by hearing others' stories about illness. Participants valued the privacy and control the technology offered, and they were more confident to make artwork without being observed. The virtual connection perhaps allowed inhibitions to be dropped and the sharing to be more candid. Being able to stay in the comfort of their own home, they could save their limited energy for other things.

In order to preserve a sense of confidentiality I suggested to participants in their Information Pack that they clear a quiet place for themselves in their home for the duration of the session. In reality, this was not always possible, and there were glimpses of participants' home life. Kate's dogs leapt across the room, barking at the postman. Their barking then set Ashley's old dog, Dasha, barking, 40 miles away. Other factors that affected the privacy and boundaries of the session were the location of the Internet point in the home, or where a spouse may bring in a cup of tea. These interruptions are not unlike working on an inpatient ward or in a patient's home environment. One occasion, a district nurse needed to collect a blood sample from Kate for her chemotherapy. Reflecting on the boundaries of the therapy space, I am reminded that these are not my spaces, yet it is important that participants communicated to the group about any planned interruptions to keep the therapy space secure and confidential.

Working with technology as a partner in therapy raises particular anxieties about managing the therapy space. When technology failed in the therapy session, I was powerless to put it right immediately, but still felt responsible for running the session, which was an uncomfortable position. In my desperation to keep a connection with Gemma, for example, I spotted a phone-conferencing machine at the other end of the table. Not having used it before, I picked up the phone and rang her number and it worked, and we could all hear each other. The relief was tremendous and a lucky co-incidence that the phone conferencing was available and provided a valuable connection from that day onwards.

Working in a rural health board where financial restrictions mean limitations to the access of psychological support, telemedicine offers a better use of resources, cutting down on travel for both health professionals and patients. It is a technology more familiar in countries such as Canada and Australia and in the realms of physical medicine. But it clearly also has applications in the provision of psychological support and therapy. Most importantly, the experience has shown that telehealth appears to offer a valuable space to connect and support people and has unique benefits for clients living in a rural area undergoing chemotherapy treatments.

As a result of the two original research projects the palliative care team was awarded funding to buy iPads for patients to use in their own homes, to link with health professionals and continue the piloted service. The funding also enables us to make a short bilingual, introductory film for patients and professionals, which demonstrates telehealth and illustrates the experiences of past clients with the intention of overcoming some of the preconceived barriers and anxieties people may have about using technology in this way. Finally, the funding will provide access to training and education sessions for the team and make it possible to continue to evaluate the care and support provided through telehealth.

Our partnership working with the researchers at the University supporting us in obtaining this funding, the palliative care team will now be able to develop new ways of providing support and care in our rural county.

## References

Bion, W.R. (1961). *Experiences in Groups*. London, Tavistock.

Dale, J.R., Williams, S.M., & Bowyer, V. (2012). What is the effect of peer support on diabetes outcomes in adults? A systematic review. *Diabetic Medicine, 29* (11), 1361–1377.

Hoey, L.M., Leropoli, S.C., White, V.M., & Jefford, M. (2007). Systematic review of peer-support programs for people with cancer. *Patient Education and Counselling, 70* (3), 315–337.

Jones, G. (2000). An art therapy group in palliative cancer care. *Nursing Times, 96* (10), 42–43.

Jones, G. (2007). Complementary and psychological therapies in a rural hospital setting. *International Journal of Palliative Nursing, 13* (4), 184–189.

Keenan, J. (2018). *The feasibility and acceptability of telehealth to support palliative care in Mid-Wales: Exploring professional perceptions and patient experiences* (Unpublished thesis), Aberystwyth University Psychology Department, Wales, UK.

National Institute for Clinical Excellence (NICE). (2004). *Supportive and Palliative Care Services for Adults with Cancer*. London: National Institute for Clinical Excellence (NICE).

Thompson, C.A., Spilsbury, K., Halt, J., Birks, Y., Barnes, C., & Adamson, J. (2007). Systematic review of information and support interventions for caregivers of people with dementia. *BMC Geriatrics, 7*, 18.

Ussher, J., Kirsten, L., Butow, P., & Sandoval, M. (2006). What do cancer support groups provide which other supportive relationships do not? The experience of peer support groups for people with cancer. *Social Science & Medicine, 62*, 2565–2576.

Winnicott, D.W. (1971). *Playing and Reality*. London, Tavistock.

# 24 Snapshot of Practice

## Mind-Body Art Grief Group

*Becky Jacobson*

## About Me

I began my studies in art therapy in 2010. Before entering into the Art Therapy master's program at The George Washington University in Washington DC, I had previously studied art and psychology at a liberal arts school, earning a BA in the Arts, and studied massage therapy at a natural health school in Auckland, NZ. Working with the body and the psyche would eventually come together and shape how I worked with clients as a therapist. Living internationally would also shape my perspectives personally and as a clinician. Later, as an art therapist, I worked with youth in South Africa and with individuals and families in hospital, hospice, bereavement, community, and private practice settings. After graduating with a master's in art therapy with counseling I had no idea I would find myself in the world of grief and loss and death and dying. However, a job opening became available specifically for an art therapist within a hospice and bereavement center. Following my work as an employee within hospice and bereavement care I decided to open my own practice. In 2015 I began offering the Mind-Body Art Grief Group, which I developed and facilitated as a contractor within a bereavement center in the city of Richmond, VA, USA.

## About the Context in Which I Work

Richmond, Virginia, USA, is a relatively small city. It is not hugely international but the city is diverse. In the area where I live hospice and bereavement centers are often connected with a hospital healthcare system. In Richmond, although it is a city of only about 227,000 people, there are actually three large healthcare systems each with their own medical hospitals and facilities. What medical services one chooses often depends on the healthcare plan they have and what services their specific healthcare plan will cover. Over the past decade healthcare in the United States has been going through many changes and has been a major focus of conflicting political views. Many families and individuals throughout the country do not have access to adequate healthcare and this has made it difficult for many to receive adequate end of life and bereavement care. Over the years those working in bereavement care throughout Richmond have formed a community of providers through a professional coalition. Every month the Bereavement Coalition meets and professionals working in hospitals, treatment centers, residential facilities, private practice, community organizations, religious organizations, and more come together. The meetings begin with a networking portion of the meeting, followed by attendee introductions and opportunity for announcements. The meeting concludes with an educational piece, which is presented by a different coalition member each month. Through these meetings I was able to connect with the director of a local bereavement center who expressed interest in hiring me as a contractor to facilitate a grief group incorporating mind-body practices and art therapy. This group was offered to the community for no-charge and was paid for by the bereavement center themselves. It was offered twice a year and each group ran for eight sessions.

## Case Example

Throughout the Mind-Body Art Group art therapy was coupled with mind-body practices, which included breathing techniques, meditation practices, yoga exercises, and more. Using this combination of therapies and practices a very special group process emerged, allowing for holistic and creative healing to occur. Through the participation in mind-body practices, art therapy, and group engagement a newfound acceptance, capacity for self-awareness, and new understandings emerged. The group members were able to understand their own responses to their losses both emotionally and physically; were able to create tangible expressions of their emotions and experiences; found their individual and collective voices; and connected with fellow group members in therapeutic and meaningful ways.

The artwork included here will highlight the personal growth experienced by one participant in particular. The following art pieces were created at the start and finish of an eight-week Mind-Body Art Grief Group offered at the bereavement center. Participants were led through a body-scan meditation and then invited to create art on a piece of paper with the outline of a body on it. Colored pencils, markers, and oil pastels were all made available for the art making. After the body-scan meditation was facilitated the participants were then directed to use the art materials available to them to fill in the body and the page in front of them in any way they saw fit. They were told that they could use whichever lines, shapes, colors, symbols, or imagery they believed would best represent their feelings and experiences during the meditation.

Figure 24.1 shows the beginning and final art pieces created by a client I will call "Betsy." Betsy was a middle-aged woman whose mother had died several months before the group began. In sharing about her first drawing Betsy explained that losing her mother was extremely painful and that her relatives would often lovingly joke that Betsy and her mother were more like sisters "always joined at the hips." As she spoke she stared at her body outline and remarked on how interesting it was that now after her mother's death she is left with not only a pain in her heart but also a pain on her hip. Through the body-scan meditation and art making she was able to connect to the pain she felt since the death of her mother, both emotionally and physically. In her second drawing, completed on the last session of the eight-session group series, Betsy stated that her body felt at peace throughout this meditation, she felt a smile on her face, and brightness around her head. She expressed a peace that has been gained throughout the eight weeks. She was still grieving the loss of her mother but she no longer felt her grief in the form of a painful hole in her heart or as a pain in her hip.

During the first session Betsy was able to share with the group how her grief affected her physically and emotionally and how she experienced her loss (verbally and visually). She was able to illustrate the special relationship she shared with her mother. Other participants in the group were able to connect and support Betsy, and each other, through this process. There were several other participants, for example, who also drew pain or emptiness in the area of the heart; they were able to see that emotionally and physically they were not alone in their experiences. In reflecting on the final art piece Betsy and other group members witnessed that, although the grieving process can seem slow and even stagnant at times, change had occurred within both their physical and emotional wellbeing. This was illustrated directly through their artwork, which offered a tangible example

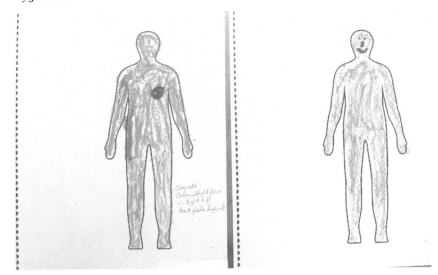

*Figure 24.1* Betsy's Artwork

of the changes that had occurred. This process was holistic, healing, and empowering for Betsy and her fellow group members.

## Advantages of Art Therapy

Art therapy allowed group members to express their stories in new and creative ways. The art images gave members tangible representations of the steps they took on their eight-week journey, individually, and collectively. The participants were able to share emotions and memories with one another in ways that words do not always allow for. In some sessions participants would share their artwork with the group with tears in their eyes; in other sessions group members would be laughing as they reminisced, through the art made, about all the good times shared with those no longer with them. The art therapy allowed for a deepened connection among the participants and a greater awareness of the Self. It additionally presented participants with a new venue for remembering and honoring their loved one who had died. Each participant was able to see, through the art they created, where he or she had been when the group first started versus where they were as the group came to an end. The art therapy strengthened the healing and transformative process.

## One Idea That Shapes My Work

In this work I am most influenced by my understanding of the mind-body connection, and its importance in the healing process. I am also inspired by the holistic approach art therapy offers as it heals both our visceral and emotional selves and our rational and cognitive selves. Taking this somatic, person-centered, holistic approach is what is most important to me. When designing each group session I ensure that the physical, emotional, mental, and spiritual needs of each participant are honored, heard, and given the opportunity to be explored and expressed. I believe this approach is necessary in empowering others to heal, grow, and transform.

# 25 Beginning at the End

*Lynda Kachurek*

The change was so subtle that it took me most of the day to discern what was different, why I felt something was off. After spending far too many months, days, weeks, hours in hospital rooms with my husband, Patrick, I was used to the rhythms and patterns of hospital life. The various doctors breezing in and out with the latest suggested treatments; the nurses and techs coming and going regularly, adjusting this piece of machinery, delivering yet another round of medication, or tending to their regular routines of taking vitals or drawing blood. But this afternoon, this somewhat quiet Sunday afternoon, I finally realized what I sensed. Every time someone came in, their question was the same: "What can we do for you?" While not uncommon for the amazingly kind staff to include my needs in their requests, today was different. They had stopped asking about what my husband needed. Oh, they still took incredible care of their patient, but no longer were they asking what they might be able to do for him. They knew, well before I figured it out, that my husband was not going to survive.

By this point, Patrick had been in a hospital or rehab center for 14 of the previous 18 months. His kidneys had completely failed, and dialysis was no longer effective. A seizure had left him unable to communicate, and he had been on the respirator for two weeks with no hope of it being removed. Doctors, unwilling to quit seeking solutions, wanted to do a tracheostomy and a colostomy, yet they were waiting for him to "get stronger" before doing an MRI to check for damage from the seizure. He was being kept sedated to alleviate his very evident pain and discomfort.

Prior to one of his operations the previous July, we had created his advanced directive, so I knew his wishes on the matter. Having been in a wheelchair for most of his life because of muscular dystrophy, he was clear about not spending time at the end of his life bound to any type of machines. After many discussions with his doctors and especially the palliative care team, I made the difficult decision to bring his suffering to an end. On Wednesday afternoon, the team removed all life support. He passed away peacefully just before dawn on Thursday, January 15, 2015, his hand in mine and surrounded by some of the most dedicated and loving nursing staff we had ever encountered.

## The Long Hallway

I remember walking off the ICU floor that morning, knowing it would be the last time I would walk that hallway, the path to the parking lot so familiar I probably could have done it blindfolded. One of the hospital chaplains walked with me to the elevator, hand on my shoulder, doing her best to offer comfort. Her comment stayed with me, though, as she reflected on what had just happened. "You know," she said softly, "the ICU nurses see some difficult moments. Hard things happen up here. And your husband's passing just made three of them cry. He must have been something very special."

I also remember thinking that day, "This is not how the story is supposed to end." In the fables of childhood, no one ever tells you what happens after "happily ever after." Nobody teaches you what to do when the fairy tale ends, but your story isn't finished.

Grieving was not something new to me. As the child of older parents, both of my grandmothers passed away while I was in grade school, as did many of my aunts and uncles. My father died suddenly right before Christmas of my senior year of high school, and my mother passed away after a two-year illness when I was 29. She had been widowed twice, each time after twenty years of marriage, and I found myself wanting to ask her a whole new set of questions as I now began the journey of widowhood myself.

But this loss was unimaginable to me and not simply because we were only 49. Patrick and I were the best of friends and well-matched partners in life from the beginning of our relationship. Friends and strangers frequently commented about how close we were. We were that couple, the ones who spent as little time apart as possible, who absolutely enjoyed each other's company and always did things together. We rarely fought, were caught holding hands or kissing regularly enough to be mistaken for honeymooners even after more than a decade of marriage, and were visibly partners that moved with the comfortable precision of long-term practice. His muscular dystrophy required him to use a power wheelchair, so we went most everywhere together and helped each other out. Many commented on how well we worked in tandem, our love and partnership truly visible even in the most daunting of circumstances. For almost twenty years, we had been constant companions, so much so that we frequently joked that our name was "PatrickandLynda" because they were always said in the same breath. Although I knew he had been getting increasingly sicker with each stay, at no time did we truly ever think that his death was actually a possibility. While all losses are painful, this loss devastated me. I didn't simply lose my husband. I lost my best friend, my soulmate, the best part of my life for the past twenty years, and any future I had ever imagined. All I could see ahead was a long dark hallway going nowhere.

## Closing Doors

Because I had missed so much time at work over the previous months, I returned to work the day after the funeral. Throwing myself back into my job helped fill the time that had been occupied with doctors and hospital visits. I hated walking back into our empty apartment, which was full of his medical equipment. All of our attempts to make things better stared me down every minute. The Hoyer lift we had gotten the week before he entered the hospital for the last time. The bedside commode surrounded by the mounds of wound care materials. Worst of all was his empty wheelchair. Even the cat avoided it.

To be honest, I don't remember a lot of what happened in February and March that year. I know now one experiences a "widow's fog," the blinding numbness of grief that shields your brain from pain as much as possible. I know I slept a lot, but at odd times. Often, I'd come home from work and sleep until late evening, then get up and live in my head until the early morning hours when I'd try to sleep again. Friends and colleagues would check in, and I would assure them things were "okay," even when they were not. It was not necessarily that I did not want their help; I simply did not know how to describe what I needed, so I chose to be left alone.

I made lists, long lists of things needing done. What about his estate? With no will, did I need to go through probate? What to do with his medical equipment? Thankfully I was a filer of papers, so I had important documents ready at hand as they were required to be mailed to this place, or presented at that one. Every tiny thing was listed, done, and then checked-off. It gave me order in a world that had lost any sense of it. As I closed my eyes one night in late February, the image in my head was once again walking down that long, dark hallway, a hallway full of doors into even darker rooms. With each step, I'd take a deep breath and pull the door closed, exhale, and move to the next. As I peered down the hallway in either direction, the doors never seemed to end. Pulling the doors closed behind me just kept going on and on into the darkness, and I realized that was my world. All I could see was darkness and all the things that had ended, all the things I had lost with his death. And even more than the incredible loss of my husband, what struck me to the core was that it also took everything I thought I was. Although I held myself together for the most part during the day at work, I was a wreck at home in the evenings and especially on weekends. Tears flowed often, long, and deep. I didn't know how to be just me anymore, and I had never liked the dark. I knew I needed help.

The hospital's bereavement center had been in touch right after he passed away, offering their services if I wanted them. The next meeting coming up was one of their regular monthly group meetings, which were always focused around a single topic, different each month. The meeting in early March was on grief and finances, as tax season was coming up the next month. I went, despite the topic, and was immediately sorry I did. At 49, I appeared to be the youngest person in the room, including the presenter, and nearly all the questions related to Social Security, Medicare, and the like. Never saying a word throughout the session, I quickly left as soon as could get out of the door.

In April, for the next meeting on the schedule, the center was starting a book group, centered on a new common reading. I registered for a place, picked up a copy of the book, and tried, but couldn't get past the first couple of pages. Thinking of going made my stomach twist. I had fallen into the habit of talking to myself and in this conversation, I reminded myself that I didn't even enjoy going to book groups for books that I really wanted to read, on topics that I really enjoyed. What was I thinking? The book remained unread, and I did not go to the session.

The darkness around me, however, deepened instead of lessened, despite the coming of spring. It seemed the more I checked things off the never-ending to-do list, the deeper into the dark hallway I traveled. I was out of ideas and unsure of what to do next. When I went in for my annual physical, my regular doctor simply asked, "So, how is your husband doing?" and I broke down in her office. Obviously concerned, she offered pharmaceutical solutions for my lack of sleep and probable depression, but I just couldn't say yes. I knew I had to find a path through this darkness and that medications were only going to slow that process down. I called the bereavement center one more time, just to see if they had other options or, if they didn't, to sign up for one-on-one counseling with one of their therapists. The kind receptionist chatted as she looked for open appointments and commented that they had a new group starting up in early May that I might be interested in joining.

"What kind of group is it?" I asked more from politeness than interest.

"It's a new kind of group for us," she responded. "It's a mind-body art therapy group. This is the first time we're offering it."

It caught my attention because I knew nothing about art therapy, and certainly had never participated in something termed mind-body anything. But it sounded more interesting than anything else I had been offered or sought out.

"Okay," I said reluctantly. "I'll give it a try."

## The Sessions

Walking into the bereavement center the first night took some willpower. I was not enthusiastic about it at all, and exceptionally wary of the "art" description. Any artistic talent in our family had belonged to my mother, and she had been the first to understand that I couldn't even draw a straight line with a ruler. I was skeptical to say the least. In the lobby, a gentleman who looked a bit younger than me was standing off to one side, his expression about as un-enthusiastic as I felt. I quickly glanced the other direction, out the doors, seriously considering leaving. But I had promised myself to give this one night, to try something different, to try anything at all that might help deal with the darkness, the emptiness. He and I both kind of shrugged our shoulders and stepped through the door.

When we got back to the classroom, the welcoming environment surrounded me like a favorite blanket. Essential oils infused the air with calming fragrance, and the therapist gave a warm welcome that was reassuringly calm as well as gentle. A grouping of chairs and a couch were on one side of the room, surrounding a coffee table, while a second set of chairs surrounded a table scattered with pens, crayons, scissors, and a host of other things. My memories of the rest of the evening center on two things. First, I remember crying a lot, feeling as though I cried through the whole session even if I didn't really. The introductions were blurry moments, although I was comforted by the fact that there were other women there who had lost their husbands in addition to people who had lost siblings, children, or parents.

What I remember most, however, was the activity we did that night. Our therapist asked us to collage two things: where we were starting from that evening, and where we wanted to go in this process. Using any or all of the abundant materials on the table—crayons, pastels, pencils, magazines, stickers, glitter, glue sticks, and scissors—we were to create something that showed where we were. Avoiding the crayons and pencils, I dove into the magazines, looking for something, anything that could possibly illustrate where my head and heart were at that particular moment. Early in one magazine was an advertisement for Walt Disney World, which happened to be our favorite place. We honeymooned there and returned as frequently as we could; I clipped out the image of Cinderella's castle and set it aside. An ad for a mobility service was in another issue, and the image of the wheelchair joined the castle on the table.

Bit by bit, images, and words were clipped and stacked next to me. Phrases like "Where Are You?" and "You're a perfect fit for each other," spoke to my heart. A large blue eye and an image of an arched doorway that reminded me of one of our wedding pictures joined the pile. When I found someone had cut a letter "K" out of a map of Ohio and it had Dayton showing on it, I gasped, stunned to find the perfect piece, as we lived in Dayton for twelve years before moving to Richmond. But the one image that did the most to demonstrate what I was feeling at that moment, what I had been feeling since the funeral, was an image from a pharmaceutical advertisement about a medication for depression that portrayed a middle-aged woman as a wind-up figure, with a large mechanical key sticking out of her hunched-over self. That single image managed to capture almost exactly what I felt like moving through my days. Get up, wind up, make it through work, slowing down once home and then stuck, hunched over, alone, until it all started again the next day.

Placed together on a random sheet of scrapbook paper, the images did what was intended, showing a graphic representation of what was going on inside of me, what I felt like, and what I was thinking at that moment. I attempted sketching a few gray clouds at the top and a couple of broken and empty hearts, but quickly abandoned the attempt at drawing in favor of the collage. I spent almost no time on the second collage, ignoring it to work on the first one, in part because the only thing I could think of that I wanted to be was "better."

When we went around the table and talked about our collages, having the images available made it much easier to talk about my feelings. I could not and had not been able to express the complex sentiments that were wrapped up tightly in the single visual image of the wind-up woman. For the first time in this process of grieving, I had been given a way to express what I was feeling deep inside in a simple and direct manner. That's not to say it was without tears, because it wasn't, but for the first time in several months, I was able to communicate what I felt, what I feared, was happening. The accepting nods of the others offered empathy and understanding. As I left that evening, I knew I would be back the next week.

Although each of our sessions would include breathing and relaxation exercises as well as suggestions for mindful living, it was always the art projects that captured my attention most. For the second week, we were asked to bring photocopies of pictures of the individual we were grieving. I arrived with a stack of printouts an inch thick, having printed off nearly every picture I could easily find on the hard drive. Asked to collage our person, I filled my sheet much as he had filled my life, to overflowing with images, memories, and things I couldn't bear leaving out like his kindergarten picture, with those prominent blue eyes, or a photo with Mickey Mouse and one with his mother. Our wedding picture was an obvious choice, and I included pictures of him with famous people he had met. A picture from his long hospital stays made it on the collage, as did the last picture we ever took together, from Thanksgiving.

As we once again shared memories while introducing each other to our loved ones via our collage work, I was fascinated with how everyone put their collages together. There were individuals who, like me, threw a large number of images together as though purging their memory banks. Several others were more restrained, some using only one or two images to tell the story of their love. Perhaps the most haunting was from the woman who had lost a young child. But as with the previous week, there was an unexpected comfort in talking via pictures; the words still came with tears, but the focus of talking about the images provided a frame where there were far fewer tears than I would have expected. Rather than emphasizing all that I had lost, this project provided a way to celebrate all that I had been given. When I left the session this week, I thought that maybe, just maybe, there was a way out of the darkness that surrounded me.

Returning the following Tuesday evening, we turned to working with words. After creating a list of descriptive words, the therapist asked us to create a haiku. Once we had crafted a haiku to our liking, she asked us to illustrate it, bringing the words to life via pictures we drew. Being poetically and artistically challenged was not to be an obstacle, she insisted. This art had nothing to do with being "good," however one defined it, but rather she encouraged us to be free of such judgments and just create. No rights or wrongs, no criticism, just create however we felt like creating. That freedom was both liberating and stifling, as I had a challenging time deciding where to end up. Did I want to write about Patrick or the loss of him? Should I explore my current feelings, or what I was hoping to work through during this process? The blank space next to the list of words I had put down waited for me, and looking around, I don't think I was the only one finding this piece a difficult challenge.

One of the images that had been in my dreams came to mind. During Patrick's last several days, we both struggled with the idea that his death was the probable outcome. His palliative care counselor had talked with him in depth that he would probably not be going home again. Before it became necessary to increase his sedation, I sought ways to ease the panic I felt in both of us and rambled through conversation after conversation to keep it at bay. I talked of things we had done, and especially trips we had enjoyed. One trip that came to mind morphed into an image that eventually helped us both; it was our first visit to Niagara Falls. We had gone there as part of a larger trip that included visiting

Toronto, and we each had favorite spots from previous trips with our respective families. His was the Ripley's Believe it or Not Museum; mine was the Maid of the Mist boat ride. During that trip, we also decided to try the tour behind the falls, a first for each of us, and something we found profoundly moving, to be behind that wall of water and hear the intense power of it.

As I spoke to him in those last days, Niagara Falls became our metaphor for the journey he was taking. I reminded him how scared he had been rolling onto the boat the first time, convinced that this time would be the one time the boat would get pulled into the falls. The brief trip delighted us both, and I teased him frequently about how by the end of the ride, he couldn't wait to go again, his fear conquered. Coupled with the excursion behind the falls, I ended up morphing that into a description of death, how we were all afraid of the unknown journey, but that once it was completed, there was joy and the realization that there was no need to be afraid. Journeying behind the falls, I continued, was something not everybody took the opportunity to do, and that such a trip would be extremely powerful. Both of us were raised in religious households, although we had not continued attending church regularly. But faced with the reality of death, a faith-based imagery was welcoming for us both.

That story became my haiku during that third week of group meetings. His journey to "the other side of the falls" was imagery that had offered us both strength during his passing, and I turned to that for this exercise.

What struck me most after this session was that while the imagery I was working with was incredibly meaningful and emotionally challenging, the combined focus of crafting the haiku and deciding how to turn it into a drawing gave my mind a creative aspect to focus on instead of the pain. Rather than only remembering the circumstances that prompted the story, my attention was centered on the creative output, on finding a way to get it

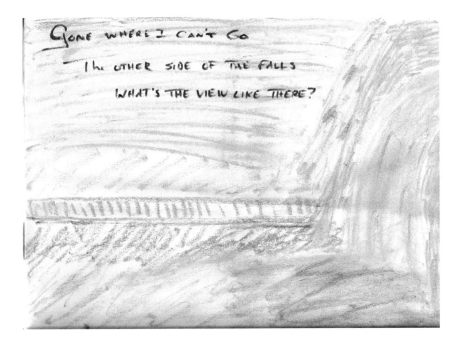

*Figure 25.1* The Other Side of the Falls

from my head to the paper as best I could. It was still painful, but that pain was lessened by producing a descriptive piece that expressed the story in a different manner than my words. Although this was more challenging for me than previous exercises, I felt it added a different dimension to my expression of grief.

For the fourth session of the therapy meeting, the group arrived to face a very large piece of drawing paper tacked to the board, running the length of most of one wall of our meeting space. The assignment for that evening was to create a group mural of the journey of grieving, and it took us all a bit of time to warm up to what things to include. Although we were by now used to the idea of sharing our pieces at the end of a session, somehow the idea of drawing in front of the group seemed to intimidate most of us. Finally, one person stepped up and drew what most of the rest had been thinking by putting a gravestone at the far left edge, the beginning of the journey. Slowly each of us stepped forward and added something to the long sheet of paper, and once we got started, it became easier to add to the creative blend that was developing on the mural. Without planning among the group, the final image, which took two sessions for us to complete, was an odd mix of *The Wizard of Oz* and *Up*. The gravestone served as the start of a makeshift yellow brick road of sorts, leading to a rather large tornado near the middle. Between those two points were the familiar story elements of the poppy field and the flying monkeys, both signs of impending danger and chaos in the story.

On the far side of the twister, once one had made their way through it, the story become more that of the house carried away by balloons over new landscapes. At the end of the paper, as we hoped with the end of our journey, was the familiar signpost pointing out that adventure was waiting just past the edge of the mural. Despite the fact that each of the participants had a unique story that brought them into the group, the mural that we completed at the half-way point of our meetings drew us together as we realized our journeys had many points of similarity. Others existed who knew what we were feeling at some level; we were not alone on this crazy unknown path.

The final third of the group sessions went by rather quickly. The sixth meeting focused on issues of health and self-care, including charting the current state of pain in the body, both emotional and physical. The next to the last evening, the seventh together, felt much like a re-centering of self. Each participant brought in a song that was a favorite or had special meaning to be played as we drew. The assignment this evening was to create a mini-journal, draw a circle on two of the pages, and then fill each circle with a self-assessment of where we felt we were at the beginning and now near the end of the group sessions. My beginning circle filled quickly with unending spirals, overlaid with color tones of deep blue. Words on the outside included "cut circles" and "outside in." In contrast, my now circle was made of softer, lightly colored lines, beginning to blend together. The title was "Blurred Lines," and the phrases alongside it included "emerging patterns," "softer edges," and "multicolored." What I had been feeling over the past weeks became apparent in the differences between the two images. I had begun to heal.

During the final meeting of the group, each participant brought back in all the art pieces created during the past seven weeks to review. It seemed several of us, including me, were surprised at the changes in the things we had made and how they had changed between the beginning and the end of the group sessions. To end our sessions, each person drew an outline of their hand, then passed the sheet from person to person so that they could add their comments or drawing. Unlike the grey-blue colors of the first week, this image danced with multicolored brightness, a reflection of the new sense of possibility I felt.

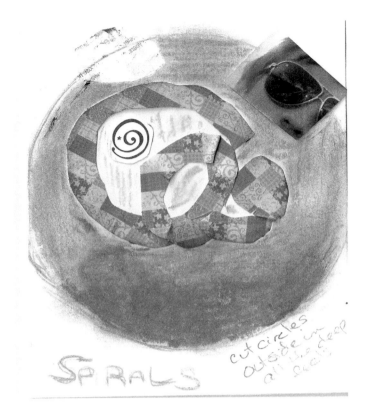

*Figure 25.2* Spirals

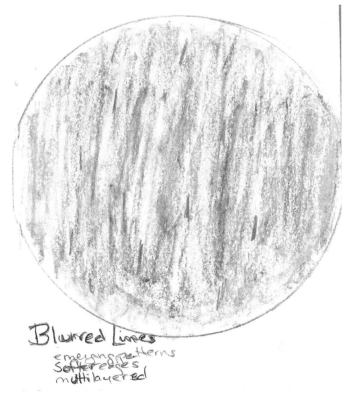

*Figure 25.3* Blurred Lines

## Summary: Opening Doors

In the nearly two years since Patrick passed away, there have been moments both of sadness and of joy. I survived the whole year of "firsts" without him, including birthdays, holidays, and our anniversary. I bought a house and moved, and I traveled for both work and vacations. When there are moments where tears fall and the darkness threatens to return, I always return to the tools that I learned from the therapist during our eight weeks of sessions. I learned to tap into different ways of expression, whether through words or pictures to help me focus on what I'm feeling and, if needed, be able to explain it to someone else. She taught me a variety of ways of being in tune with my emotional and physical self, to be mindful of body and soul, as well as a way of readjusting my focus.

When we were each asked to summarize our experience of the group sessions, I used the analogy of doors to explain mine. I started the program aware of only the darkness that surrounded me and all the things I had lost, all the doors I was pulling closed in my life. Over the course of the eight weeks of sessions, I found ways to express my grief in concrete forms that allowed me to better understand and accept those feelings. I could look forward, see the darkness lift, and become aware that a whole set of doorways lay ahead, just waiting for me to decide which ones to open. It may not have been the happily-ever-after I had believed in, but there was a story out there for me to discover, learning how to blend the wife that I was with the widow I became, and discovering the woman, the survivor, that I am.

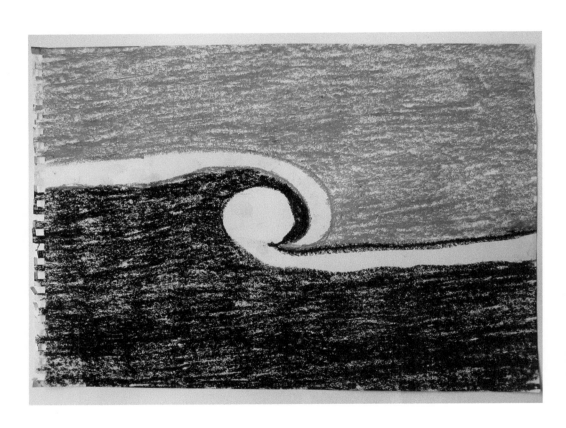

# Section Three

# Art Therapy for Cross-Cultural Encounters, National Tragedies and Disenfranchised Grief

In this section we explore the global and cultural influences that shape our understanding of illness, dying and death and recognise the strengths and limitations of the UK and US models of art therapy. The value of art therapy to address unacknowledged grief is a key theme of the chapters.

In Snapshot of Practice 26, from United Arab Emirates, Sara Powell shows how visual exploration impacts a young boy, revealing anxieties around loss and bereavement at the root of worrying behavioural symptoms. David E. Gussak (Chapter 27) and Emma Allen (Chapter 28) present the anticipatory grieving of those excluded from mainstream society through incarceration in the US and UK. Gussak gives a theoretical overview of the issues facing individuals incarcerated in the USA, while Allen provides a UK perspective on her work in a high secure hospital with men detained for their criminal offences being treated for mental illnesses, while also living with terminal disease.

Disenfranchised grief is also explored in Chapter 29, where Rachel Mims offers a personal account of becoming disabled following a physically demanding job as a soldier in the US Army. Alongside this, Jacqueline Jones presents clinical examples of art therapy with veterans with traumatic brain injury and post-traumatic stress disorder. This chapter differentiates non-complicated and complicated grief, and the disenfranchised grief of service men and women.

Addressing the complex power dynamics that manifest in cross-cultural art therapy, several contributors acknowledge the importance of the art therapist locating her own cultural starting point. Anxieties about the negative associations with colonialism are raised in Chapter 35 by British therapists Cooke et al. Despite their worries, it is clear that a significant mutually beneficial connection developed between patients in India and London through their intervention of art therapy quilts. New Zealand art therapist Jennie Halliday (Chapter 33) writes about the adjustments she had to make in order to meaningfully engage with her male Māori patient. Her account of the Māori approach to health has much in common with Cicely Saunders' model of Total Pain.

Art therapists' contribution to mental wellbeing in the face of national trauma is detailed by Hayley Berman and Nataly Woollett (Chapter 34). They describe the HIV and AIDS crisis in South Africa, highlighting the traumatic effect of recurrent bereavements upon health and social care professionals and present their response to this overwhelming need; an art therapy mental health intervention for community counsellors who support people infected with and affected by HIV. The impact of using art therapy as a response to national calamity in another part of the world can be found in Deborah Green's chapter (31). This calamity is a natural disaster; the 2011 earthquakes in New Zealand's South Island. Green presents a powerful phenomenological exploration of personal loss reawakened by these events, alongside a unique innovative art therapy practice—'quake-arts therapy'. The ability of sudden unexpected events to trigger memories and action are further illustrated by Todd Stonnell in Chapter 30. This presentation of the incremental impact of gun crime on a young man growing up in the USA shows Stonnell mobilising his skills as an art therapist to create an outdoor pop-up event within his LGBTQ community.

In the final Snapshot of Practice (32), British art therapist Hilary Rapp presents her experiences of researching art therapy in Singapore with a Chinese population; highlighting once again the cross-cultural limitations and opportunities for art therapy at the end of life.

The contributions in this section highlight 'double awareness'—the potential art therapy can have to connect our intimate 'inner world' reflections with the large-scale outer experiences of the world in which we live. They prompt us to recall the foundations of the profession, forged in the aftermath of World War II and serve as a reminder that through continued reflective practice, innovation, creativity and authentic engagement between professionals and their clients, art therapy will develop to meet the needs of people experiencing loss in a diverse and changing world.

# 26 Snapshot of Practice

## Private Practice Art Therapy in Dubai

*Sara Powell*

### About Me

My name is Sara Powell and I am from United Kingdom. I have spent many years in the Middle East and Asia. I am the founder of the Art Therapy International Centre (ATIC), a psychological and counselling centre, which specialises in art(s) therapies. ATIC was first established in Singapore in 2010 (co-founder) and subsequently Dubai in 2015 as a sole proprietor, the latter after moving back to Dubai in 2015. I received my MA in Art Therapy from LASALLE University, Singapore and am currently a registered member of the Australian New Zealand and Asian Creative Arts Therapy Association (ANZACATA). I have since provided art therapy to children, adolescents, adults, the elderly, families, and couples and have facilitated a variety of therapy groups. Additionally, I have been fortunate to work with government agencies, NGO's and a variety of medical, education and rehabilitative organisations. I specialise in supporting women and children with varied challenges.

### About the Context in Which I Work

The Emirate of Dubai is a spectacular place and is one of seven Emirates that makes up the United Arab Emirates (U.A.E.). The U.A.E. is geographically situated within the Arabian Gulf in the Middle East. Dubai is a progressive and modern city steeped in rich Arab traditions and culture. The local population in the U.A.E. are Muslim, which, as with many religions, has a big impact on the populace's daily lives, as well as on their culture and values. As a clinician, the differences between cultures and religions must be taken into account when providing therapeutic sessions. Islamic beliefs are woven into everyday life and are a huge source of strength when supporting grief and bereavement; this must be taken into consideration before an effective therapeutic plan is formulated and implemented. The UAE is also home to an increasing number of multinationals, boasting an extensive expatriate population. It is a harmonious country, respectful of all its guests and the diversity they bring and share. It is also especially beneficial for the art therapist to recognise cultural diversity when working with varied ethnicities, cultures and religious beliefs of those who reside in the U.A.E.

Art Therapy is still in its infantile stages in Dubai and in the Middle East region, and ATIC is the first and presently the only art therapy centre (a Social Impact company) licenced in Dubai. It is therefore our understanding that therapists of ATIC are the only qualified art therapists practicing in Dubai. As it stands, art therapy is an extremely new concept and not yet fully integrated within the holistic frameworks of the social care sector. The U.A.E. is already well regarded and respected for its medical sector and continues to familiarise the community and develop a comprehensive medical system inclusive of mental healthcare. Consequently, in the absence of art therapy in the medical sector setting, it provides an opportunity for interaction with many populations within the private practice sector. On one hand, this can be advantageous, as it allows practitioners to create a unique non-threatening space dedicated to the practice of art-based therapy in a non-clinical setting. And on the other hand, it is a disadvantage as there is a distinct possibility that grief, loss and bereavement support may be delayed (in the form of art therapy) as art therapists are not currently utilised within the hospital settings. However, there is an existing grief support structure within the hospitals catering for the community to manage grief from an emotional perspective but currently this does not include Art Therapeutic services. Added to this, it is also the intention to provide art therapy at selected hospitals shortly and if that materialises, it would be a huge step in integration of art therapy into medical settings and help assist wider recognition of art and expressive therapeutic services in U.A.E and probably the region.

## Case Example

Art therapy is yet to be fully integrated into palliative care specifically. Art therapy is primarily offered in the form of private practice and therefore the support afforded to those with a terminal illness is compromised. However, within private practice we readily support grief in all its forms, in addition to supporting children with a variety of chronic illnesses and rare genetic diseases.

Sam (identity concealed), is a nearly seven-year-old boy and an expatriate of Arab descent. He lives with his mother, stepfather and soon a baby brother. He was referred for art therapy due to behavioural difficulties at school (particularly with peers, he displayed frequent aggressive outbursts); as a result of this, he had become socially withdrawn. He was also having symptomology in line with separation anxiety. He was unable to sleep by himself or go to the bathroom alone. These symptoms had been observed for over nine months and were exacerbated when his mother announced her pregnancy. Sam's biological father passed away when he was a few months old; however, Sam and his stepfather appeared to have a good relationship, with his stepfather slotting into the father figure role. Sam had a number of evaluation sessions followed by a total of eight sessions. Sam's artwork at the beginning of treatment was heavily rooted in fantasy, metaphors and symbolism, focussing primarily around a fear of death.

This art piece (Figure 26.1) is a reflective artwork I did depicting Sam's artwork and process, of a 'mummy and a daddy'. Sam was keen to explore the medium of paint which allowed him to regress; investing heavily in creating a 'mummy' while producing this artwork (right side of the page). She had three sets of arms to separately care for and cuddle a daddy, a son and a baby. Through the depiction of multiple arms, Sam was able to express his family dynamic with a baby sibling on the way. The three sets of arms ensured his mother's ability to perhaps provide equal amounts of affection. It allowed him to form a sense of control and integrate his evolving family dynamic, seeing his mother as more than just 'his'; although, there was a slight reluctance to fully share her. The left side depicts how Sam attempted to paint a father. He needed to paint over the incomplete figure and smeared it with paint in an aggressive manner, as 'the dad (had) died'. This perhaps was Sam's way of dually processing his father's passing and his absence from his life, as well as his desire to remove his stepfather in order to have his mother to himself and limit a connection between the two parents and the new baby. Children as young as six months can exhibit grief reactions in response to separation, affecting attachment (Bowlby, 1982). Childhood bereavement has also been associated with increasing susceptibility to development of psychiatric disorders (Dowdney, 2000). Families with one of the parents

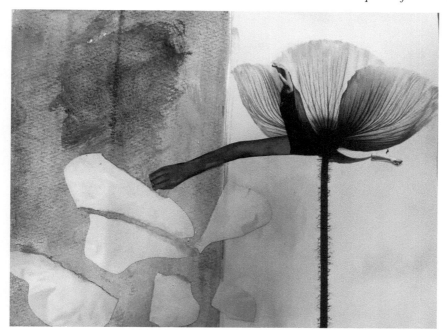

*Figure 26.1* Mummy and Daddy Plant—A Reflective Artwork

remarrying or having another child can bring about new challenges, major stressors which may be interpreted for some children as a traumatic transition (Nichols, 1985). This may also be further exacerbated in expatriate families where they are away from their extended families.

At the beginning of therapy Sam found it difficult to be separated from his mother. Sam was exhibiting high levels of distress when separated from his mother, indicating a high level of anxiety and fear. This was perhaps rooted with a fear of losing another parent.

Later through his artwork, the use of fantasy and metaphors reduced and through his narrative story he was able to relate his current symptoms to the death of his father; perhaps this revelation came about as a result of his new sibling, allowing for the restructuring of his concept of family to include his stepfather and brother, along with himself and his mother. Figure 1.2 is a reflective art piece I did capturing Sam's ability to integrate all family members within the house (mother, father and baby). His father was symbolically represented and described to be in the sky with one foot on the roof of the house. At the beginning, Sam's artwork was incomplete and unfinished, depicting a portion of his family while excluding newer additions, embodying and exposing his grief in his art. His later art still didn't fully depict the entirety of his new family; however, the narrative explained their inclusion in an art piece far removed from fantasy and make-believe and more grounded in reality. Treatment focussed on developing identity, and resiliency. Resolved grief can result in growth and increased strength, in addition, art therapies processing and supporting grief are considered appropriate as a preventive measure (Raymer and McIntyre, 1987). We focussed on lessening anxieties and reinforcing the fact that he would not be taken away from his mother (helping him manage the birth of his brother and the family). We worked on identity, incorporating his father and making scrap books and a memory box, in order to help preserve the memory of his father. Towards the end of the sessions Sam's artwork represented his new sense of safety and belonging; fear of

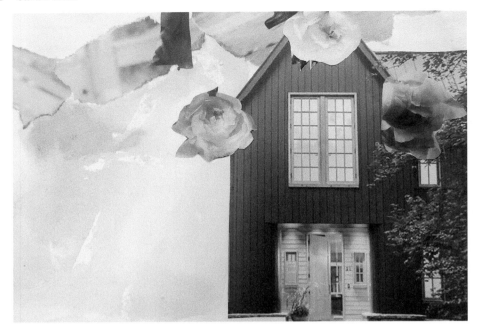

*Figure 26.2* My House—A Reflective Artwork

death was no longer infiltrating his artwork. As the grief was addressed the symptoms diminished and he felt able to connect and be a part of his family. The school counsellor reported Sam's angry outbursts had reduced at school.

## Advantages of Art Therapy in My Context

Due to the nature of art therapy, it is perfectly suited for the cultural hotpot prevalent in U.A.E. If we were to rely on purely verbal-based therapeutic practices, we would struggle to be able to cater to the massively diverse population in the U.A.E., as not all residents speak a common language, hindering their ability to accurately verbalise their inner thoughts and feelings. Additionally, we are able to support non-verbal populations, as art transcends language barriers and facilitates individuals to express themselves through non-verbal means, highlighting thoughts and feelings that they may otherwise lack the capabilities to convey verbally. Added to this, many are arguably able to express themselves more openly and freely through the medium of art, exposing and giving shape to their emotional and mental status, which they may feel constrained or uncomfortable to discuss verbally. This overarching ability underscores art therapy's unique and robust approach in tackling cultural diversity and even religious divide as it allows participants to express themselves to the fullest without inhibition, constraints and weight that words may carry. Many who use the medium of art to express themselves in a therapeutic setting often reveal a deeper level about themselves than they may consciously intend, and in so doing, provide art therapists with further insight into individuals' inner world and their challenges. Availing such information equips the therapist with evidence-based material illuminating a path towards an appropriate support/treatment plan.

## One Idea That Shapes My Work

The desire to help those in need on a global scale. Although, this may sound lofty and idealistic, I have found that art therapy has provided me with the strength and the tools necessary to take small steps towards that goal. Granted, it is unrealistic to believe one can help everyone, but by setting the bar as high as possible, it propels me to do and hopefully achieve more. Art therapy has allowed me to travel to many countries providing the same level of therapeutic care, irrespective of language barriers or cultural differences. The ability to provide therapy without the use of words is truly inspiring and arguably a unique and universal language whose mastery overarches the gaps and differences in language, ethnicity, culture, genders, etc. Desire and drive to help others and passion for understanding the uniqueness of the mind led me to become an art therapist. It is a resourceful and rewarding profession on many levels and I do hope I can continue to reach more countries and communities internationally.

## References

Bowlby, J. (1982). Attachment and loss: Retrospect and prospect. *American Journal of Orthopsychiatry, 52*(4), 664.

Dowdney, L. (2000). Annotation: Childhood bereavement following parental death. *The Journal of Child Psychology and Psychiatry and Allied Disciplines, 41*(7), 819–830.

Nichols, W. C. (1985). Family therapy with children of divorce. *Journal of Psychotherapy & The Family, 1*(3), 55–68.

Raymer, M., & McIntyre, B. B. (1987). An art support group for bereaved children and adolescents. *Art Therapy, 4*(1), 27–35.

# 27 Art Therapy in Prison Hospice

## A Compassionate Bridge

*David E. Gussak*

In an environment where identity is stripped away, where survival of the fittest reigns and weakness is preyed upon, the notion of dying within prison walls is especially egregious. In a quote from Byock (2002, p. 107) the author writes, "Dying in prison is what inmates fear most . . . spending their last hours in agony, alone, separated from family outside and from friends within . . ." As our prison population continues to expand and age, with longer sentences and limited use of compassionate release (Ratcliff, 2000), prisons are finding themselves responsible for the end of life stages for their wards. Fortunately, some correctional facilities are responding, developing hospice units and programs.

Art therapy has been found to provide a sense of identity, social connection and improving mood inside the prison walls (Gussak, 2007, 2009). It has also been seen as a valuable tool in working with those who are dying (Barrington, 2016; Bolton, 2008; Givens, 2008). Together, art therapy may provide a sense of re-humanization, a renewed identity and an opportunity for atonement and authentic connection with others that may otherwise be missing for those dying inside. This brief exploratory essay will first provide an overview of the issues of hospice care with a prison population. Next, it will outline the benefits of art therapy with the prison population, followed by an examination and application on how art therapy can be used to bolster a sense of value, purpose, and lasting permanence amongst the forgotten dying.

## Dying in Prison—A Double Loss

It seems obvious that end-of-life attention for prison inmates should maintain the same degree of unconditional care, responsiveness, authenticity, and relational development as it would in any hospice setting for its patients. However, in an environment where the population is objectified and dehumanized in order to maintain order and security (Fox, 1997; Gussak, December, 2016b), providing special attention to those who are dying seems antithetical. Yet the fear of those inside remains the same as those outside—"[d]ying alone, in pain, without social, familial, and spiritual supports, is the terrifying end that many prisoners . . . fear. Unfortunately, it is too often the reality they experience" (Dubler & Heyman, 1998). What makes this worse is they are dying with the derogatory and shameful label of inmate intact, with little opportunity for atonement or forgiveness (Craig & Craig, 1999).

The number of elderly inmates and those dying inside is increasing. Overcrowding coupled with lengthy prison sentences have made for a greying, more ill population. Despite the facilities' best efforts, prisons are not exactly conducive to good health. "Prison inmates, as a group, experience greater disease burden and worse health outcomes than community-dwelling adults" (Cloyes, Rosenkranz, Berry, Supiano, Routt, Shannon-Dorcy & Llanque, 2016). This population suffers from higher likelihood of infectious diseases, chronic illness, higher rate of cancer, and more mental health and substance use disorders. Cognitive and physical dysfunctions result from the lack of accommodation and difficulties of adaptability for the aging population. As a result:

> Correctional health programs . . . will be required to address the need for end-of-life care for an exponentially growing number of inmates. How to adequately address this need, and provide constitutionally mandated and humane care while balancing security and custodial demands will become an increasingly pressing problem for those . . . that have not already initiated . . . end of life care.
>
> (Cloyes et al., 2016, p. 390)

While some perceive inmates as less than deserving of such care, some philosophically believe that all should be shown mercy (Rich, 2013).

Over the past several decades, institutions around the country have developed various methods of hospice care. In the early 1990s, soon after I began working at California's Correctional Medical Facility [CMF] as an art therapist, Dr. Kubler-Ross, renowned psychologist and author of the book On *Death and Dying*, was coming to visit. She was to take a tour of our facility's fairly new hospice treatment center. She had visited the prison some time before and chastised the medical staff for not developing proper end of life resources despite it being the state's medical prison. Since then, CMF developed its own system, relying on medical staff to provide medicinal comfort and volunteering inmates to provide human attention. She was quite satisfied with how much more advanced CMF was since last she visited. I remember quite clearly Dr. Kubler-Ross describing how important it was to maintain and "give back" dignity to those who had long lost it.

Hoffman and Dickenson (2011) indicated that by 2011 sixty-nine such programs existed that provided different degrees of palliative care. Cloyes et al. (2016) conducted an in-depth qualitative grounded theory study at Louisiana State Penitentiary, which holds the longest continuously running prison hospice program in the United States. Long considered a model of sustainable hospice programs inside the walls, the authors discovered that there were five essential categories that were the foundation of a sustainable program: *Patient-centered care, a comprehensive inmate volunteer model, safety and security, shared values* and *teamwork*. While not sacrificing security, subscribing to this model relies on a humanistic and humanizing understanding unusual for the prison environment. Such characteristics correspond to the very nature of art therapy as an intervention in the prison milieu.

## Redeveloping a Humanized Sense of Self: Art Therapy in Prison

Creative expression is a natural byproduct of the prison subculture, emerging from the instinctual impulses, specifically aggression, sexuality, and the need for escape, already prevalent in the institutionally restrained and vapid environment (Fox, 1997; Gussak, 1997, 2016a). Dissanayake (1992) linked the need to express art through the libidinal impulses of sexuality and aggression through shared primal needs of expression, bonding, and release. For one to survive, even thrive, such impulses have to be discharged. But, releasing those impulses in this subculture can have undesirable consequences such as negative incident reports, time added onto one's sentence, or even solitary confinement, as such behaviors are seen as antithetical to the correctional mission of security. Contrarily, creative expression is more socially acceptable as a means to sublimate these primitive, instinctual, and, sometimes destructive reactions (Kramer, 1993; Rank, 1932; Rubin, 1984). The act of creating also allows the inmate to "escape" for a few moments or hours into his or her own created world; it provides a necessary diversion (Gussak,

1997; Gussak & Cohen-Liebman, 2001; Hall, 1997). It is not a coincidence that early empirical studies examining the effectiveness of art in prison populations demonstrated that art-making decreased recidivism (California Arts in Corrections, 1987) and the number of disciplinary reports written on inmates who participated in an Arts-in-Corrections program (Brewster, 1983). Thus, creating art may provide a safer, less volatile outlet for inmates.

In addition, I have come to realize that art making provides an opportunity for the inmate to create a new identity above that of simply "inmate." Again, one of the ways prisons control their populations is by objectifying the inmates—it is easier to control those who are seen as inferior or subhuman (Fox, 1997). Essentially, they are stripped of their identity, labeled with numbers, and are forced to wear the same uniform. While seen as essential for ensuring security, such dynamics are detrimental to rehabilitation. Eventually this may result in a pervasive sense of helplessness and loss.

Art provides an opportunity to reinforce individual identity and helps define or shape a sense of self (Gussak, 2006); it may even provide an opportunity for each to redefine himself. To ultimately cause a positive transformation or change, inmates, through art making, may be able to "remain human in an inhuman environment" (Brown, 2002, p. 28). One of the most challenging obstacles within the institution is to assist the inmate in rising above the detrimental labels imposed, and to eventually assist him in developing a distinct and unique identity capable of thriving independently. In so doing, the very factors that can contribute to a sense of loss and hopelessness can be alleviated. A sense of identity and worth, even pleasure, can help assuage such helplessness, pervasive in the institution.

Art may also provide a bridge between the outside and the inside culture, underscoring for those "outside" that those in prison are indeed real people. Those inside are oftentimes forgotten by the outside culture. As well, their societal and familial relationships are put on hold, and at times, denied, making them even further removed. Such barriers from their loved ones diminish their sense of belonging. However, art therapy provides an opportunity to re-engage with others, and become a more active member of a group. As well, art making gives them something else to be known for—they take on the role of a "creator" and in a sense, develop a new self-[re]creation. During this process the inmate can reconcile lost meaning and correspondence with the outside world in the therapeutic environment.

Whereas the inmate is locked inside, their art may "exit" the walls. Such art, when viewed by others, reflects the very humanity of the creator. In turn, this allows societal members to recognize those who create inside as real people, those with a purpose, those with an opportunity to contribute to the greater culture. As a result, the factors that contribute to their loss of identity may be reversed. For example, in 2008, the Florida Department of Cultural Affairs hosted a gallery show of inmate art. Those inmates whose artwork was to be exhibited expressed feelings of engagement and value; family members of the inmates whose work was on display reflected how proud they were. Community members, who would otherwise not acknowledge the marginalized members of their own society, marveled at the creations on the walls. The art became a mediator and mirror for those inside, thus allowing a connection between the two cultures. Yet, while previous publications have long stressed the benefits of art therapy with general and psychiatric prison populations, no publication has really underscored how such services can assist end of life care inside.

## Bringing It All Together: Art Therapy in Prison Hospice Care

Art therapy clearly benefits those who require end-of-life care. Givens (2008) believed that focusing on the art of those whom she visited in their own home provided a sense of presence, acceptance, and an exchange of ideas and worth. This, in turn, reinforces the importance and dignity of the person who is dying; it honors their endeavors. Bell (1998) indicated that art making allows the dying patient to communicate his or her "feelings of what may seem unfathomable despair and uncertainty" (p. 95). It provides an opportunity to safely reflect on their own lives. Safrai (2013) reinforced that art can help transition from a sense of isolation into connection to the larger world when the art can be discussed with others. In fact, she recognized that art making might even empower and enable confidence and a renewed sense of equanimity. Kelly (1999) stated that the "intense feelings evoked by facing one's mortality propel many people to seek relief through a search for wholeness, healing . . . and making peace with the world" (p. 139). Barrington (2016) emphasized that art therapists are uniquely equipped to work with those who are dying. The very narrative quality of the art making provides a visual voice to what needs to be expressed, providing a permanent record of their story.

Additionally, art therapists who engage from a social justice perspective should reach out and assist those that are marginalized and disenfranchised (Barrington, 2016). To be successful, the clinician understands that he or she is not there to "fix the client" but rather to simply be present, validate, and accept what the client has to offer; in short, to recognize that every story is important. I believe that nowhere is this more true than in prison settings.

It needs to be underscored, however, that the hospice in prison is fundamentally different than those outside. Once a person enters hospice care in the community, the understanding is that he or she only has months to live. However, prison hospice allows an inmate to enter its program with a considerably longer term of survival; in some cases, an inmate may be in prison hospice several times longer (Cloyes et al., 2016). Cloyes et al. (2015) noted this might be related to the enhanced, comprehensive care being used, which, in turn, reduces signs and symptoms of patients. In addition, only 14% of hospice patients in the Louisiana State prison hospice died within 7 days of admission as compared to the 35% percent of community patients—so they are living longer once admitted, as well.

Less than 16% of community-hospice patients were 64 years of age or younger on admission. In contrast, 82% of prison hospice patients in the Louisiana State Prison system were under age 64; Cloyes et al. (2015) posit this is due to an enhanced continuity of care in the prison setting as all healthcare is provided under one roof, so delays in admission are less common. Furthermore, the stigma associated with admission to end-of-life care could be less common in prison settings as the programs are often well accepted among the offenders. When discussing this phenomenon with a doctoral social work student conducting research on the benefits of hospice services in prison, she indicated that the length of stay in her facility was as much as ten times longer than those indicated in Cloyes' review; she attributed this to the many levels of care represented in the facility, i.e., acute, skilled-nursing, and end-of-life (S. prost, personal communication, February 13, 2017).

As a result, as they have more time and physical energy as compared to those in hospice outside, there is an enhanced opportunity to take advantage of various therapeutic opportunities to fully process the ramifications of dying in prison. Such therapeutic programs, taken to their logical conclusion, would include art therapy along with the skilled nursing, social work and psychological counseling services already offered. The following are the reasons *why* art therapy should be provided in prison hospice care.

### It Provides a Voice to the Anxiety of Dying Alone

As previous publications have revealed, the subculture of the prison is not conducive to voicing one's weaknesses and vulnerabilities, given the risk of someone taking advantage of him (Gussak & Cohen-Liebman, 2001). Over time, the inmate has a tendency to internalize this, making it a challenge to learn how to express anxiety and fear. One of the benefits of art and art therapy is that such vulnerabilities can be expressed without others recognizing it as such ( Gussak, 2016b). The inmate in hospice care can take advantage of the expressive nature of the material to finally give voice to that which they fear most— disintegration of self, loss of identity, and of being forgotten. These can include drawings that focus on feeling states, materials that lend themselves to more fluid and emotional expression, and media that require more manipulation such as clay or plasticine. This, in turn, can contain the energy through catharsis and sublimation.

### It Provides a Sense of Value and Worth, Living on Beyond the Death of the Inmate

The very act of creating re-humanizes the dehumanized. While the institution is focused on removing a sense of value and worth to better control its wards, art making reinstalls merit and accomplishment. What is more, while there exists the existential angst and anxiety that one will simply disappear, leaving nothing behind, the inmate in hospice care may take solace in knowing that a piece of him may continue long after he is gone. Even though the inmate will not be able to exit the walls prior to his death and spend his final moments with loved ones, there is comfort in knowing that the art he creates will make it out and provide a bridge to the living. It reconnects him to loved ones, allowing him to die with a sense of connection and belonging. This can include art directives that focus on life review, inside/outside boxes that contain memory objects and symbols, or simple manipulations or collages of photographs and images associated with family and life experiences.

### Accepting the art from the inmate makes him feel that he is, contrary to what he has experienced inside, accepted for who he is

Ultimately, this one seems to be the most powerful. Within the confines of the institution, the inmate maintains his label, and in essence, becomes his crime. Such derogatory labels make it almost impossible to succeed, and perpetuates the sense of self-loathing and worthlessness. Yet, when an inmate makes an art piece that is received and celebrated by someone for its intrinsic value, then by extension, the inmate who created the piece is accepted. As the piece symbolizes the very essence of all this person is, he is that much closer to accepting himself. In addition, the piece may also provide atonement. The piece may reflect or contain the very shame and regret the inmate wishes to express but has been unable to put into words. Accepting such a piece allows for closure. These can include directives that focus on self-image and unique identity, such as white-paper sculptures (Gussak, 2016a), mask making or illustrated messages to victims or even loved ones, to provide closure and sense of acceptance and responsibility.

## Creating the Bridge

The institutional dynamics of isolation, dehumanization, and security through dominance runs counter to the compassionate and connecting goals of end of life care. However, hospice programs such as those found at the Louisiana Correctional Institution and the Correctional Medical Facility in California have successfully integrated such programs into their correctional mindset. They have demonstrated, through a change in the subculture, and through pragmatic developments such as an inmate volunteer model [in which inmates from general population work on the hospice units and provide direct care], along with philosophical and epistemological shifts towards patient-centered care, shared values and teamwork, that safety and security do not have to be sacrificed to provide empathetic support. In addition, the programs benefit all members of the institutional system, not just those who are dying. Wright and Bronstein (2007) indicated that by developing compassionate life care in prison, the institutional dynamics change from an "Us vs Them" mentality to one of collective support and recognition of inclusivity.

Inmates who work as caregivers are valued by the medical and correctional staff for the selfless interventions they provide. The inmates that offer care encounter a transformative experience in which they embrace the value of their services and recognize their contributions to the betterment of their subculture (Cloyes, Berry, Reblin, Clayton & Ellington, 2012). The inmate caregivers become members of the interdisciplinary team, providing them worth and sense of identity as well. This, in turn, results in a decrease in incident reports and need for security, ultimately resulting in indirect cost benefits; thus, hospice care in prison is both compassionate *and* cost effective (S. Prost, personal communication, January 31, 2017). Adding art therapy to the program's structure will only enhance the care provided, and improve not only the care of the inmate but the entire system.

Art therapy and hospice care simply make sense; the nature of the art materials and selected directives lends itself to expressing and relieving the strong emotions associated with end of life angst. The products of such sessions provide an opportunity for life review and connection with others, a sense that something can be left behind. Certain experientials provide an opportunity for healing and can reduce the sense of isolation. In turn, the inmates and staff who provide the care on the hospice units can use the art as a way to reach those they are caring for, relying on art to help strengthen the necessary relationships. Ultimately, art therapy can provide a compassionate bridge between those who are dying inside to those living outside.

## References

Barrington, K. (2016). Art therapy and thanatology. In D. Gussak & M. Rosal (Eds.), *The Wiley-Blackwell handbook of art therapy* (pp. 282–291). Oxford, UK: Wiley-Blackwell Publishers.

Bell, S. (1998). Will the kitchen table do? Art therapy in the community. In M. Pratt & M. J. M. Wood (Eds.), *Art therapy in palliative care: The creative response* (pp. 88–101). New York, NY: Routledge.

Bolton, G. (2008). Introduction: Dying, bereavement and the healing arts. In G. Bolton (Ed.), *Dying, bereavement and the healing arts* (pp. 13–21). Philadelphia, PA: Jessica Kingsley.

Brewster. (1983). *An evaluation of the arts-in-corrections program of the California Department of Corrections.* San Jose: San Jose State University.

Brown, M. (2002). *Insider Art.* Winchester, UK: Waterside Press.

Byock, I. R. (2002). Dying well in corrections: Why should we care? *Journal of Correctional Health Care,* 12, 27–35.

California Arts in Corrections. (1987). *Research synopsis on parole outcomes for Arts-in-Corrections participants paroled December, 1980-February, 1987.* Sacramento, CA: Author.

Cloyes, K. G., Berry, P. H., Martz, K., & Supiano, K. (2015). Characteristics of prison hospice patients: Medical history, hospice care, and end-of-life symptom prevalence. *Journal of Correctional Health Care,* 21(3), 298–308.

Cloyes, K. G., Berry, P. H., Reblin, M., Clayton, M., & Ellington, L. (2012). Exploring communication patterns among hospice nurses and family caregivers a content analysis of in-home speech interactions. *Journal of Hospice & Palliative Nursing,* 14(6), 426–437. doi:10.1097/NJH.0b013e318251598b

Cloyes, K. G., Rosenkranz, S. J., Berry, P. H., Supiano, K. P., Routt, M., Shannon-Dorcy, K., & Llanque, S. M. (2016). Essential elements of an effective prison hospice program. *American Journal of Hospice and Palliative Medicine,* 33(4), 390–402. doi:10.1177/1049909115574491

Craig, C. L., & Craig, C. E. (1999). Prison hospice: An unlikely success. *American Journal of Hospice & Palliative Care,* 16(6), 725–729.

Dissanayake, E. (1992). *Homoaestheticus: Where art comes from and why.* New York, NY: The Free Press.

Dubler, N. N., & Heymann, B. (1998). End-of-life care in prisons and jails. In M. Puisis (Ed.), *Clinical practice in correctional medicine* (pp. 355–364). St. Louis, MO: C. V. Mosby.

Fox, W. M. (1997). The hidden weapon: Psychodynamics of forensic institutions. In D. Gussak & E. Virshup (Eds.), *Drawing time: Art therapy in prisons and other correctional settings* (pp. 43–55). Chicago, IL: Magnolia Street Publishers.

Givens, S. J. (2008). Home hospice art therapy: Re-storying the therapist as an invited guest. *Art therapy: Journal of the American Art Therapy Association, 25*(3), 134–136.

Gussak, D. (1997). Breaking through barriers: Advantages of art therapy in prison. In D. Gussak & E. Virshup (Eds.), *Drawing time: Art therapy in prisons and other correctional settings* (pp. 1–12). Chicago, IL: Magnolia Street Publishers.

Gussak, D. (2006). The effects of art therapy with prison inmates: A follow-up study. *The Arts in Psychotherapy, 33*, 188–198.

Gussak, D. (2007). The effectiveness of art therapy in reducing depression in prison populations. *International Journal of Offender Therapy and Comparative Criminology, 5*(4), 444–460.

Gussak, D. (2009). Comparing the effectiveness of art therapy on depression and locus of control of male and female inmates. *The Arts in Psychotherapy, 36*(4), 202–207.

Gussak, D. E. (2016a). Art therapy in the prison milieu. In D. Gussak & M. Rosal (Eds.), *The Wiley-Blackwell handbook of art therapy* (pp. 478–486). Oxford, UK: Wiley-Blackwell Publishers.

Gussak, D. E. (2016b, December). *Rehumanizing thru art-Pressing on with the discourse* [Blogpost]. Retrieved from www.psychologytoday.com/blog/art-trial/201612/re-humanizing-thru-art-pressing-the-discourse

Gussak, D., & Cohen-Liebman, M. S. (2001). Investigation vs. intervention: Forensic art therapy and art therapy in forensic settings. *The American Journal of Art Therapy, 40*(2), 123–135.

Hall, N. (1997). Creativity & incarceration: The purpose of art in a prison culture. In D. Gussak & E. Virshup (Eds.), *Drawing time: Art therapy in prisons and other correctional settings* (pp. 25–41). Chicago: Magnolia Street Publishers.

Hoffman, H. C., & Dickinson, G. E. (2011). Characteristics of prison hospice programs in the United States. *American Journal of Hospice and Palliative Medicine, 28*(4), 245–252. doi:10.1177/1049909110381884

Kelly, C. R. (1999). Transformations: Visual arts and hospice care. In S. L. Bertman (Ed.), *Grief and the healing arts: Creativity as therapy* (pp. 139–144). Amityville, NY: Baywood.

Kramer, E. (1993). *Art as therapy with children* (2nd ed.). Chicago, IL: Magnolia Street Publishers.

Rank, O. (1932). *Art and artist.* New York: W.W. Norton.

Ratcliff, M. (2000). Dying inside the walls. *Journal of Palliative Medicine, 3*(4), 509–511. doi:10.1089/jpm.2000.3.4.509

Rich, B. (2013). Justice, mercy, and the terminally ill prisoner. *Cambridge Quarterly of Healthcare Ethics, 22*(4), 382–388. doi:10.1017/S0963180113000236

Rubin, J. (1984). *The art of art therapy.* New York: Brunner/Mazel.

Safrai, M. B. (2013). Art therapy in hospice: A catalyst for insight and healing. *Art Therapy: Journal of the American Art Therapy Association, 30*(3), 122–129. doi:10.1080/07421656.2013.819283

Wright, K. N., & Bronstein, L. (2007). Creating decent prisons: A serendipitous finding about prison hospice. *Journal of Offender Rehabilitation, 44*(4), 1–16.

# 28 Killing Time

## The Dying Art Therapy Group in a High Secure Hospital

*Emma Allen*

"Do we kill time, or does time ultimately kill us?" (Liccione, 2018). Grave and immediate risk to self and others, such as homicide, along with additional mental health needs, detains many men into old age in one of three high secure hospitals (HSH) in the UK. The psychiatric hospital detains patients under the Mental Health Act (1983, amended in 2007) who fulfil the criteria for "treatment under conditions of high security on account of their dangerous, violent or criminal propensities" (NHS Act 2006), are classified as having a mental illness, intellectual disability disorder and/or a personality or psychopathic disorder, and referred from the criminal justice system, the courts, prisons, or mental health services.

The HSH houses both the living and the dying. Risk and sentencing can be life-long, and admission and offending brings difficult endings and beginnings. Bereavement is defined as a state of loss, often triggering anger and a grief reaction that manifests in a set of behaviours known as mourning, which can result in murderous behaviour. Bereavement means to be "be bereft, robbed, deprived and left desolate, alone, forlorn and disconsolate" (Simon, 1996, p. 124) and is amalgamated with emotions such as denial and can resurface through displacement and projection. Inhibited grief provokes "intense and curious rage" or precipitates severe depression (Kübler-Ross, 1970; Raphael, 1984, p. 60); particularly in the elderly (Murray Parkes, 1996). In older-adult lives, integrity, self-efficacy, social engagement, and other components of self-esteem and stress reduction are all considered important issues that affect physical and socio-emotional health, but it is often the place where one lives near the end of life that is often disregarded (Sokolec, 2016). Bereavement in the HSH is multi-layered; grieving the loss of self, health, mental and physical well-being, as well as freedom and of being a part of society and the outside world. There is an additional loss of status, role and belonging through residence in the HSH, which has now become 'home'. Many patients have lost all contact with family and the hospital is often perceived as the 'end of the line'. Fears of dying in this setting, and the subsequent stigma attached to it, are often expressed behind the secure fencing where the ultimate threat for some can be to die in confinement. Paradoxically, death is often perceived as a 'way out'; an escape from incarceration, mental illness and the past, but, it is dying and loss of control that is feared most (Byers, 1998). In addressing the ageing forensic population, (Sturge, 2018), where many prisoners and offender-patients are detained into their old age due to the length of their sentence, the HSH rehabilitation villa now lies demolished where patients who are wheelchair bound or severely physically disabled or unwell have now moved onto a physical health ward that offers an 'end of life' suite. Being witness to the dismantling and destruction of the villa, along with supporting patients as they grieve their loss of home and experience significant changes forced upon them in the HSH, has all paralleled that of murder and mourning.

This chapter reminisces to the time when an 'open' art therapy group was offered for many years to those residing on the physical healthcare, rehabilitation villa, in the HSH mental health directorate. Group members included men who had committed homicide as a result of bereavement and loss, and suffering with schizophrenia and life-threatening illnesses or disabilities at that time. Some group members include those who have since passed away (in the HSH) and those who have since moved on. For those who are at risk of re-offending (violence and aggression, or harm to self and others) will never reduce, even until death, forensic, palliative, end-of-life care can be offered in long-standing art therapy groups. Art therapy provides those with life-threatening conditions the opportunity to adjust to the effect of their diagnoses and accept the way in which this has changed their life, their body image and appearance, whilst also managing pain (Wood, 1998), and in forensic settings, art therapy allows patients to reflect upon their incarceration, regret, remorse, shame or guilt for offending; exploring complex emotional responses to institutionalised, hospital life and locating a deep sense of compassion for self and others.

Rather than just 'killing time', the art therapy group provided sufficient time for emotional expression and symbolic re-enactments in image-making; working through complex fears, grieving and outrage, and in coming to terms with physiological and psychological change. Imagery from three patients are included, along with the art therapist's artwork that was made in group sessions. Psychological themes around disempowerment, deterioration, helplessness, failure, loss and fears of being forgotten, and unresolved conflicts are all considered and explored from the 'group-as-a-whole' (Skaife & Huet, 1998). Images of illness, delusions, grandiosity, paranoia, or avoidance are also explored where death anxieties were shared. This group vignette also aims to address the difficulties of 'burn-out syndrome' and 'devaluing countertransference' responses in the art therapist (where the value of the work can often be dismissed as 'low-key' or lacking significant change), along with challenging fatigue and lethargy, redundancy and helplessness in the transference. Art therapy groups "can be empowering and containing at a time when body and mind are disintegrating" (Byers, 1998, p. 130). For those who have been life-threatening to others, image-making alongside peers provides an opportunity to gain self-insight into relationship difficulties, offending behaviours and risk. Visual aspects of reminiscing (Butler, 1963) create a vehicle for 'life review' (Ravid-Horesh, 2004), allowing issues of loss that evoke anger to be addressed safely, and for recovery from loss to begin.

## Life on the Rehabilitation Villa

Long stay inpatients that have an average of staying for seven and a half years in the HSH, are often institutionalised and require therapists to hold and sustain hope for recovery in this challenging setting (Rutherford & Duggan, 2007; Hughes & Cormac, 2013). The ward-based day care input for the rehabilitation villa provided a service to elderly male adult patients who had enduring mental health needs and physical health problems, with the aim of enhancing patients' well-being through meaningful activity in a safe, supportive and respectful environment. Villas in the hospital grounds were popular with patients due to their separation from the main hospital building, and for their difference in style of location (surrounded by gardens for ground privilege and the opportunity to spend time outdoors). Villas like this also offered a 'step-down' or progression from the block-wards and offered a unique preparation for lower secure settings and regional secure units (RSU). The villa differed from other wards in that it housed bedrooms on the ground floor, and assisted in the healthcare of the terminally ill or disabled patient. The villa even had its own resident cat that retired along with staff once the villa closed.

## The Villa Art Therapy Group: A Sense of Loss

Long-term art therapy groups for hospitalised inpatients aim towards decreasing their sense of isolation, and alleviate hospital anxiety (Yalom, 1985). They can also act as a 'refuge' from the depersonalising aspects of large institutions and provide a unique space in which to express unspeakable feelings. An 'Open Studio Model' (Foulkes, 1991) art therapy group was offered weekly on the villa for over five years. The group had originally been offered by two art therapists before me, and already had its core members: Billy, Harry and Abdul, with the addition of Gerald and Fred who joined during my facilitation; making most sessions to be made up of five patients. Patients were invited into the group each morning after breakfast. Due to the tendencies for these men to retreat to their side-rooms to rest, it was important to capture some time to invite them in before they left. Patients were always advised that they would be able to come into the room for part or all of the session, according to their personal preference and physical needs. The art therapist's role, as 'group conductor', was to pay attention to both verbal and non-verbal aspects: supporting group members to share whatever came to mind and in being 'spontaneous' so that feelings could be shared. No directions were ever given, needed or necessary; autonomy, or perceived autonomy and control were crucial for these men. The slow-open model encouraged time for self-reflection to consider '*here and now*' dynamics and to find meaning in patterns that emerged in the imagery and discussions.

Being 'given' a long-term-habitual group felt daunting; how would the group tolerate change, a new therapist and what would my role be if the group didn't need me? I quickly discovered that the group had formed its own identity (and group cohesion) and was able to adapt well to new facilitation, but would never forget the previous 'deaths' of therapists leaving the group and hospital. Patients would continuously ask, year after year, enquiring into the welfare of the therapists of the past (perhaps checking they hadn't died); 'clinging on' to the old way of life, and experiencing symbolic difficulty around mortality and institutional living. In addition to these losses, the consultant was also retiring at that time. The sounds of ill-health such as heavy breathing, coughing and wheezing often filled the space and sometimes patients would fall asleep or appear drowsy. Many of the group were suffering with schizophrenia and it would be important to assist these men in their ways of relating to one another in a healthy way, without paranoia.

### The Core Members

The five core group members, and residents on the villa were all elderly, aged into their late seventies and appeared much older than their years. They had all been at the HSH for many years under a mental health act section for hospital treatment and each had physical health needs. They all had difficulties in engaging in offence related treatments and had offence histories related to bereavement and homicide.

### Billy

Billy was the 'leader' of the group, a prolific and violent sex offender in his youth and suffering with psychosis. He had been in a serious car crash in the past and was very frail through his physical disabilities. He had suffered significant injuries and brain damage where he was sometimes delusional and grandiose, and often believed he was having sexual relationships with famous popstars.

## Gerald

Gerald attended the group whilst he was admitted to the physical healthcare ward and during the time he was wheelchair bound after falling and breaking his leg. He was suffering with prolonged and enduring paranoid schizophrenia; believing he was wrongly detained, and had delusional beliefs that his food was being poisoned. His mobility issues and physical limitations caused significant amounts of stress to him where he had bitten and attacked staff when experiencing pain. Gerald had an extensive history of violent and sexual offences (against female partners) and had been in prison since he was eighteen years old. After attending the group, he entered individual art therapy work with me when he moved to a personality disorder ward for assessment.

## Harry

Harry was diagnosed with paranoid schizophrenia after committing homicide, having murdered his wife during divorce proceedings. Harry was a 'co-leader' with Billy (who he'd known whilst in prison) in the group, but liked to identify as the 'joker'. Harry eventually progressed onto an RSU after the group had ended.

## Abdul

Abdul had also attempted homicide by making explosives following a marriage breakdown and was later diagnosed with paranoid schizophrenia and suffering with chronic obstructive pulmonary disease (COPD) which he later died from. He was the verbally 'silent' member of the group who often preferred to entirely focus upon image-making, but would often alert the group to his life-threatening illness from coughing and wheezing, often evoking concern.

## Fred

Fred had been diagnosed with persistent delusional and schizoaffective disorder and had extensive physical health needs, poor mobility and was wheelchair bound. He was suffering with prostate cancer, diabetes and also required triple heart bypass surgery. Fred's past offending had included extensive threats to kill others whilst in possession of firearms. Whilst in a low secure setting, he had arranged to kill his consultant. Fred also presented with antisocial personality difficulties and was fixated by delusions that this doctor was deliberately jeopardising his progress and keeping him in the HSH. His engagement difficulties, and the high risk he presented to this doctor, resulted in his telephone and mail being monitored and was considered high risk to the doctor 'until the day he can no longer write'. Fred declined to engage with psychology, and was deemed treatment-resistant but did attend the art therapy group on three occasions, during a time that he was awaiting heart surgery. His high risk was taken to the grave, with Fred eventually passing away with heart failure.

## Beginnings: "Do you think you'll stay?"

The need for consistency was paramount for holding and containing death anxieties. Patients would routinely sit in their usual seats, bringing with them their mugs of tea to have alongside them. It was important for me to keep bringing the same materials, and to place these in the 'correct place' as instructed by the previous therapist during handover, and from the men themselves. I quickly discovered that any small changes had a detrimental impact, where patients would fear loss or change. Very rarely were any images completed in the time and they seemed to reflect something symbolic about needing to 'hold on' to the group, and to their existence, identity and sense of self. The group would usually begin by each member obtaining their own portfolio of work, as patients would often wish to continue working on images for a number of weeks. Having the artwork present at all times was a visual way of installing hope and building trust that the group was continuing and living and was not going to die any time soon. Questions from the group often arose upon the security and future of the group's continuity: would the group die too? Patients would also enquire into my earnings, and ask if I was paid well and valued. Being a younger female, I evoked memories of and story-telling from their relationships with their mothers, wives, or daughters. The men often spoke of wanting to be 'gentleman-like' and 'not swear'. Harry would often create repetitive imagery of his home he shared with his wife. Traumatic responses, as well as bereavement, may occur in homicide perpetrators where treatment should assist patients to adapt to the changes that the killing brought (Papanastassiou et al., 2004).

Age was a prominent theme. Patients often tried to ask or guess my age, perceiving me to be much younger or a 'student'; often showing concern for how temporary I might be, and whether I would leave, asking, "Do you think you'll stay?" Their ongoing preoccupation with the group dying persisted. Patients would show their concern and sensitivity to illness or injury. Whilst wearing an adhesive bandage on my finger, and when my car broke down, (and the group cancelled at short notice) the group feared the worst in that I was dying, or abandoning them. I often wondered if the dynamic and risk of becoming the partner that had left them in the past would play out in the transference. In addition to being new, there was an additional complex transference of low self-worth, inadequacy and failure, where I often felt that I hadn't 'done enough' for the group. It was important for the group to show me that they were not childish, weak, or incapable. Themes of endurance and suffering, expressions of failing and being a failure and acknowledging a passivity and loss of control in their lives as additional forms of grieving took place.

Occupational loss was also prominent where past employment, professions and money was often spoken about and worth and value an ongoing theme. Sharing memories of their past 'capabilities' and occupational successes allowed them to consider some successes in life, and not focus upon their failings or offence (which was discouraged in the group to maintain confidentiality). They often enquired into my own experiences of the HSH; did I like it enough to stay, or was I thinking about leaving? They wanted to leave, did I too? I often needed to reassure them that I had no plans to leave, (particularly as I had only just started). Informing them of this suggested that there was a need to not only survive the tests, but to also be alongside and a joint member of the group in their admission and long stay; we were all in for the long-run. These patients later identified that they had felt abandoned after two previous art therapists and were concerned it had been a rejection; much like many of their relationship breakdowns with women.

## "How Time Flies"—Ghosts and Fears of Being Forgotten

*Our experience of time is at the heart of what it means to exist.*

(Langdridge, 2007, p. 30)

The group often reflected upon the length of time in incarceration, and upon the 'Hospital Time' as being separate to the actual passing of time; time passing slowly, things happening or changing, being non-existent, or, in stark contrast, that things would immediately happen like a sudden death. Time is paradoxically precious, yet cruel. Time is punishment for the offender-patient and is captured by the art therapy image. On one occasion, Billy asked if Abdul was going to draw all the flags of the world and that if so, 'you'll die'. The risk of completing was symbolic of reaching the very end of life. Billy indicated that Abdul wouldn't achieve this and would die before finishing, suggesting that he had already taken so long to draw the flags he had done so far and that he may not ever complete it.

The clock from the wall was often drawn around for a shape for patients to colour in, and time was always of unconscious significance. One group topic was about 'how time flies' where the group were unsure as to whether this was a good thing or not. The whole group reflected upon this and I made an image for them to look at on this theme (Figure 28.4). Billy spoke as he drew, saying that "It's a terrifying feeling that I may grow old in here" which created a feeling of sadness. Projected fears of being forgotten were powerful in the group. Gerald seemed preoccupied by the homeless during winter and wondered how they would survive in the cold enquiring with the group; "They'd die out there wouldn't they?" The group hoped that charities would open their doors for them and they continued to ask me to remind them to attend each week. They didn't want to be forgotten, or rejected. Many patients would become preoccupied by the thought that their artwork would be 'taken away', or 'lost'. Patients often joked they were making 'weirdo pictures' which paralleled their own feelings of inadequacy and failure. Gerald often considered his images weren't 'worth' keeping and seemed bemused by my suggestion to keep them, particularly his ghost-like man, showing the group: 'Look at the state of him!' (Figure 28.1). The constant presence of their past artwork allowed a deeper containment; to know that they were being held in mind. Increasing self-respect is important in groups with the elderly; reaffirming the self-value that society has taken away. This was done through respecting and valuing their artwork. The group would often thank me for 'saving' or rescuing their artwork (advising them not to dispose of imagery) and showing them their worth.

The group often explored thoughts and feelings surrounding health and medical problems. There were many concerns raised over loss of hair, fears for each other's health, and comments upon each other's likelihood of death and there were many moments of reminiscence of those who had died in their life. Gerald's drawings often expressed fears that he was losing himself, and would die in high secure (Figure 28.1). Ghosts and shadows were a popular topic. They sometimes joked that *they* were ghosts. Gerald considered trees in hot countries being dehydrated only to be drowned with rain that would be too hard to endure. The group often talked about their belief in ghosts and sightings of 'shadows' on the villa. Often patients would feel frustrated with their experiences being assumed psychotic. My questions to the group were often responded to in good humour. I once asked if they had seen anything strange during their time in the HSH where ghost sightings are sometimes talked about. Harry told me 'Yes—him!' and pointed to Billy—everyone burst out laughing. Billy often described the hospital as an old people's home. The group often relied upon humour as a way of coping with bereavement and loss. This often presented itself in self-deprecation in both patients and staff, and within the image. Gerald passed the drawing over to me and told me that 'here's another failure', whilst Harry informed the group of how everything had been decided for him at a tribunal and that he had 'said nothing'. From an existential viewpoint, imagery such as these (Figures 28.1 & 28.2) depict the fundamental crisis of bereavement; not from the loss of others, but the loss of self (Charmaz, 1980).

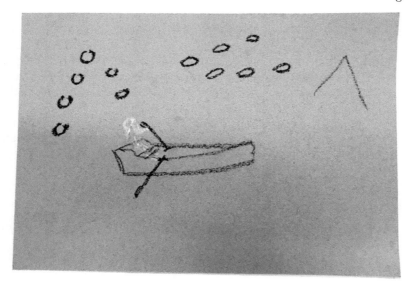

*Figure 28.1* Look at the State of Him! ('Gerald')

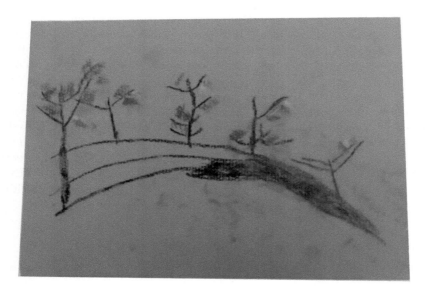

*Figure 28.2* Waiting for Heart Surgery ('Fred')

## Images of Reminiscence and Life Review

Spontaneous images of the group often arise in art therapy that are often linked to pre-occupations with their lives in and outside the HSH. Themes would arise spontaneously from either a group member or the art therapist. The emphasis of the group was upon encouraging members to 'be' and do for themselves; allowing them to set their own pace. Art therapy provides symbolic experiences that help shift the patients view of themselves and the world; guiding and encouraging patients to review the entirety of their life (pre and post offending) and invite patients to address all areas of thought, feeling and action which patients can intuitively feel of importance (Weishaar, 1999). In art therapy, the imagery progression and reflective diary of their time in HSH provides a therapeutic framework and visual life review (Erikson et al., 1986; Butler, 1963). Life reviews evoke reminiscence (Zeiger, 1975), personal adjustment and awareness of an imminent end of life (Butler, 1963), and in addition, are considered effective for memory loss and schizophrenia (Weishaar, 1999).

## Unexpected Death from Unnatural Causes: "How can anyone Shoot Someone Dead?"

*Because we don't know how death is experienced we invent hypotheses that are inevitably limited by our own way of seeing things.*

(Simon, 1996, p. 96)

Death in the HSH not only reminds us of our own mortality but of the victims that have been killed. Murder, at the hands of an offender, was an additional complex layer to the topic of death and dying. Many members of the group had been involved in murder, or attempted murder, but for Billy, being the odd one out as a sex offender, often blurted out the question: 'How can anyone shoot someone dead?' to which an uncomfortable silence would follow. Making each other's offence history known (in this case Harry's index offence) breaks confidentiality and poses risks to patients from each other. Sometimes this felt uncomfortable and inappropriately direct. Billy also picked up on the fact that Fred was dying and on one occasion shouted out that 'He'll beat me to it!', as if dying would be an achievement, an escape or a competition. Although Fred didn't respond or react, patients were often advised to consider other people's feelings in the group and to install a sense of empathy to one another overall. An additional complexity to the group was the impact of the deaths they had caused themselves. There is a synergism of trauma and loss that takes place in bereavement after homicide (Rynearson & McCreery, 1993) and I would suggest that the perpetrator can also become traumatised by the death he has caused himself, which added a complex layer to the psychodynamic contributions in the group around guilt and endings, rejection and abandonment.

## "Struggling to Survive"—Images of Illness and Disintegration

Art therapy groups with the elderly facilitate the expression and exploration of 'being old' and resistances or insecurities to artistic ability can result in the opening up of both negative and positive feelings. Image-making is not pathological but represents the individual's state of mind (Simon, 1996). Concentration and psychological mindedness would drift, whilst pastels and charcoals would smudge, fade and obliterate. Images would inspire and influence other imagery made, and often a sense of copying one another or repetition took place. Abdul often made repetitive abstract patterns that he said were due to being Muslim, and unable to produce imagery of his God's creations. Many other patients would produce repetitive imagery, which can also indicate an arrest in the development of the psyche; stuck and unable to move forward or psychologically progress. Patients can become attached to their mental illness where recovery or wellness can become a threat to identity, initiating a process of mourning (Sandison, 1994).

Many images seemed to disintegrate over time, becoming fainter in colour the more the men became physically weaker over time. Trees were a predominant theme for the majority of the group, (e.g. Figure 28.2) including myself, the art therapist (Figures 28.4 &Figure 28.5). Symbolising life and growth and symbolic of inner development, they convey individuals' 'felt image' of themselves and are symbolic representations of the self, the human body and individuation. It is suggested that those who are physically unwell or disabled often produce broken or damaged trees that allude to traumatic life histories (e.g. Rankin, 1994), and can indicate changes in self-image over time (Isaksson et al., 2009). Drawn trees were often described as 'looking dead' or incomplete. Fred created his trees whilst awaiting heart surgery and described them as 'struggling to survive', similar to himself. What started out as a potentially dark and bleak landscape of dying trees, had colourful autumnal leaves added to them, similar to what was happening outside and a symbolic reminder of the fall. The trees seem to disintegrate, and lead into a point of nothingness, perhaps a journey towards death. Fred later returned to the image, adding colour and potentially hope to the frightening prospect of heart surgery. Figure 28.2, a reflective piece, seems to summarise themes of disintegration. Fred was noticeably defensive and abrupt after the group commented upon his image, sarcastically thanking them for their 'input', which made the group laugh. He spoke of his pending operation and of his understandable feelings of angst and anxiety. He sat with his eyes closed for some time before finally leaving. I wished him well for his operation, which he replied with "Well, if it doesn't it doesn't". Fred left his work unfinished and for me to clear away, and was not ever seen again.

## "Dying Inside": Spiritual Beliefs, Regret, Forgiveness, and 'Killing' Guilt

*I have to think about religion all the time as I'm past it.*

('Billy')

Transpersonal or existential issues can be contained within the therapeutic relationship (Hughes & Cormac, 2013) and within the image. For Billy, art therapy was a spiritual task in seeking renewal and redemption, informing the group that he "had to think about religion all the time as I'm past it". Billy would often draw crosses whilst talking about death and made an image he worked on for weeks reflecting on 'good and evil' and 'yin and yang' (Figure 28.3). Billy shared an idea about how people who have near-death experiences go down a tunnel and see their loved ones who have a message to bring back to the world and to their loved ones. He seemed to be attempting to exorcise his guilt in order for psychological rebirth and transformation. It also seemed to hold the metaphor of the group dynamic around the death of attachment.

When forensic patients are provided a mirror into themselves and into the past, many seek forgiveness and turn to religious or spiritual beliefs in search for meaning and re-evaluation of their lives (Wood, 1998). The threat of death threatens the individual patient's belief systems and challenges their sense of personal meaning and self-worth (Wood, 1998). Although many men in the group had killed, they were now facing their own imminent, natural death and ending, assisting in shifting their thinking around the brutality of their crime. Regret, guilt and shame around their offending can safely emerge pictorially and without explanation; "seeking absolution without confronting the offence" (Hughes & Cormac, 2013, p. 71). Crosses, like trees, are symbolic of life, crucifixion, punishment and suffering, suggesting feelings of redemption. Image-making can be a cathartic confession-making, revealing inner fears, fantasies or delusions.

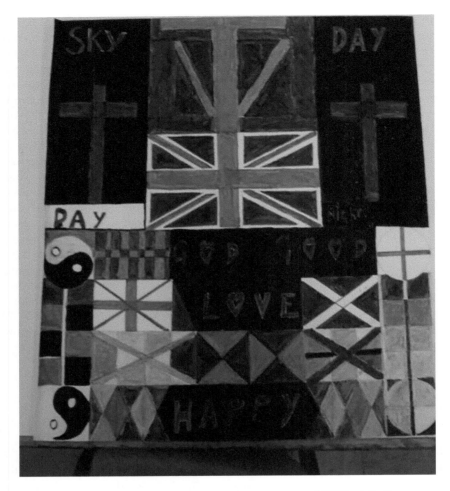

*Figure 28.3* Dying Inside: Spiritual Beliefs, Regret, Forgiveness, and 'Killing' Guilt

The grieving often search for lost people or places, attempting to resolve past conflicts (Byers, 1998). The group often spoke about loved ones who were not alive anymore, or unable to visit them. Tormented by disturbing and distressing paranoid delusions, forensic patients can express the unspeakable in a safer way; the group provided the opportunity to explore their hospitalisation and criminogenic past. Yalom (1985) suggested that psychiatric patients can be assisted to understand how their behaviours prevent them from developing anticipated interpersonal relationships. Perhaps the confrontation to their own mortality enabled these patients to grieve their own mistakes. Patients suffering with schizophrenia often have impaired attention levels, and difficulties with paranoia. Death anxiety, life regrets, religious and spiritual coping and philosophical reflections where death proposes existential challenges to patients at the end of life are common. Interventions that attempt to improve patient self-worth, or appease destructive life regrets through meaningful life review (Butler, 1963), that affirm sources of spiritual meaning (Breitbart et al., 2004), or to forgive self and others (Enright & Fitzgibbons, 2000) could lessen regrets and reduce death anxiety (Neimeyer et al., 2011).

Art therapy aims to address all of these factors where image-making eases the confrontation to physical and psychological suffering and growing old in forensic settings. Religious beliefs can aid dying anxieties; evoke comforting emotions; offer strength, empowerment and control; facilitate self-acceptance and reduce self-blame and emotional burden of illness, relieving fear and uncertainty of death (Siegel & Schrimshaw, 2002). Patients believed they had been sacrificed and spoke of near-death experiences. Restoring a sense of dignity and identity affected by their experience of life in the HSH was important, along with exploring or expressing the ways in which some control could be resumed, along with not focusing entirely upon their physical or medical condition. Paradoxically, there were also many incomplete pictures that represented fears of dying (e.g. Fred's trees, Figure 28.2) and emerged in my own artwork. Perhaps the armchair represents the elderly patient, and the dog, myself, the therapist as a faithful companion (Figure 28.5). Patients may often feel that they are waiting to die and releasing painful emotions provides psychological rehabilitation. The patient's personality and their accustomed way of viewing the world and coping with difficulties influences how they cope with death and dying; not only is there fear, anger and depression in bereavement, but it can also be accompanied with a 'bargaining'; accepting a sacrifice in the expectation of a reward (Murray Parkes, 1998).

## Endings: Disempowerment and Redundancy ('Killing Off the Group')

Offending is a disempowering experience where there is a loss of role and place in society. The group was not 'dying out' due to a lack of motivation but there was a deadness in the group. Offered over a number of years, with the same participants and repeated imagery being produced, there was a repetitive, but consistent autonomy. I often felt redundant and not needed; a helplessness in the transference-constellation. This countertransference of redundancy was illustrated in my imagery (e.g. Figure 28.4) with an empty chair representing a sense of anticipated loss (Figure 28.5). There was often the multi-disciplinary opinion that the villa patients needed 'new life' and I recognised my 'burnt-out' feelings with the group in that I wanted it to 'die out'. The group were often preoccupied by concerns that the art materials would run out and I wondered if this paralleled their concern for me losing interest in them. On a deeper level, this dynamic may have symbolised unconscious fears of change and a sense of guilt of offending against, or harming others. Perhaps they were unconsciously afraid of offending against me.

Countertransference is a powerful tool in understanding and empathising that the group were expressing deep responses to their own mortality. Therapists often block out their ability to empathise with the elderly due to being at a different stage of life which might explain this projective identification of wanting to 'kill off' the group to avoid despair and anxiety. The sleepiness of the patients, however, that I initially had felt frustrated by, had not entirely been avoidance, but a sign of ill-health and in 'shutting down'. It seems important to encourage therapists not to over-analyse sleepiness, or always consider it transference-related, but to be compassionate and understand it as a physical symptom; forensic patients are human, and when unwell, need to rest—we cannot pathologise everything.

Perhaps my frustrations and agitation were with ageing and to cut the group dead would be to manage these feelings and escape from them. I certainly felt guilty and ashamed that I wanted to be free of the group. Processing complex countertransference took place through a series of images made both in and outside of the group through reflective

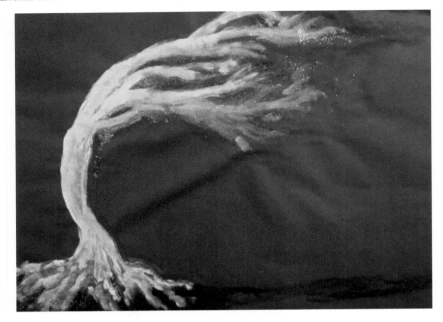

*Figure 28.4* How Time Flies (Art Therapist)

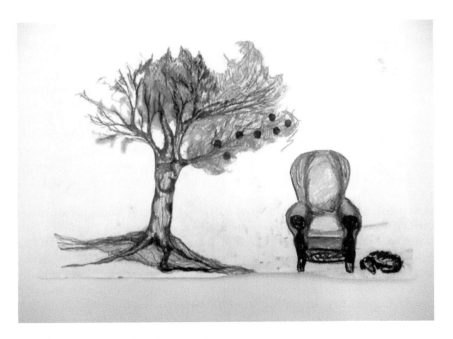

*Figure 28.5* The Waiting Room (Art Therapist)

practice. Figure 28.4 helped identify my fatigue and frustration at the slow pace and seem-ing lack of change. My countertransference became embedded in feelings associated with death where I remember telling colleagues 'The group is dying a death—it has to end soon!' What I failed to realise is that the consistency of the group and my responses to it, were the vehicles to change itself. My reaction felt offensive, destructive and punitive, but also necessary to try to enforce a change or a 'break' in the status quo. It is important that therapists do not succumb to ageist doubts and assume that elderly patients cannot psycho-dynamically change and work effectively in the 'here and now' (Byers, 1998). Paradoxically, expectations of change can be unrealistic and detrimental to forensic mental health where primitive anxieties need to be contained. My role was predominantly one of consistent containment, and whilst it is important to challenge burn-out responses, it is also important to have hope and compassion.

## Mourning the Death of the Villa

Continuing to facilitate the group during a time where the villa was preparing to move back into the main hospital and into a 'block ward', the group also died a death. The group has taken some time to be re-established, and as Billy recently pointed out: 'They've all died, haven't they?' The group has long since died, along with the villa that contained it; now demolished, leaving a void in the hospital grounds of what parallels the psychological grieving process. Whilst writing this chapter, I also seemed to 'lose' my work many times and seemed to be acting out a grieving process for the patients I had once worked with; feeling anger and frustration to sadness and despair. Suffering unexpected losses can be traumatic if unprepared. Major losses in themselves can contribute towards both physical and psychiatric illness, and anger and shame complicate bereavement.

## Conclusion: Life After Death

Beginnings and endings, life and death, are all prominent in the HSH—a place that can, sometimes, be a home for life. Forensic inpatients confront physical, emotional, internal and external change—in a state of bereavement, whether near to their end of life or not, unresolved grief and bereavement issues lie within those who are incarcerated and separated from society, where there is a loss of freedom, control, well-being and health. The closure and demolition of the rehabilitation villa brought additional difficult change, and feelings that paralleled that of murder and mourning, where patients still mourn the loss and death of the villa. Hope, creativity and quality of life are essential, particularly when forensic populations, including staff, are ageing and the stigma of living and dying within the walls of an infamous HSH has an overwhelming affect. The closer an offender is to death, the more focused he may be upon unresolved conflicts from the past; the index offence. There is trauma and loss in complicated grief and bereavement after homicide; even in the killer himself. Bereavement and loss can evoke anger, even homicide and pathological mourning takes place in those who have murdered and can be symbolically felt in the process of image extermination. Images contained group themes on the trauma of ageing, and fears of death and dying; art therapy assisted in exploring these on both verbal and non-verbal levels. Additional support was provided to these men from the art therapist making images alongside.

It is the making of art that proves our human existence, our living as opposed to dying, but also exposes hidden truths, unrealised potential and an inner sense of redundancy and failure. Therapy can thereby feel life-long, similar to the offender-patient's admission and a testing of the forensic art therapist's perseverance can also be commonplace, who is in danger of 'burn-out syndrome', or feeling redundant during group cohesiveness where intolerable feelings and internal suffering can often be transferred onto the therapist in order to manage them.

Diary and 'life review' imagery, which contained complex themes around reminiscence, fragility, bereavement and loss, all marked time in the psychiatric hospital, reflecting upon the past, and increasing self-awareness, acceptance and identity. Images also acted as transitional objects; providing a psychological, inner confrontation to the self and asserting meaning through metaphor. Releasing emotions not only provided psychological rehabilitation and enabled physiological and psychological pain management, but through a form of repetition, patients were able to deal with life behind the fence and with life and death anxieties. Humorous self-deprecation was also important for these men who found talking about their health too hard to put into words, but often revealed their grieving processes in personal imagery. Accepting the difference between past and present self, disempowerment, deterioration, helplessness, failure, lethargy, bereavement, loss, (and loss of self, masculinity and sexuality) and mortality were all considered and explored both as a group 'as-a-whole' and for each individual.

Art therapy groups enable visible communication as a mode of memory retrieval, self-regulation and social interaction. Releasing incarcerated emotions through image-making is not just an activity-based therapy, but one that increases self-worth by stimulating creativity and reducing risk or acting-out behaviours. These men were not just *'killing time'* but were philosophically confronting and accepting the past, present and future. Group treatments prevent a withdrawal into isolation, and allow a space for hope, compassion for self and others, trust, containment and a sense of belonging; offering empathy, dignity and respect and maintaining stability near the end of their lives in high secure.

## Acknowledgements

This chapter is dedicated to the villa that once stood, and to the long-stay forensic psychiatric inpatients who attended the group during 2009–2014. It is in memory of 'Abdul' and 'Fred', and my thanks go to the patients, and to the hospital, who gave consent for the work and for imagery to be included. All names have been changed and some information has been omitted to protect individual's identity.

## References

Breitbart, W., Gibson, C., and Poppito, S.R. (2004). Psychotherapeutic interventions at the end of life: A focus on meaning and spirituality. *Canadian Journal of Psychiatry*, 49, 366–372.

Butler, R.N. (1963). The life review: An interpretation of reminiscence in the aged. *Psychiatry: Journal for the Study of Interpersonal Processes*, 26, 65–76.

Byers, A. (1998). 'Candles Slowly Burning', Chapter 6 in Skaife, S. and Huet, V. (eds.) *Art Psychotherapy Groups, Between Pictures and Words*, London: Routledge.

Charmaz, K. (1980). *The Social Reality of Death: Death in Contemporary America*. Reading, MA: Addison-Wesley.

Department of Health. (1983, 2007). *Mental Health Act*. London: HMSO.

Department of Health. (2006). *National Health Service Act*. London: HMSO.

Enright, R.D., and Fitzgibbons, R. (2000). *Helping Clients Forgive: An Empirical Guide for Resolving Anger and Restoring Hope*. Washington, DC: American Psychological Association.

Erikson, E., Erikson, J., and Krivnick, H. (1986). *Vital Involvement in Old Age*. New York: W.W. Norton.

Foulkes, S.H. (1991, first published 1975). *Group Analytic Psychotherapy: Method and Principles*. London: Karnac.

Hughes, P., and Cormac, I. (2013). 'Music Therapy with Long-stay In-patients: Communication Issues and Collaboration with the Clinical Team', Chapter 3 in Compton Dickinson, S., Odell-Miller, H. and Adlam, J. (eds.) *Forensic Music Therapy, a Treatment for Men and Women in Secure Hospital Settings*, London: Jessica Kingsley Publishers.

Isaksson, C., Norlén, A-K., Englund, B., and Lindqvist, R. (2009). Changes in self-image as seen in tree paintings. *The Arts in Psychotherapy*, 36, 304–312, Elsevier.

Kübler-Ross, E. (1970). *On Death and Dying*. London: Routledge.

Langdridge, D. (2007). *Phenomenological Psychology: Theory, Research and Method*. Harlow: Pearson Education.

Liccione, A. (2018). *Iz Quotes*. Available at https://izquotes.com/author/anthony-liccione/3

Murray Parkes, C. (1996). *Bereavement: Studies of Grief in Adult Life*, New Edition. London: Penguin Books Ltd.

Murray Parkes, C. (1998). 'The Dying Adult', Chapter 10 in Murray Parkes, C. and Markus, A. (eds.) *Coping with Loss*, London: BMJ Books.

Neimeyer, R.A., Currier, J.M., Coleman, R., Tomer, A., and Samuel, E. (2011). Confronting suffering and death at the end of life: The impact of religiosity, psychosocial factors, and life regret among hospice patients. *Death Studies*, 35, 777–800, Routledge, Taylor & Francis Group.

Papanastassiou, M., Waldron, G., Boyle, J., and Chesterman, L.P. (2004). Post-traumatic stress Disorder in mentally ill perpetrators of homicide. *The Journal of Forensic Psychiatry & Psychology*, 15 (1), March, 66–75, Taylor & Francis Ltd.

Rankin, A.M.A. (1994). Tree drawings and trauma indicators: A comparison of past research with current findings from the diagnostic drawing series. *Art Therapy: Journal of the American Art Therapy Association*, 11 (2), 127–130.

Raphael, B. (1984). *The Anatomy of Bereavement: A Handbook for the Caring Professions*. London: Hutchinson.

Ravid-Horesh, R.H. (2004). "A temporary guest": The use of art therapy in life review with an elderly woman. *The Arts in Psychotherapy*, 31, 303–319.

Rutherford, M., and Duggan, S. (2007). *Forensic Mental Health Services: Facts and Figures*. London: The Sainsbury Centre for Mental Health.

Rynearson, E.K., and McCreery, J.M. (1993). Bereavement after homicide: A synergism of trauma and loss. *The American Journal of Psychiatry, Washington*, 150 (2), February, 258–261.

Sandison, R. (1994). Working with schizophrenics individually and in groups: Understanding the psychotic process. *Group Analysis*, 27, 393–406.

Siegel, K., and Schrimshaw, E.W. (2002). The perceived benefits of religious and spiritual coping among older adults living with HIV/AIDS. *Journal for the Scientific Study of Religion*, 41 (1), 91–102. DOI: 10.1111/1468–5906.00103

Simon, R.M. (1996). *Symbolic Images in Art as Therapy*. London: Routledge.

Skaife, S., and Huet, V. (1998). *Art Psychotherapy Groups, Between Pictures and Words*. London: Routledge.

Sokolec, J. (2016). The meaning of "place" to older adults. *Clinical Social Work Journal*, 44 (2), June 2017, 160–169. DOI 10.1007/s10615-015-0545-2

Sturge, G. (2018). *UK Prison Population Statistics*. Briefing Paper Number CBP-04334, 23 July, House of Commons Library.

Weishaar, K. (1999). The visual life review as a therapeutic art framework with the terminally ill. *The Arts in Psychotherapy*, 26 (3), 173–184, USA: Elsevier Science Ltd.

Wood, M. (1998). 'What Is Palliative Care?' Chapter in Pratt, M. and Wood, M. (eds.). *Art Therapy in Palliative Care, the Creative Response*, London: Routledge.

Yalom, I. (1985). *The Theory and Practice of Group Psychotherapy* (1st ed., 1975). New York: Basic Books.

Zeiger, B. (1975). Life review in art therapy with the aged. *American Journal of Art Therapy*, 15, 47–51.

# 29 Disenfranchised Grief

## The Impact of Grief in the Military

*Rachel Mims and Jacqueline Jones*

*The views expressed in this chapter are those of the authors and do not reflect the official policy of the Department of Defense, or the U.S. Government.*

The following chapter details the personal and professional experiences of two art therapists. Rachel is a U.S. Army veteran and an art therapist who has worked with student veterans and dependents. Jackie has worked with service members and veterans in recovery from traumatic brain injury, post-traumatic stress, and other mental and physical health issues. In the following chapter, Rachel will discuss her personal experience with disenfranchised grief and Jackie will describe how she addresses disenfranchised grief when working with her clients.

### Introduction: Rachel's Story

My life changed dramatically when I was 28. My job in the Army as a PATRIOT Missile Launcher Operator Maintainer was very physically demanding. I had to run, climb, lift, and carry while doing crew drills and wearing about 40 lbs of Army gear. Eight years of this job and other physical demands in the Army led me to have problems with my hip, which necessitated surgery. During my 30 days of convalescent leave before returning to work, I was isolated and lonely. I turned to art and began to see how it allowed for emotions to be transferred onto paper or canvas.

After my leave, I continued to do art on my own to keep myself positive when my recovery did not go as planned. I was told that I would be fully recovered after several months of physical therapy, but at that time I still needed a cane to walk. My career as a soldier revolved around my ability to carry out the physical requirements of my job, but I was not getting any stronger. The military did its best to help me. I went to physical therapy for several years and participated in programs such as water therapy and pain management. None of these programs increased my strength physically, and none of them addressed the mental and emotional issues I was dealing with as a result of my disability. Military units depend on each member's contribution in order to accomplish missions; when someone is hurt or unable to do his/her job, he/she is almost instantaneously devalued. Not only were my peers and supervisors viewing me as a liability, but also my personal sense of identity was being challenged. If I was not a soldier, who was I? Could I even stay in the Army?

This unexpected, life altering change left me with many questions that remained unanswered. I was given treatment aimed at addressing only my physical needs; no one thought to see if my sudden physical disability was causing me emotional difficulty. Emotions are not welcome in the military, so I could not discuss my feelings with my supervisors. I was stationed far away from home too, so I was unable to turn to my family for support. I was experiencing disenfranchised grief; I was mourning a loss that was not recognized by others. For over two years after my surgery, I dealt with this change in ability and the loss of my identity as a soldier; I struggled both mentally and physically trying to figure out how to live my new life. Even now, 7 years post-surgery I still grieve what I lost.

My experience in the military is not uncommon; many others have experienced a loss of ability that resulted in a sudden change in position within their unit, a change to their identity, and a change in how others perceived them. Military culture focuses on accomplishment of the mission and selfless service; this often results in a less than 100% healthy individual being viewed as a liability, and thus being treated poorly. Many service members are unable to empathize with those who have experienced a loss such as mine. As was the case in my own experience, many doctors focus solely on physical recovery and even clinicians may not be aware of the grief process that is occurring.

My experiences in the military are not unique. This chapter will review current literature as it pertains to grief work with veterans and military service members. The mental and physical health impacts of combat will be discussed. Then, the ways in which service members and veterans experience disenfranchised grief will be detailed. Literature pertaining to the treatment of grief within this population will be examined with an emphasis on the use of art therapy. Lastly, Jackie, an art therapist currently working with military service members, will detail how she has utilized art therapy to aid veterans who have suffered losses due to their time in service.

## Literature Review

The following section will review literature that discusses grief and loss within this population. First, the impacts of combat will be examined, including physical and mental health wounds sustained by those with combat experience. Then, disenfranchised grief and how it may occur within military service members and veterans will be discussed. Lastly, treating grief and loss among this population will be detailed with special emphasis on utilizing the creative arts in treatment.

## The Impacts of Combat

As of 2011, approximately 2.6 million living veterans have participated in the Iraq and Afghanistan wars (U.S. Government Accountability Office, 2011). Of these veterans, 52,337 were wounded as a result of deployment for Operation Iraqi Freedom (OIF), Operation Enduring Freedom (OEF), or Operation New Dawn (OND) (U.S. Department of Defense, 2016). Additionally, many service members have returned from deployment with "invisible wounds" such as post-traumatic stress disorder (PSTD), anxiety, depression, substance abuse and traumatic brain injury (TBI) (Tanielian, Jaycox, Adamson & Metscher, 2008).). Both visible and invisible wounds can result in a loss of ability, which may cause a grief reaction.

While some individuals may return from deployment without any of these wounds, they may still be grieving losses due to their combat experience. In a survey of Army and Marine Corps infantry units, Hoge et al. (2004) found that 43% of Army infantrymen that served in Afghanistan and 86% of those who served in Iraq knew someone who was seriously injured or killed; a total of 87% of Marine Corps infantrymen who served in Iraq had experienced this as well. Additionally, many of these service members saw dead bodies or human remains, handled or uncovered human remains, and/or saw dead or seriously injured Americans. Similar numbers were found when Currier and Holland (2012) examined combat loss and found that 68% of those who participated in the National Vietnam Veterans Readjustment Study reported that a close personal friend had died during Vietnam.

Veterans are clearly subject to experience situations that may result in grief, but is this something about which clinicians need to be concerned? Several researchers have found data that suggest focusing on this topic is necessary. Toblin et al. (2012) examined how grief impacted the physical health of infantry soldiers returning from combat. Over 1,500 soldiers were surveyed and 21.3% were struggling with grief over the loss of someone close. Results showed that difficulty coping with grief significantly contributed to poor general health, missed work, increased medical visits, and an increased amount of somatic symptoms. Fatigue, sleep problems, headaches, musculoskeletal pain, and back pain were the top five physical symptoms reported by respondents. Additionally, the researchers found that grief resulted in occupational impairment.

Grief not only impacts physical health, it also impacts mental health. Psychosocial adjustment of women amputees was examined by Cater (2012). She found that in addition to pain, amputation resulted in body image issues and grief issues; furthermore, each of the women in the study had to re-build her self-image and life based on her "new normal." Currier and Holland (2012) found that Vietnam veterans who had experienced combat loss had increased difficulties adjusting post deployment as well as increased trauma symptoms. Results of this study showed that veterans who experienced combat loss were more likely to experience increased health problems, family issues and/or financial issues as well as functional impairments.

Grief due to combat loss also affects the mental health of those who were deployed to Iraq and Afghanistan. Hoge et al. (2004) found that the prevalence of PTSD was strongly related to experiences such as knowing someone who was killed or handling dead bodies. Additionally, being wounded or injured, situations that can result in grief, were significantly associated with PTSD. Those who have experienced combat loss also more frequently reported stress and depression symptoms (Chapman et al., 2012).

Some researchers have looked into the differences between healthy and normative grief processes and grief that is considered complicated, or prolonged. Ott (2003) examined the differences between noncomplicated grief (NCG) and complicated grief (CG) in a sample of 112 widows and widowers. Results showed that those whose Inventory of Complicated Grief scores placed them in the CG Group experienced a decrease in mental health as well as an increase in social, family, health, self-management and work/home roles issues which resulted in a decreased level of functioning as compared to the NCG group. Boelen and Prigerson (2007) examined data from 346 mourners and found similar results; prolonged grief disorder was "distinct from depression and anxiety and to be predictive of reduced quality of life and mental health" (p. 444). Similarly, Bonanno et al. (2007) compared grief, depression, and PTSD symptoms and found that grief was a unique forecaster of functioning.

Combat experiences can result in both physical and mental health issues, including grief, which may become complicated or prolonged due to the circumstances of the losses. Additionally, veterans, and service members are likely to experience another type of grief. The following section will detail disenfranchised grief and how it may occur within veterans and service members. The consequences of disenfranchised grief will also be discussed.

## Disenfranchised Grief

All people experience grief; however, different cultures experience grief differently. Cultural norms dictate who is allowed to grieve, how a grieving individual should behave and think, which losses are acceptable to grieve, and who can support the grieving individual (Doka, 2002). When these norms deny individuals the right to grieve, disenfranchised grief can occur; Doka (2002) identified the several categories of loss that often result in disenfranchised grief. First, a relationship may not be recognized as significant. Corr (2002) points out that "disenfranchised relationships include associations that are well accepted in theory but whose full implications are not appreciated in practice or in particular instances" (p. 43). Military service members may experience this type of disenfranchised grief upon death of a member of their unit. Military service members often feel that the members of their units are their families/brothers/sisters; thus the relationship may be much more meaningful and impactful than non-military members may understand.

The second category of loss that can result in disenfranchised grief is loss that is not acknowledged, or recognized as significant (Doka, 2002). Military service members who have suffered serious wounds/injuries may fall into this category if others around them are focused solely on how lucky the individual is to be alive or on moving forward with life. This type of disenfranchised grief may also be experienced by those with invisible wounds; for instance, PTSD and TBI can dramatically change one's life in unexpected and unappreciated ways which would result in grieving parts of oneself one has lost. Doka (2002) also points out that losses often result in other changes such as losing friends, losing a job, or being unable to participate in one's favorite activities; these secondary losses can result in additional grief.

The way in which an individual grieves can also cause grief to be disenfranchised (Doka, 2002). Individuals whose natural grieving style is different from the norm of their culture are likely to experience disenfranchised grief. This may be the case for individuals in the military who are unable to hold in or hide their emotions as is in line with military culture (Reger et al., 2008). Barbant (2002) points out that a culture's grieving rules become part of an individual's identity; thus, even after leaving the military, a veteran may still suffer disenfranchised grief as a result of the belief that he/she should "suck it up" (Reger et al., 2008).

Loss experienced during combat is especially likely to result in grief that is disenfranchised due to the nature of the combat environment and the culture of the military. Thornton and Zanich (2002) conducted an empirical assessment of disenfranchised grief and found that those who experience it are less likely to seek help. The authors also pointed out that many caregivers may not recognize that social support for disenfranchised grief is necessary. There is clearly a need for counselors who are aware of the unique situations faced by service members and veterans and for treatments to aid those who are impacted, but are effective treatments available?

## Treating Grief and Loss in Veterans and Service Members

Keenan, Lumley, and Schneider (2014) wrote about a program for veterans that addressed grief as the result of losing a loved one and the guilt and shame that resulted from causing harm to others. The authors utilized a group therapy program with three phases that aimed to foster connections to others and to one's self. Psychoeducation was the focus of phase one and facilitators presented on topics such as depression, sleep issues, anger, stress, and anxiety management. The purpose of this phase was to increase the veterans' understanding of their emotions and symptoms while enhancing their stress management skills. During phase two veterans discussed their traumas in detail and developed a trauma narrative; the authors pointed out that veterans typically shared milder traumas first and then progressed toward more distressing trauma over time. As part of phase two, veterans wrote a letter to someone they lost or harmed and then read it to the group. The final phase of the group, phase three, was focused on providing the veterans with the tools necessary to move forward in their lives. Topics discussed during phase three included spirituality, finding meaning, community involvement and relationships. Additionally, the group was encouraged to meet for peer support on alternating weeks.

This three-phase program was conducted for over two years, and Keenan et al. (2014) found that nine veterans made an optimal size for the trauma group in phase two. The authors reported no identified need to sort groups based on gender, military occupational specialty, generation, or rank. The authors also suggested that such a group should be co-facilitated which would benefit both the group members and the therapists.

Keenan et al. (2014) found that veterans benefited from this program in different ways. One Vietnam veteran was able to move from fearing sleep due to nightmares that involved witnessing a friend die, to looking forward to sleep because of a newfound ability to dream about the good times with his friend. Some veterans who participated in the program utilized their letters in a ritual or ceremony. One veteran in particular, conducted a burial ceremony of the victim of his "first kill"; during the ceremony he said a prayer and burned his letter.

There currently appears to be a general lack of research on treating grief and loss in veterans or military service members. Art therapy has often been used to aid those suffering from trauma because it offers the opportunity for nonverbal expression (Johnson, 2000) and allows for containment of traumatic material within an object or image (Collie et al., 2006). This type of expression can be quite beneficial for veterans and military service members who come from a culture that encourages emotional suppression (Reger et al., 2008). As a result, some practitioners have already begun utilizing art therapy to treat grief and loss among this population.

## Using the Creative Arts in Treatment

Art based methods were utilized by Artra (2014) to examine how improvement in PTSD symptoms corresponded with changes in moral injury and complicated grief. Each of the eight male combat veteran participants created 11 pieces of art and a story over the course of a five-day retreat. Art created by the participants included papier maché, clay sculptures, sand tray, collage, the creation of a shield, and several types of drawings. The retreat aimed to assist in meaning making for loss of personal self, loss of others, and loss of sense of soul. Results of this study showed that clinically significant improvements in PTSD can occur while an individual is grieving loved ones and recovering a sense of soul; these improvements corresponded with breakthroughs in identity.

As a means of processing grief that resulted from the events of September 11, 2001, Haeseler (2002) guided veterans in the creation of a memorial mosaic. Veterans were provided with blank 4" × 4" tiles upon which they painted a variety of scenes. These tiles were arranged in a checkerboard pattern on a 54" × 42" plywood base with a frame. Veterans utilized broken tile, stones, shells, and found objects to fill in the remaining spaces of the mosaic. On March 11, 2002, a public dedication ceremony was held. Haeseler (2002) pointed out that many veterans, who normally had difficulty tolerating emotional expression or dealing with large groups of people, participated in this event. Veterans that participated in this project felt that it helped them express their sympathies, distract them from their pain, move past the experience, and keep those who perished alive.

At the National Intrepid Center of Excellence (NICoE), The Healing Art Program utilizes many forms of alternative treatments, including art therapy, to treat military service members with PTSD or TBI (NICoE, n.d.). The program involves a four-week group art therapy curriculum. Participants create masks to depict their "warrior" selves, complete expressive writing exercises, write postcards to former participants, and make montage paintings about their past, present, and future. Walker (n.d.), the Healing Arts Program Coordinator, reported that grief/guilt and death were among the reoccurring themes that service members depicted when creating their masks. Participants reported that the art therapy program helped them develop hope for the future while also increasing insight into and awareness of problems.

Scrapbooking as an intervention has not yet been used with veterans or service members but has many beneficial aspects such as allowing for organization of words and images, paralleling the reconstructive nature of the healing process, and allowing for the telling of personal stories while simultaneously aiding in remembrance. Kohut (2011) assisted clients in the creation of scrapbooks in order to address grief and loss. The scrapbooking bereavement group was conducted over a four-week period. The clients of this group found that creating scrapbooks resulted in a sense of control as well as providing a means for self-expression. Additionally, it provided a way to heal while also memorializing their loved one. Many of the participants reported looking at the scrapbook as well as sharing it with friends or family. Although Kohut's (2011) participants were not veterans or military service members, scrapbooking and similar interventions such as collage, have the potential to be beneficial for this population.

## Summary

The VA estimates that as of September 30, 2016, there are over 2.9 million living Operation Iraqi Freedom (OIF)/Operation Enduring Freedom (OEF)/Operation New Dawn (OND) veterans (U.S. Department of Veterans Affairs, 2016). These veterans, along with those who served before them, have had many experiences that place them at risk for experiencing loss and developing physical and mental health issues which may result in disenfranchised grief. Different treatment methods have been used to address grief within this population: narrative therapy, group therapy, and the creative arts. Overall, however, there is a lack of research and academic writing on the treatment of disenfranchised grief with service members. The following section will detail the work of an art therapist who has used an intervention developed specifically for the treatment of grief and loss among this population.

## Addressing Disenfranchised Grief With Service Members: Jackie's Approach

As the art therapist at Intrepid Spirit One (ISO), the National Intrepid Center of Excellence satellite at Fort Belvoir, I provide art therapy to active duty service members in rehabilitative treatment for TBI and psychological health conditions, such as PTSD. Most of the patients I treat deal with chronic issues that have built up over time as the service members continued to push forward, "sucking it up." For some, this manifests primarily as cognitive impairments; patients may not be able to process and retain information they read as successfully as they used to. For some, this manifests primarily as physical pain and inability; service members may not be able to perform physical tasks that they could before, and may not be physically able to work out with the same intensity as before. For some, this manifests primarily as psychologically rooted changes in behaviors; patients may report difficulties with functioning in daily life and in their relationships due to an inability to control their emotions and reactions when triggered by elements in their environments, or difficulty connecting with others after learning to become emotionally numb in order to keep going and be successful at work. For most, the cognitive, physical, and emotional effects are intertwined and exacerbate one another. For all, the toll that these effects take on one's identity is profound, especially in the military where service members are expected to operate like elite, fail proof machines.

> *"I don't want to accept my new normal."*
> *"Who am I if I'm not a soldier?"*
> *"I can't run anymore, I can't find another outlet."*
> *"I watched my best friend die and I had to keep going, get back into the fight."*
> *"I couldn't go to his funeral, I was still deployed."*

I have witnessed patients struggle first with mourning significant losses of one's own sense of self, career, and comrades, and second with feeling invalidated, unheard; these remarkable losses were routinely disenfranchised. The following intervention was initially developed in direct response to this commonly shared issue and has been integrated as a standard component of the art therapy program at ISO.

## Celebration/Commemoration Boxes

Service members are invited to create a box or container in which the outside of the box celebrates aspects of career and self and the inside of the box commemorates or memorializes aspects of career, self, and/or buddies lost. When selecting their containers, they are asked to consider the quantity and size of any items that they may have at home that have been saved and held onto throughout their career. Perhaps the items were significant so they were saved, but for various reasons kept hidden, or maybe just need a place. Patients are provided prompts for additional options, such as approaching the box as positives on the outside, negatives on the inside, or aspects of pride on the outside, things they don't show publicly on the inside; utilizing the inside to create a grieving space; to work on the outside and inside in the order of their choice; to use a special container from home; to incorporate any personal photographs.

This project allows service members to acknowledge and celebrate prideful aspects of career and self, which they report are slighted or ignored when they are told to simply accept their new normal and move on. At the same time, it also provides the space for expression of negative or complicated thoughts and feelings they may have in reaction to their experiences. The open/close nature of a box makes for a safe place for grieving, an appropriate place to keep items that have been saved but warrant the protection that the walls of the box provide and allow for a shift of control, as it can be opened and closed as the service member desires. The inside of the container frequently becomes a special memorial space, which service members express appreciating since many lack the ability to visit gravesites or places where people died. The box enables service members to acknowledge coexisting positives and negatives, such as displaying points of pride while processing feelings of shame, guilt, anger, and sadness. Finally, the box ultimately becomes a conduit for the integration of aspects of career, self, and comrades lost into life moving forward.

## Case Example: Salinas

Salinas is a 31-year-old married Hispanic male, active duty Petty Officer 1st Class in the Navy (PO1), working as a journalist. As a result of exposure to several traumatic events throughout his Navy career and significant injuries sustained when he fell down a ladder well of a ship, he receives rehabilitative treatment for symptoms of several diagnoses, including sequela of diffuse traumatic brain injury with loss of consciousness of unspecified duration, post-traumatic stress disorder, and chronic pain throughout his body. He reported personality change after his fall in 2011, stating that he is hypervigilant, easily frustrated, irritable, isolative, "no longer a nice gentleman," and is constantly accompanied by pain, his "unwanted visitor."

Salinas was referred to art therapy as part of his interdisciplinary treatment plan at ISO. When he was directed to create his celebration/commemoration box as he engaged in the structured art therapy groups, he initially approached the project intending to use the outside to represent celebratory aspects of his career in the Navy while the inside would enable him to express his emotions regarding being pulled from performing certain duties that would have allowed him to achieve certain merits and advance in his career, due to the injuries he had sustained on the job. Salinas worked on the box for eight sessions that spanned a duration of nine months, because he was often unable to attend outpatient appointments in order to undergo various surgeries or attend other appointments in preparation for medical retirement. During initial sessions working on the box, Salinas had printed several personal photos of himself as a sailor in moments he enjoyed on ship, in operating rooms post surgeries, with his family, and of ships and aircraft that were meaningful to him. When he revisited the project several months later, he experienced a paradigm shift when deciding which photos to include on the outside versus the inside of the box. He verbalized feeling a shift from "Seeing this made me feel mopey because I can never have that again to being like 'hey!' I had this experience in my life!'" He changed his perception of career goals he was no longer able to pursue from examples of personal failure to achievements "that just didn't happen." He brought in coins he received throughout his career, explained the meaning of each, and chose to keep the most significant inside the box. When he completed his work, he shared that the box helped him shift from feeling intense negative emotions when thinking about retiring from the Navy to being able to think and talk about it "as if [he] were making a sandwich," in a more matter of fact manner, with greater acceptance.

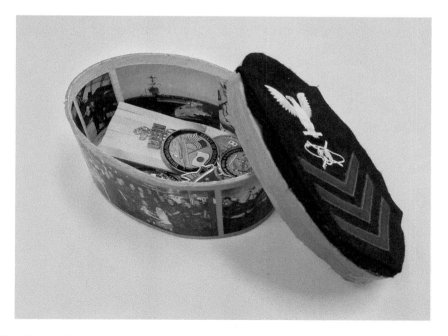

*Figure 29.1* Salinas' Box

## Case Example: Bjorn

Bjorn is a 29-year-old married Caucasian male, active duty Army Sergeant who worked as a Practical Nurse and deployed twice to Afghanistan with the infantry as a Combat Medic. During his first deployment he was exposed to firefights at least once a week, and had many close calls with improvised explosive devices (IEDs). During his second deployment he was exposed to blasts by IEDs and rocket propelled grenades (RPGs) two to three times per week. There were a couple of noted incidents in which rockets landed within 10 feet of Bjorn, but as the combat medic he shook off any disorientation as quickly as possible and pressed on. Bjorn was referred to ISO where he engaged in interdisciplinary treatment (in which multiple disciplines work cooperatively to assess and treat) for the diagnoses that resulted from his combat experience, to include: traumatic brain injury, post-traumatic stress disorder, chronic pain, migraines, and anxiety.

Bjorn began his celebration/commemoration box by creating a sculptural depiction of the Afghan mountainscape on top of the box lid, which he stated represented his sense of accomplishment. He painted the outer walls with a camouflage motif and affixed meaningful objects from deployment to the outside and inside of his box. Bjorn utilized the outside/inside aspects of the container to represent the concept of beauty versus reality. The outside includes representations of his unit and battalion as well as the Afghan mountains, as even in bad situations, beauty could be found in the mountains. On the inside of the box, Bjorn included a Domo stuffed toy that a battle buddy had started using as a platoon mascot, as well as the memorial bracelet for this same comrade who died in 2009. Bjorn placed another significant memorial bracelet as well as a meaningful coin and piece of camo netting on the inside as well. The inside lid contains an Army combat uniform (ACU) pattern with blood painted on top to show how uniforms get bloody in reality.

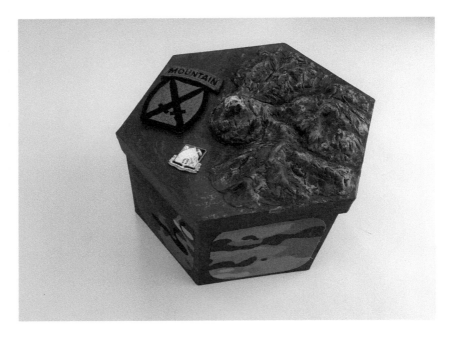

*Figure 29.2* Bjorn's Box (Exterior)

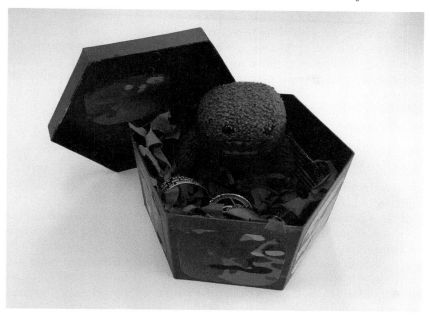

*Figure 29.3* Bjorn's Box (Interior)

Bjorn expressed enjoyment in his creative approach to the container, and content-ment that he was able to create a special place for the significant objects he had saved throughout his career. The box allowed Bjorn to process the duality of positive and nega-tive thoughts and feelings related to his deployment experiences as well as establish a memorial space for comrades who were killed in action (KIA) with whom he was close. Afterwards, Bjorn's continued work in art therapy focused on improving mood and sup-porting him as he created a plan for his next career. He moved from a depressed state to one of hope and excitement for the future.

## Additional Approaches to Address Disenfranchised Grief

In addition to the celebration/commemoration box which is typically created during a series of structured art therapy groups, service members have used a variety of approaches in individual art therapy sessions at ISO to process grief that has been disenfranchised or otherwise complicated. Once the circumstances and effects of someone's loss are dis-cussed and examined by the patient and art therapist, an intervention, or idea for art process or product, is identified as appropriate to promote bereavement, processing, and healing. Examples of these approaches include the creation of: memorial stones (memo-rial collages on the undersides of flat-bottom glass beads); memorial books (handmade books in which each page becomes the canvas for expressive artwork reflecting on individ-uals who have died); Intensive Trauma Therapy (series of images that compose a Graphic Narrative of scenes drawn in accordance to stages in the Instinctual Trauma Response) (Gantt & Tinnin, 2009); compilation of memorial tiles (tiles created for each deceased individual laid together); sculptures of Kevlar helmet, boot, and rifle combat cross memo-rials created to grieve specific individuals; drawn, painted, or sculpted portraits of the deceased; series of past, present, and future self-portrait drawings; and artwork made at the culmination of one's career.

Providing service members with the opportunity to grieve losses of aspects of self, career, and comrades through visually self-expressive and creative means makes a profound impact on their recovery. The artwork created allows individuals to experience a sense of release, to recover positive aspects related to self, career, or comrades that have been consequentially figuratively buried with the intentionally suppressed negative aspects, to create tangible objects that honor the deceased or recognize traits of one's past, to move from avoidance to acceptance, and to integrate the losses into themselves in ways that enable them to move forward.

## Coming Full Circle: Rachel's Box

To have a better understanding of what Jackie's clients experience, I (Rachel) completed a box project to address my own experience with disenfranchised grief. I wanted to approach the box project with as much open-mindedness as possible, so, although I had previously heard about the project, I did not read the preceding case examples until after I had completed my own box. Truthfully, I was a little hesitant about completing this project; I think this is important to note because I have had seven years to deal with my grief and loss—it is not as "fresh" as that of a newly injured or discharged service member. I completed the box project over the course of several days. I began by using gesso on the outside of the box and then painting it green, brown, and black in a battle dress uniform type of camouflage pattern. The inside of the box was white and I left it as such.

I tried my best to imagine what it would have been like to create this box when I was newly injured or after I had realized that I was not going to get back to "normal;" I was unable to run, jump, and climb—things that were required to say in the Army. Even as few as four years ago I probably would have had a much more negative approach to this project; Like Salinas, I would have had the "this is what I have lost" mindset. It has taken many years and a lot of self-care and self-discovery to see the positives of my experience.

I utilized collage to fill the inside of the box first. I included things such as the word "soldier" and a picture of combat boots to signify the fact that I lost my ability to be in the Army. I also included things like "leader of the pack" which I used to signify the feeling I had when I was first injured, that I could no longer be a leader.

On the outside of the box I focused on the positive things I gained from being in the military. I am proud of being an Army veteran and I made sure to include it on my box. I also made note of the fact that the Army was a part of my journey, "a once-in-a-lifetime experience," and resulted in "lasting memories." Additionally, I noted the personal dedication and determination that I developed while in the military. Even though I completed my box project seven years after my surgery, I still benefitted from this project and I am proud of what I created.

## Summary

The box project aids individuals in reframing their loss and in processing their grief. They are able to acknowledge what they have lost while also focusing on what they get to keep as a result of their experience. The benefits of the box don't end with the finishing artistic touch. More often than not, service members place their boxes on display at home or at work. The containers then provide tangible objects to aid in their communication with others about their experiences, act as daily reminders of what they've gotten to figuratively carry forward, and often become miniature memorial grounds to be visited conveniently and privately. The creation of the box promotes processing of disenfranchised or complicated grief, and the finished product continues to provide support for the ever-evolving experience with grief.

# References

Artra, I. P. (2014). Transparent assessment: Discovering authentic meanings made by combat veterans. *Journal of Constructivist Psychology, 27*(3), 211–235, doi: 10.1080/10720537.2014.904704

Barbant, S. (2002). A closer look at Doka's grieving rules. In Doka, K. J. (Ed.), *Disenfranchised grief: New directions, challenges, and strategies for practice* (pp. 23–38). Champaign, IL: Research Press.

Boelen, P. A., & Prigerson, H. G. (2007). The influence of symptoms of prolonged grief disorder, depression, and anxiety on quality of life among bereaved adults: A prospective study. *European Archives of Psychiatry and Clinical Neuroscience, 257*, 444–452, doi: 10.1007/s00406-007-0744-0

Bonanno, G. A., Neria, Y., Mancini, A., Coifam, K. G., Litz, B., & Insel, B. (2007). Is there more to complicated grief than depression and posttraumatic stress disorder? A test of incremental validity. *Journal of Abnormal Psychology, 116*(2), 342–351, doi: 10.1037/0021–843X.116.2.342

Cater, J. K. (2012). Traumatic amputation: Psychosocial adjustment of six Army women to loss of one or more limbs. *Journal of Rehabilitation Research and Development, 49*(10), 1443–1456, doi: 10.1682/JRRD.2011.12.0228

Chapman, P., Elnitsky, C., Thurman, R., Spehar, A., & Siddharthan, K. (2012). Exploring combat-related loss and behavioral health among OEF/OIF veterans with chromic PTSD and mTBI. *Traumatology, 19*(2), 154–157, doi: 10.1177/1534765612457220

Collie, K., Backos, A., Malchiodi, C., & Spiegel, D. (2006). Art therapy for combat-related PTSD: Recommendations for research and practice. *Art Therapy: Journal of the American Art Therapy Association, 23*(4), 157–165.

Corr, C. A. (2002). Revisiting the concept of disenfranchised grief. In Doka, K. J. (Ed.), *Disenfranchised grief: New directions, challenges, and strategies for practice* (pp. 39–60). Champaign, IL: Research Press.

Currier, J. M., & Holland, J. M. (2012). Examining the role of combat loss among Vietnam war veterans. *Journal of Traumatic Stress, 25*, 102–105, doi: 10.1002/jts.21655

Doka, K. J. (2002). Introduction. In Doka, K. J. (Ed.), *Disenfranchised grief: New directions, challenges, and strategies for practice* (pp. 5–22). Champaign, IL: Research Press.

Gantt, L., & Tinnin, L.W. (2009). Support for a neurobiological view of trauma with implications for art therapy. *The Arts in Psychotherapy, 36*, 148–153, doi: 10.1016/j.aip.2008.12.005

Haeseler, M. P. (2002). In remembrance: September 11, 2001. *Art Therapy, 19*(3), 123–124, doi: 10.1080/07421656.2002.10129407

Hoge, C. W., Castro, C. A., Messer, S. C., McGurk, D., Cotting, D. I., & Koffman, R. L. (2004). Combat duty in Iraq and Afghanistan, mental health problems and barriers to care. *New England Journal of Medicine, 351*, 13–22.

Johnson, D. R. (2000). Creative therapies. In Foa, E., Keane, T., Friedman, M., & Cohen, A. (Eds.), *Effective treatments for PTSD: Practice guidelines form the international society for traumatic stress studies*. New York: The Guilford Press.

Keenan, M. J., Lumley, V. A., & Schneider, R. B. (2014). A group therapy approach to treating combat posttraumatic stress disorder: Interpersonal reconnection through letter writing. *Psychotherapy, 51*(4), 546–554, doi: 10.1037/a0036025

Kohut, M. (2011). Marking art from memories: Honoring deceased loved ones through a scrapbooking bereavement group. *Art Therapy: Journal of the American Art Therapy Association, 28*(3), 123–131, doi: 10.1080/07421656.2011.599731

National Intrepid Center of Excellence. (n.d.). *The NICoE Healing Arts Program*, retrieved from www.nicoe.capmed.mil/Shared%20Documents/Healing%20Arts%20Program(AEM)_Fact%20 Sheet%20FINAL2_2012%2006%2018.pdf

Ott, C. H. (2003). The impact of complicated grief on mental and physical health and various points in the bereavement progress. *Death Studies, 27*, 249–272, doi: 10.1080/07481180390137044

Reger, M. A., Etherage, J. R., Reger, G. M., & Gahm, G. A. (2008). Civilian psychologists in an Army culture: The ethical challenge of cultural competence. *Military Psychology, 20*, 21–35, doi: 10.1080/08995600701753144

Tanielian, T., Jaycox, L. H., Adamson, D. M., & Metscher, K. N. (2008). Introduction. In Tanielian, T. and Jaycox, L. H. (Eds.), *Invisible wounds of war: Psychological and cognitive injuries, their consequences, and services to assist recovery* (pp. 3–18). Santa Monica, CA: RAND Corporation.

Thornton, G., & Zanich, M. L. (2002). Empirical assessment of disenfranchised grief: 1989–2000. In Doka, K. J. (Ed.), *Disenfranchised grief: New directions, challenges, and strategies for practice* (pp. 79–89). Champaign, IL: Research Press.

Toblin, R. L., Riviere, L. A., Thomas, J. L., Adler, A. B., Kok, B. C., & Hoge, C.W. (2012). Grief and physical health outcomes in U.S. soldiers returning from combat, *Journal of Affective Disorders, 136,* 469–475, doi: 10.1016/j.jad.2011.10.048

U.S. Department of Defense. (2016). *Casualty.* Retrieved from www.defense.gov/casualty.pdf

U.S. Department of Veterans Affairs. (2016). *Veteran population.* Retrieved from www.va.gov/vetdata/veteran_population.asp

U.S. Government Accountability Office. (2011). *VA mental health: Number of veterans receiving care, barriers faced, and efforts to increase access* (GAO-12-12). Retrieved from www.gao.gov/assets/590/585743.pdf

Walker, M. S. (n.d.). *Art therapy programming at the National Intrepid Center of Excellence (NICoE).* Retrieved from www.arttherapy.org/upload/toolkitmedicalsettings/intrepedcenter.pdf

# 30  Feeling the Pulse

## An Art Therapist's Response to Tragedy

*Todd C. Stonnell*

Do you remember where you were when you received the news of the terrorist attacks in New York on September 11? When details of 9/11 began to emerge, I remember sitting in my tenth-grade history class, probably drifting off into some daydream, as usual; another student walked into the room and whispered to my teacher the details of the events that had just transpired; awestruck and tearful, my teacher repeated this information to us. A cold sensation of fear and confusion filled my body, as I immediately thought of my family and the harm that could befall them. I cried to my mother on the phone when I got home, praying someone would hurry to our house and ease my tension. Fast forward to June thirteenth, 2016. We find me sitting in a pew at an LGBTQ (Lesbian, Gay, Bisexual, Transgender, Queer/Questioning)-friendly church in Richmond, a rare occasion for me. On this day, something had pulled me into the building. A member of the congregation greeted everyone graciously and began to cry as she relayed the information of a shooting that had occurred in a gay nightclub in Orlando, Florida. I had not watched the news or read anything on social media before entering the church doors that morning, so I was completely oblivious to these details. I felt nauseated at the sheer fact that such an occurrence took place, but I also felt curious if it happened to be the same night club at which my friends and I had danced a few years back; my curiosity was confirmed when I received a text that read: "Did you hear about Pulse?"

Terrorism and acts of violence invite us to dig within ourselves to make sense of the world around us, as well as our place within it. Most of the time we are left with the pangs of sheer senselessness of these actions, as well as uncertainty of what to do with those feelings. What many of us lack, and may never achieve, is the complete understanding of what it meant for the victims of these tragedies, as well as those who were directly impacted in the aftermath of the event. We weren't there. We didn't have to worry about losing our lives in that moment or be forced to fight for our own survival or for that of a loved one. This lack of understanding is not our fault, but it does it does mean that we as outsiders are granted the privilege of distance; therefore, it may be easy to push these feelings aside or push them into something else. For many people this energy defaults to denial that the events even happened, choosing to place emphasis on conspiracy or rationalization, instead of the painful realities of loss; pair this with a fear that can spill over into generalizations of cultures and groups, leading to avoidance or hatred of those considered to be "other" than what is familiar. For others, the feelings of sadness and fear become so intense that they do not know what to do and they become stagnated in grief. With so many methods of reaction and response, what does this ultimately mean for me specifically as a caregiver? As a therapist, do I hold a specific responsibility to the community following such events? What is my role in all of this?

I start this exploration outside of the role of a therapist, beginning first as a student in high school, as described previously. With very little training or experience in empathy, nor the confidence or pull to action, my approach was very different at first. I will explore how these shifts in both my roles, as well as my identity, colored my experience in processing what was occurring. Take for instance the tragedies at Virginia Tech on April 16, 2007; on this day, a student at the Virginia Polytechnic Institute and State University in Blacksburg, Virginia shot and killed 32 of his classmates and teachers, wounding 17 others, before taking his own life. When this occurred, I was a sophomore in college, living on campus at Longwood University in Farmville, Virginia. I remember lying down onto my bed between classes, fully intending on taking a nap and naïve to the attacks that had just taken place. Only a few minutes after I rested my head upon my pillow, I received a text from a friend asking if I had heard about the events at Tech. It stood out to me because it felt extremely intimate, and I felt more vulnerable than I had as a high school student on 9/11; I kept hearing the phrase "it could have been me, it could have been someone I know and love."

The shootings at Sandy Hook Elementary in 2012 hit me in a more unique way. This tragedy took place in Newtown, Connecticut, in which a lone gunman entered Sandy Hook Elementary and opened fire into various hallways and classrooms; in total 28 people were killed, including 20 children. The mere mention of *children* being murdered in a school, an elementary school of all places, stirred my immediate concern for my then-six-year-old nephew. It was nearly impossible to wrap my brain around the possibility that someone could be driven to that extreme. By placing the image of my nephew into the context of this tragedy, I felt overwhelmed with grief for something that had not even transpired. I had a morbid image of him walking into his school and not coming back out. I could not let this happen! Again, I heard that fearful voice, but this time it asked: "What can I do about it?" However, this voice sounded slightly less shaky than it had before, because at this point, I was gaining more of an awareness that I could just maybe have a role in healing. During this time, I was interning at a residential school for youth who were struggling with emotional and behavioral issues. A few of the students would bring up the events of Sandy Hook in their individual sessions with me, and I noticed a varying level of concern, ranging from paralyzing fear to mild indifference. We spent time processing their emotions, and I attempted to nurture a sense of safety, as a few of them were afraid that something like that could happen there. I witnessed these kids work through some puzzling questions and seek a degree of resilience within themselves, which in turn empowered me to do the same.

Following the Pulse shootings in Orlando, Florida, a familiar sense of vulnerability swept over me; however, this time it felt strangely more personal. Much like the previous example at Sandy Hook, the shooter worked alone, entering the Pulse Nightclub, a local gay establishment in Orlando; he began to fill the rooms with gunfire, striking down over a hundred people. Ultimately 50 individuals lost their lives in this incident, representing a wide range of cultural backgrounds, especially people of color. I am a gay man who, for the most part, can keep this element of my identity to myself, and sometimes, it can feel prudent to do so. I have faced threats of violence while holding my boyfriend's hand, stared into the awe-struck eyes of those who seem confused by my attire, and I have been called "fag" on many, many occasions. I had danced in Pulse before, having the time of my life with my friends. It felt safe there—we were welcomed to dance and kiss and, hell, even dance upside down if we wanted. It was a place where the affection offered to someone of the same sex would not be regarded as an alien call to arms. It was a painful and agonizing reality that someone could invade this space of security and rip it to pieces.

This brings me to one of the most painful challenges that I find myself tackling in the wake of violence, which is the deeply complicated consideration of the goodness of people. Ever since I was a kid, I recall feeling a deeply rooted desire to stubbornly see the kindness in everyone, clinging to that candy-coated, technicolored version of the world. Through this lens, evil is easily spotted by the presence of green flames, pointy horns, a hellish laugh and maybe a wise-cracking minion for extra measure. This is always sharply contrasted by the valiant hero or heroine flying or teleporting in to save the day, representing all that is good. Sadly, good and evil do not come in such blatant and recognizable packages, evil instead taking on more insidiously good-natured disguises or just becoming easily ignored from a passive glance. It isn't until something terrible occurs that this mask of glitter melts away to reveal a more tarnished and cruel reality. Despite my awareness of this, I still long to be surprised, and I count on the universe to say, "Yes, Todd, evil can easily be spotted and vanquished, and it will never return. You were right all along." While I wait with anticipation for this message to arrive, I should instead seek and explore that gray area in between these two extremes. This has been further challenged through my experience as a therapist; I forge a more grounded approach to what both good and bad truly entail, especially when explored through the eyes of my clients.

My therapeutic approach is very strengths-based, and I currently offer art therapy services to people who are struggling with addiction. The diagnosis of addiction comes with its own layers of stigma, guilt, shame, and self-hatred. I join these patients in the middle of a story in which they think so lowly of themselves, a war waging within them, with little hope that they will find personal victory over their inner villains. I have heard stories from my patients that have shaken me to the core, but I have never fully wavered in my hope for the goodness in these individuals. Together we explore their strengths, passions, and further reconnect to their values. What this has instilled in me is a mindset that maybe there are no good people and bad people, only people who do good things and bad things. It is this message that I hope to pass to my clients, hoping that they can find the goodness within, nurturing, and empowering this side of themselves to truly change their paths. It is through this that perhaps they can create a schism between their authentic identities and the maladaptive behaviors that have defined them in the past.

It is when this work is placed within the context of terrorism and violence that it becomes complicated for me. All of this learning and clarity in goodness and badness can become skewed as if on a television screen with poor reception. If not completely faltered, there are parts of me that become agitated in response to events on the news. Take for instance the Pulse shootings. As mentioned earlier, this tragedy struck the part of me connected to the LGBTQ community. Because of this, I became more sensitive to other communities from which homosexuality is judged and condemned. The sensitivity I experienced at that time made me hypervigilant towards comments made by clients that hinted at a similar mindset. At the time this had the potential to color my experience with these individuals, either closing me off to the work we did together, or driving the energy to instill a message that, despite my differences with them, our work could still be productive. We could both grow from this experience. I had to and continue to view the therapeutic work as an avenue for greater change, rippling outward through our small interactions. These intimate moments grant minor changes at a time, paving a path through judgment, and potentially they may spark further shifts beyond the art therapy studio.

Reflecting further on Pulse in particular, I want to further consider its place in deeper shifts in my therapeutic and personal work. Pulse coincided with my own journey toward finding my voice and an ongoing fight with my inner critic, who had become overwhelming and distracting. I was experiencing a frustrating period of insecurity, and felt like the

*Little Mermaid*, a siren princess left voiceless in a world she didn't understand; I yearned to be heard, yet was not aware of what I wanted to say. I ultimately asked my patients how they felt about the events in Orlando, a seemingly desperate and selfish attempt to process my rawness with them. I supported my actions by considering my audience, which was made up of people whose professions also placed them in caregiving roles; they must also be struggling with this, right? I recognized the wounded caregiver inside of myself, possibly craving some validation and support from the patients. By realizing this, I knew that I was seeking something that they would not be able to provide, nor should they be expected to. I had to pull myself back to reality and do what I ask the patients to do every day: explore and nurture new resources for healing and growth.

Right around this time, a local LGBTQ advocacy group held a vigil in honor of those affected by the Pulse shootings. What really stood out to me about this was the sheer number of people who showed up; the chairs offered inside were completely full, and the crowd overflowed into the parking lot behind the building. There had to be hundreds of people around me. I was overwhelmed with emotion. Following the vigil, I went home and created some artwork—something I may have benefited from much earlier. The art I created was meant to reflect on the event and capture my feelings into something more tangible. I picked up some oil pastels and began to apply color to the paper. I began with red, faded into orange and continued moving along the spectrum of a rainbow. I wanted to trace the course of the events that had transpired, and what I hoped for the community to which I belong. I wanted to imagine the viewer looking at a heart rate monitor and watching the peaks and valleys form along the screen. The line began as relatively even paced, moving steadily up and down. The pulse began to quicken, capturing the fear and uncertainty that the victims may have experienced during the debacle. This line began to dip downward and flatline; this was how I felt the perpetrator, as well as many others wanted us to feel: broken, lifeless, powerless. The line rocketed upward, an illustration of the energy to overcome the tragedy and to fuel the fire within each of us to come together and seek change. I enveloped the image in yellow and red flames to represent the phoenix-like rebirth and fierceness that I hoped would be sparked into action by the LGBTQ community, especially people of color, as well as any others who suffered from this event or any event like it.

Upon completion of this piece (Figure 30.1), I quickly realized that it simply was not enough to focus the already-gathering energy inside of me. I felt more pulled towards initiating connection with other people in a way that was empowering, offering a truly safe space, reclaiming this feeling that was stolen from the community that night. Truth be told, I did not feel safe. I took this time to process my own feelings of safety, recognizing the need to resolve this if I wanted to stand as an example of safety for others. As a therapist, this is one of our main responsibilities: to provide a safe place for exploration and discovery. I realized that maybe I would need to create a space like this with the sole purpose of reclaiming this sense of security and pass it along from there.

I reached out to my friend and colleague about my hope to organize an event for the community. We agreed to create Prayer Flags, on which participants could express a wish or a hope, either focused on the victims of Pulse, or for the greater population. These Prayer Flags drew inspiration from a practice hailing from the Tibetan, Chinese, Persian, and Indian cultures, in which multi-colored flags (each representing a different element) are adorned with Buddhist prayers, mantras, and symbols of peace and power. The movements of the flags are meant to harmonize with the wind and earth to send the messages scribed on the fabric into the world. We decided to personalize the approach for our flags to give them the space to reflect on their own feelings, their own hopes for the future, while being surrounded by support. This would eventually lead to a collective piece as we

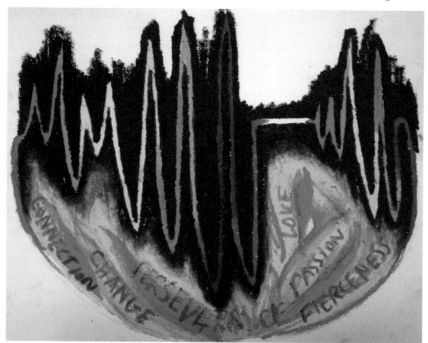

*Figure 30.1* Quickening Pulse, by Todd C. Stonnell

would hang the flags together on a string, with hopes that the wind would catch these feelings and carry them to where they could be absorbed by someone who may need them.

What followed was a quick week of preparation and a gathering of supplies. I bought some fabric and collected other scraps that I had hoarded over time, leftovers from projects of the past. My colleague and I also wanted to offer thread, paints, and markers for further embellishments. We decided to hold the event in a local park to take advantage of the beautiful weather and nurture the sense of openness that I hoped would be conveyed through the process. However, a barrage of catastrophic thoughts began to enter my mind, causing me to waver in my attempts in spreading the word about the event. I wondered how far-reaching I really wanted to event to be. I questioned if I should make a completely public event page on Facebook? Should I make flyers? Or should I mainly invite people I know, and let the word spread from there? My work with patients takes place very privately and safely within a secure residential facility; this allows for a high degree of control of most situations, especially the intervention of any outside intolerance or cruelty. In an awkward transition to public activism, I feared that if left too open to the public, that I may be putting the group in harm's way, again considering the extreme actions of others. I felt silly and, to be honest, I felt angry that I even had this thought at all. Why should I be nervous of violence occurring at an art making event in the park? Shortly after, I wondered if it was really that unfounded. I wanted to protect those who may attend this event, and I was not willing to risk their safety at all. I ultimately kept the event rather small scale, sharing it on the Facebook pages LGBTQ organizations in the Richmond area.

On the day of the event, my colleague and I met and took note of all the materials that we would provide to the participants. We arrived at the park and arranged everything in a manner that would be easily accessible to everyone. In a wonderful moment of serendipity, the same LGBTQ-friendly church mentioned in the opening of this chapter was holding their Sunday service in a shelter just a short stroll away from our picnic table. I shyly approached the group following their service and asked to make an announcement regarding our event next door. One of the members of the congregation enthusiastically greeted me and called out to the rest of the group for me to pass along my invitation.

People slowly began to trickle into our work area, and I offered instructions as they gathered. At this point, about two people had joined our intimate group, and they had already begun to dig into the collection of buttons, fabric scraps, thread, and other assorted materials that were scattered along both the table and onto blankets on the ground. We were maybe overprepared, either expecting a large group of people to arrive, or possibly only two or three. Either way, I expected the event to be successful. Slowly but surely more people began to join in, eventually filling our picnic table. It remained relatively intimate throughout the few hours, and participants remained present for most of the time allotted. A few of those who arrived were friends of mine, including some old friends who I had not seen in ages. Others were complete strangers, who heard of the event through word of mouth. I was thankful to see members of the nearby congregation drift over to us, mainly to offer a donation, but we did have some individuals join in the art making. Some members of the group appeared timid at first, putting most of their attention into the work, but I noticed a shift in the energy midway, and people began to be more interactive, sharing personal details and stories.

Once everyone settled into their spaces and began working on their own flags, I decided to join in on the process. For the duration of the event, I reflected on the words that my neighbor had offered me, following a brief and spontaneous interaction. Her words: "Love harder, hug more" echoed in my mind over and over. The meeting began as a random knock on my door, followed by her expression of support and condolences; she then hugged me as tightly as her frail frame could muster before parting. With this memory fresh on my mind, I placed a blue scrap of fabric onto the cotton and cut out large, purple letters: L, V, E, H, U, and G. I sorted through the buttons and pulled out the largest one that I could find to be an O. I organized the letters and buttons onto the fabric to spell out the words LOVE and HUG; underneath these I wrote the words: *harder* and *tighter.* "Love harder, Hug tighter." These words drifted in and out of my thoughts all day in the shaky voice of my neighbor, like the emotional closing lines of a Disney movie. This phrase reminded me of things that I take for granted much of the time. I thought about moments when I could be more affectionate with my significant other, times when I could express my love to my friends and family way more than I do, as well as new methods to do so. I added a collection of rainbow-colored ribbon as an attempt to add more movement to the flag; I wanted to capture and spread the energy that I hoped would fuel our healing. After the glue had time to dry, I held up my flag to check in on my progress. It was wonderful to see the ribbon flutter in response to the wind, a joyful and poignant ballet of colors (Figure 30.2). As someone who finds great strength from nature, it was more moving for me to see wind, one of nature's most powerful forces, send my message beyond the blanket on which I sat.

I looked up from my work many times, and I eavesdropped on the musings and interactions within the group and watched as everyone added to their creations. The timidity that I witnessed earlier had nearly dissipated completely, and people began to speak more about the work they were creating. They were all very curious about one another's pieces and asked several questions regarding the choices they made.

The flags varied in their content, ranging from completely abstract, with different patterned fabric beautifully arranged together, to flags including images and words of hope and growth. Despite the seemingly central focus of the exercise, several themes emerged among the various pieces. I noticed a theme of personal and collective empowerment, a refusal to remain "broken" (Figure 30.3); instead the artists seem to be acknowledging and embracing their own strength, as well as hope that others would find and nurture their own. Some participants included images of union and love, specifically illustrated by a linked chain of human figures, while another featured a cutout of the state of Florida surrounded by a rainbow of colors; the artist wrote the statement "Love is love is love is love" next to the cutout. In both flags, I noticed elements of protection or security, as the cutout people appeared to be forming a barrier, standing as one and ready to face anything together. Also, the rainbow around the image of Florida appeared almost as a collective, unified shield for the inhabitants of the state, or perhaps it was an aura of hope to fend off threats of hatred.

Following our art making and discussion, we welcomed the participants to pin their flags onto a ribbon that my colleague attached between two trees. Placed side by side, the flags fit almost perfectly on the length of the ribbon. We watched as the flags danced with the wind, and I shared my observations with the group. We took some time to quietly reflect on our process and watch the movement of their pieces together. It was in this moment that I remembered what my goal for this project really was. This was indeed a time for people to gather in this safe, warm environment not just to express how they were feeling, but also to empower them to do something with these feelings. It was not a time simply to mourn and grieve—it was a time granted to them to be with strangers and friends alike, and remember that they are not alone in this. It was important for me to emphasize this power of connection, illustrated in this resulting creation, made up of their unique and strong pieces now moving into action. The image of movement and progression can be incredibly motivating, especially when we feel stagnated; when paired with the messages of hope, love, and resilience as illustrated on these flags, we had created

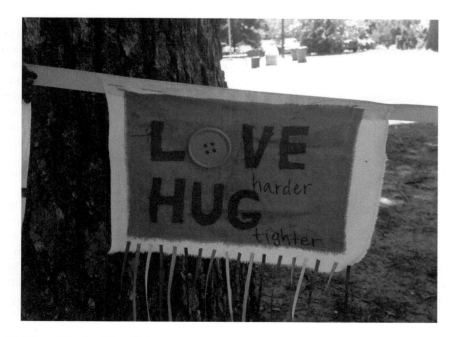

*Figure 30.2* Love Harder, Hug Tighter, by Todd C. Stonnell

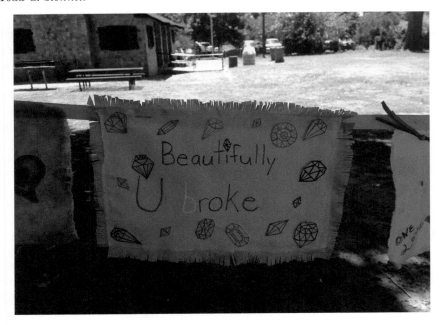

*Figure 30.3* Beautifully Unbroken, by Workshop Participant

something that, even if we were the only ones that saw it, had the power to celebrate life and honor that time together.

In reflecting on the progression from each of these events, I notice a shift in how I process both their wide-ranging consequences, as well as my place in context to them. During 9/11 I was a teenager, and I mostly experienced fear and confusion in response; my understanding of the world was becoming more open, but I was mainly focused on the angst-laden horizon right in front of me. By the time the Virginia Tech tragedy occurred, I found more of a place among the college community, so this event seemed more real to me and more intimate. When paired with the concern for my friends, I remember this striking deeper within me and pushing me to emphasize the importance of my bonds with them. Sandy Hook was similar, but instead, it felt like my nephew, someone so completely vulnerable, yet the least likely target for violence, could be in some way taken away from me. A more realized activist spirit had awoken in response, but I don't think I quite knew what I could reasonably do, other than express my love and affection to my nephew and keep him safe in any way I could. This brings us to Pulse, by which time I was prepared to act; I was fed up with these things I was seeing going on in the world.

The perspective I offer in this chapter is that of someone still learning about himself, especially in relation to a world that, despite many amazing shifts and changes, still contains glaring examples of hate and violence. I continue to explore the role of a caregiver following trauma and violence, recognizing the importance for self-nurturance and kindness before this care can be directed outward. I feel that it is easy for caregivers to become energized during times of great tragedy and sadness. We want to encourage those in need, as well as empower them to move forward, and perhaps they gain the ability to provide this for others. I also think that it is natural for this energy to become overwhelming, even transforming into a feeling of helplessness as we absorb the scope and depth of the wounds in the community. As I have stepped more fully into the role of a therapist,

I cannot say that this has completely transformed one hundred percent; I don't run into a phone booth and run out with hands full of colored pencils or tubes of paint, prepared to save the world. I do, however have enough awareness to know that despite my limits, I possess strengths that may serve to offer safety and comfort for others. This begins with sorting out my own feelings, acknowledging the pain, the stigma, as well as taking notice of any bias that may have been stirred up from the news. Building upon this theme, I feel my art therapy approach reflects a personal revitalization and reflects what power this resurgence can offer. Such simple gestures can have the same, if not greater effect as those that serve to save the world in one fell swoop. When we have these shorter, more intimate moments, the hope is that they take what they experienced, renewed, and energized themselves, then pass that along. This passing of power has the potential to ripple into a more formidable force, strengthening individual voices to join in on the chorus for change. This is my wish to those either finding their way into a caregiving role, or trying to simply be kind to themselves: explore the voice you possess, listen to its fears, let others hear what it has to say; through this connection both within ourselves and without, great change is possible, even in the wake of great tragedy.

## Acknowledgement

All artwork shown here was made for public display, and all participants were made aware of this prior to the start of the workshop. Figure 30.1 and Figure 30.2 are my own.

# 31 Communitas and Soul-Healing

## Arts Therapy Within the Loss-upon-Loss of Natural Disaster

*Deborah Green*

*It's 2011. Earthquakes are riding rampant through Lyttelton, my hometown on New Zealand's South Island. As I'm grappling to provide arts therapy within this context of loss-upon-loss, this memory from 2006 nudges for attention . . .*

*I'm in my garden—well, less garden and more untamed dancing green wilderness—attempting to impose some order on how this lushness encroaches on our weathered cedar-pole house. I've music filling my body through headphones and am shiny in the thick summer sun as I pull weeds, cut back vines and tend my illicit arum lilies stolen from a neighbour's verge. I float adrift in a wash of sensation, when suddenly my sea-anchor is snared by a song. 'The Sound of White' by Missy Higgins feels like it's directed to someone not present . . .*

*. . . and I suddenly I'm thinking of m, my dead husband . . .*

*. . . I'm talking to my dead husband . . .*

*Not aloud. Quietly. Internally. And this seems natural, alive, connected. As I open myself to this, I feel something touch me, briefly, warmly, calmly.*

*Just a simple sense of: 'I'm here'.*

*I don't jerk away. I don't question. I simply accept and keep talking. My face is wet and I'm sitting in the rich dark soil with my muddy hands limp, open, palms-up in my lap. The conversation continues. I tell m how sad I am about his suicide, how angry, how sorry and regretful, how much I miss him, how grateful I am that he's dead, how confused this makes me, how I wish I could've done things so differently.*

*Again, I feel the fleeting but deep brush of connection without judgment: 'I know'.*

*I spend the afternoon in the garden, Sebastian and Lilu swirling about my feet, climbing tree ferns, calling low Siamese-meows to me through the purple haze between the leaves. I taste the bitter edges of sceptical-me attempting to infiltrate the warm mix and I ask her to wait, allowing myself to linger within this golden moment. I extend the conversation to include my dead mother, calling her in and feeling her arrive. Again, I well with tears and layered feelings. Dad's presence causes less conflict and more regret as my relationship with him was simpler, more about missed opportunities than warring senses.*

These tussles with my own losses and reconnections have formed a living spine running through what I call my 'quake-arts therapy' practice. Let me paint you a picture of the context that birthed this practice: In the dark-before-dawn of 4 September 2010, an earthquake measuring magnitude 7.1 on the Richter scale thundered through the province of Canterbury, New Zealand. Viewed as a miracle quake, this tremor did substantial damage but killed no-one. On 22 February 2011, just after midday a magnitude 6.3 aftershock struck. This time Christchurch city, only 10 km from the shallow quake epicentre near Lyttelton, was vigorously shaken. One hundred and eighty-five people lost their lives and almost 7000 suffered injuries—at least 280 were treated for major trauma at Christchurch Hospital. Massive damage was done to buildings, roads, the infrastructure and surrounding hills. I was in the city during this quake, in a building that was badly damaged. I emerged into dust and distress to join the stream of quake-shaken people trying to get home—which for me meant a steeply treacherous slog on foot over the Port Hills to Lyttelton, Christchurch's Harbour-town.

A swarm of large aftershocks followed this February quake. In June 2011, a 6.4 aftershock struck and another rated 6 in December 2011 causing further damage and dismay. Most recently, in November 2016, a quake measuring 7.8 caused massive landslips and gouged open our sense of terror. Since September 2010, approximately 11,000 detectable aftershocks (more than 670 measuring magnitude 4 and over) have rattled the region, in excess of 1300 public buildings and 7000 residential homes have either already been or need to be demolished, and economists have estimated it will cost over $40 billion and will take New Zealand between 50 to 100 years to recover (Canterbury Quake Live, 2017; McSaveney, 2014).

As the only registered arts therapist within the city, I felt a grave responsibility to provide arts therapy for my fellow quake-shaken Cantabrians. This work was particularly challenging however because, like my clients, I too was struggling as a result of the quakes: I was working from a shed in my garden because my work-studio in town was earthquake damaged; like many of my clients, the circumstances awoke earlier woundedness in me; and I was working largely in a small town of which I am a known resident. As I write these obstacles baldly in black and white, I again wonder how and why I didn't simply fold my hands and allow others to provide therapy. . . . And yet, in this sentence lies part of the answer. Who were these 'others'? Yes, there were many lovely words of encouragement from around the world and some generous souls briefly visited us to run a session or two. The need was, however, too great and the time frame too large. And so, within these ongoing extenuating circumstances, we locals looked after each other. The saying coined by

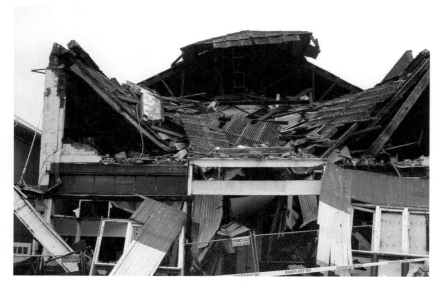

*Figure 31.1* Lyttelton Quake Damage (Green, February 2011)

Arthur Ashe encapsulates our response: "We started where we were, we used what we had and we did what we could." Those with extra water left filled bottles on the sidewalk; those with food shared with those who were hungry; the fit and strong righted fallen furniture and shored up teetering chimneys for the frail; those with space offered bed and board to those whose homes were uninhabitable. Creative artists also took to the streets, filling vacant lots post-demolition with dancefloors, gardens, performance-stages; painting huge brightly coloured murals on evacuated buildings; transforming broken shards into glorious public mosaics; placing row-upon-row of white chairs to commemorate those the quakes claimed.

I contributed what I could by journeying with groups and individual clients of all ages as we used multi-modal creative processes to express, explore and endure. Within three weeks of the devastating February quake, I began work with over 300 primary school pupils by conducting 'My Favourite Place' group workshops in Lyttelton Harbour area schools (Green, 2012). This led to my participation in developing the theatre piece 'Tremor' and I facilitated the postcard creation initiative, 'We are not alone/You are not alone', between Lyttelton West School and various quake- and tsunami-affected Japanese groups.

I established 'The eARThquake Therapy Initiative' to raise funds for arts therapy provision and my work expanded to include group sessions with several organisations including the Salvation Army, Women's Centre, Refugee Support, Christchurch Anxiety Support and the New Zealand Association of Counsellors. I worked with groups of teenagers battling cancer, trainee General Practitioners (GPs), and counsellors and care-workers who were struggling to cope. I was especially honoured to run a creative process with the staff of Relationships Aotearoa who had been in the CTV building when it collapsed, claiming 115 lives.

Whenever I facilitated one-off group-sessions, I offered ongoing individual therapy for those requiring further care. Several families accepted my offer using funds from the Lions Charitable Trust; I received funded referrals from the Salvation Army, Canteen and several GPs and I saw clients for free or raised funds to cover costs through the Lyttelton

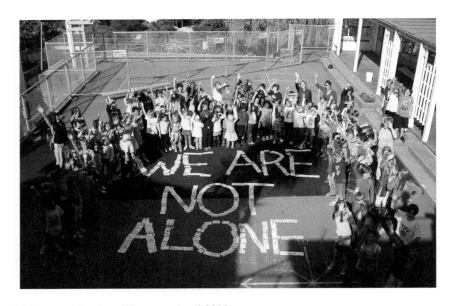

*Figure 31.2* Postcard Project (Herman, April 2011)

Saturday Garage Sale. I also accepted a year-long contract with the Canterbury District Health Board (CDHB) to work with earthquake-affected children.

Under this umbrella of quake-arts therapy, my work that focussed specifically on grief generally took two forms: for some clients (and me), the quakes wrenched open past sorrows; for others, the quakes grated alongside new non-quake losses . . . all further complicated by our broader quake context of loss-upon-loss: familiar places, homes, routines, schools/places-of-work were gone; friends and family moved away, neighbourhoods, relationships and marriages fragmented; and many lost a sense of inner trust and safety, their belief in their own capacity to respond and endure shaken and torn.

> *She uses her tangy-dark sense of humour to engage me . . . and to slide away from the grief bringing her through my door. Today, however, this grief will not be silenced. In front of her is an engorged page-hogging blue teardrop, bulging and distended, suspended breathlessly, painfully, precariously above a row of black jagged saw-toothed rocks . . . rocks that shout to their fellow razor-edged boulders that exploded free from the crags above Lyttelton and thundered down into people and homes below.*
>
> *She pulls back from this demanding image. It's caught her by surprise, travelling down her arms and through her hands onto the page. This tremulous tear fills both of us, pushing the air from our lungs and crushing our guts. She elaborates: the teardrop smells of wax and burning rubber; it wails high and thin like a power-cable taking unbearable strain; it's raw meat in the back of her throat; on her skin, it's a heat-rash; she enacts its movement as a knee-bending back-bowing weight. I know she's nudging towards making a joke to again scamper from this deep pain . . .*
>
> *. . . and I gently nudge back—inviting her to trust the safety of this space, of our relationship, of the arts that don't come to harm her—and to stay present. To be curious and gentle with this big soft-bellied tear.*

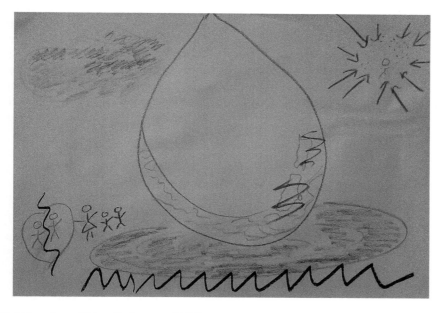

*Figure 31.3* Teardrop (Client-L, January 2012)

*So, we sit and breathe and let the tear be seen and heard and companioned. And I ask, 'What's this tear most afraid of?' 'That when it breaks, it'll never stop, it'll cry and cry and cry,' and her voice cracks and the real tears begin.*

*Finally.*

*We sit. She sobs deeply, wrenchingly, her whole body arched in agony, her breath jerking in wracking shudders. I wait, present with her, holding the space, breathing deeply into her sorrow, tears warm on my own cheeks. I quietly shift my chair and gently place my shoulder against hers. I'm not restraining, I'm being with. She leans towards me and cries on, but now her breath flows more easily—the wretched tightness, the gasping, the stuttering, is smoothing into loose fluid sadness.*

*Her dad is gone. Suddenly and unexpectedly. And she can't be there with her mother and brother, so far away, to share, to process, to remember and grieve. She has to be here, battling the quake-aftermath, keeping it together, working, caring for her young family, making school lunches and giving soothing bedtimes kisses to small souls rattled by midnight aftershocks.*

*As she quietens, we look down at her chalk image. Her tears have blurred the jagged line of hungry rocks into rounded pebbles. So, now we speak different words, words of wonder that she cried and cried and cried . . . and then she stopped.*

*I know our journey has truly begun when she says: 'Maybe now I can let go and cry and believe the agony can wash through me like a tide and I won't break on the rocks below'.*

This layering of loss, grief and instability has led me to call our quake-context 'enduring liminality' (Green, 2016). Anthropologist Victor Turner (1969) coined 'liminality' to describe the central mutable stage of ritual he discovered when studying tribal rites-of-passage in Africa (incidentally my birth-continent). Liminality is bounded by a separation from normalcy on one side and a hoped-for re-incorporation into a new normalcy at the other. This transitional betwixt-and-betweenness acts as a fertile metaphor to illuminate the disruptions of the earthquakes, the complex losses they directly caused and indirectly evoked, as well as the potentially transformative process of therapy. This liminal lens reveals relevant characteristics that help unravel my quake-arts therapy. Liminality casts me as both neophyte and shaman accompanying my clients as we journey through the uncertainties and possibilities opened by the quakes. Liminality is multiplicit—just as there is no single route through liminality, "[t]here is no single way to grieve and no single definition of 'normal' grief" (Hart, 2012, p. 145). And, especially relevant to those for whom grieving became a central feature of our quake healing—liminality emphasises *soul* and evokes *communitas* (E. Turner, 2004). In this chapter, I use arts- and fiction-based research processes (McNiff, 2013; Leavy, 2013), to re-imagine therapeutic moments as a way to ponder the crucial roles played by soul and communitas within my quake-arts therapy grief work.

## Liminality and Soul

*When evening begins to haze the trees and vines and ferns and the Morepork-owls start to shuffle and hoot from the deepening shadows, I move inside to the yellow-light. Tiredness settles in and my resolve against unpicking this numinous afternoon of connection with my loved and lost ones weakens.*

*In stalks my analytical mind.*

*Yet something's shifted. Rather than a pitched battle, the afternoon-sun-séance-softened-me sits down with the intellect-armoured-me for a deep conference.*

> *The self that needs reasons-and-evidence puts forward a rush of arguments against the sensations and events that unfolded this day. My sacred-circle-dancing-self offers her insights. Both listen. Other parts of me emerge tentatively from the shadows within and join the discussion, slowly growing in trust that they won't be shouted down or shamed.*
>
> *The listening is deep.*
>
> *I begin to know a new way of being with myself, with the many bits that make up me. Parts of me truly believe this afternoon I communed with the guiding-spirits of my lost ones. Other parts think I'm succumbing to myth and marketing. Yet other bits decide my imagination calls my dead mother, father and husband into being and this honours their memory and my need for these relationships to continue. All of these differing views sit with each other.*
>
> *The jostling, finger-pointing, tongue-pulling, one-upmanship of my previous way-of-being is absent. I experience soulful internal* communitas *and am allowed to be all of these without having to choose only one stance, self or belief.*
>
> *I find peace for the first time in a long time. It's not a permanent state-of-being, but I can now sometimes find my way there when needed by remembering to appreciate there are places within us all and spaces between us that we may not reach through intellect, spaces-and-places that spirit and soul may be better suited to illuminating through the arts. In talking to those on the other side, I offer myself the suggestion that this isn't all, there is more, that the small scurryings that make up my life and the lives of many I work with are just that, small scratchings on the face of a larger tale that has a rhythm of its own. These conversations aren't held in the absence of the selves that deride and scoff—these nay-sayers are called into presence alongside the ghosts of my mother and father and husband.*
>
> *This opens me to my Circle-of-Self, to listening intently for all voices and ideas and opinions, to calling into the shadows, to being patient, to loving even the most prickly and poisonous parts of myself and my clients.*

Liminality evokes the "medium in which we all live that is permeable from person to person" (E. Turner, 2004, p. 99). Therapeutic processes that take place within enduring liminality thus call for an approach that leans into this connective permeability and attends to soul-wounds. But what does this word 'soul' mean and how did my quake-arts therapy become soul-based? Mid-2011, in the thick of my burgeoning quake-work, my grapple to locate my arts therapy practice was at its zenith. With the clarity of hindsight, I now characterise this as a false dichotomy between my soul and my intellect which caused a struggle between my embrace of the arts' creative mystery and my felt-obligation to follow medicalised trauma theories framed by psychology and neurobiology. I'd internalised how these science-based and soul-based orientations are often set in opposition, creating a tension that radiates throughout the profession of arts therapy (McNiff, 1998). In my therapeutic practice, this emerged as friction between the cognitively focussed, discursive, analytical and pre-planned processes I felt I should be implementing and the way I was actually employing an innately playful, non-directive approach to honour the pre-verbal embodied distress expressed by my clients.

I grasped this nettle in supervision and experienced a sense of homecoming. I reconnected with Hillman (1983); McNiff (2004); and Halprin (2003), all of whom privilege creative soul-making. I followed suit and, without rejecting the science-based approach, I invited it to become the chorus and re/placed soul-building through imaginative poiesis centre-stage within my therapeutic practice. In addition, I steadily became aware that my early exposure to evangelical Christianity, then traditional Zulu and Xhosa spirituality and now to Māori worldviews, had shaped a wide-open attitude to soul. Traditional Western belief systems grounded in Christianity tend to view the soul as the central singular essence of each individual. These individuals are fundamentally whole creatures who inhabit an ordered world. Through this lens, traumatic events and losses fragment this world and the beings within it, suggesting therapy should be about restoring order. My sense-of-soul takes flight beyond this. I embrace Stephen Levine's (2009) view of humans as intrinsically multiplicit and contradictory—calling for a bereavement-therapy that focuses on a sense-of-soul which may not respond well to linear and/or reductive processes that impose order. Conceptions of soul that infuse my work are inclusive, resonant with Gendlin's (1997) characterisation of humans as an 'ever open edge'—a large, numinous-self extending beyond the biological brain which is merely the substratum or filter that allows this more-than self to encounter the world. Through this lens, soul becomes a gestalt, a halo forging connections between and radiating out beyond mind/body/affect (Gendlin, 1997). Soul resonates with concepts of life force, the energy that courses through all things—what the Eastern philosophies call 'chi' (McNiff, 2004); the Māori call 'mauri' (NZETC, 2016); and French philosopher Bergson coined as 'élan vital' (Merriam-Webster, 2017). Framed in this post-postmodern way, soul may be eternal or merely temporal; collective/universal or purely individual; religious, secular or experientially derived; capable of wholeness or intrinsically fragmented; or it may be all of these entwined in complex both-and-*and* ways that thoughts and words can't fully capture.

Soul-building therapy thus becomes firstly a quest to discover how soul is characterised for each individual client. This then informs the grief-healing that follows. This healing may not be about chugging through predictable stages, or about attempts to return to a former (possibly delusional) wholeness. "There are no set stages or tasks that need to be worked through or accomplished. We merely need to live the experience" (Rogers, 2011, p. 21). Healing for grieving souls invites creative bespoke processes, involving expression and connection, to re/build emotional limberness and loss-embracing growth.

*His mother is angry with me. She sits stiffly at the studio table while he's wretchedly hunched between us. Up until now he's been the angry one, brought to me to 'help him deal with his unreasonable rages'. Together we've indulged in what I've come to call 'imagical play', inviting the imaginative magic of unfettered imagery to help us find new ways to be with his rage—we've created wild scribbles and flung clay and done stamping-dances to express the unnamed fury; and we've blown bubbles and hummed and used watercolours to invite calm. And finally, during the previous session, several of his creations—in which parts where scratched out or left inexplicably blank—were gifted with meaning: He mentioned his Nana's death. He spoke in a whisper, afraid I'd chastise him. I gently queried this—he disclosed he'd been told not to dwell on it, that it was better to just move on.*

*He turned a pale freckled face to me, 'But I can't. I loved her and I miss her.'*

*Wow.*

*So, he told me all about her. He then chose colours and I poured small mounds of salt onto white pages. He steadily ground a coloured chalk pastel into each salt-mound. At first his jerky movements created teeth-gritting grating crunching that felt like anger. But he steadily slowed into fluid circular rhythms as the colours infused the salt. Into a small glass bottle, he poured pink for her humour, yellow for her smartness and green for her generosity. He held this to the light and we sat quietly. He then described the windowsill in his bedroom where this memory-bottle will live. He finished our time by creating a song asking her to always be with him. He left smiling.*

*I felt pleased with us.*

*But not for long. His mother emailed, enraged that I'd 'reopened the wounds', that we were just 'messing about with arty-farty stuff' when I should be teaching him 'anger-management strategies'.*

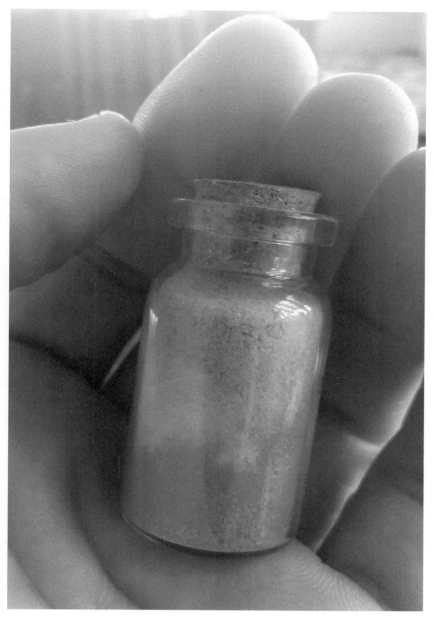

*Figure 31.4* Memory-bottle; Reconstruction (Green, July 2017)

*Now we sit together. Breathing deeply, I invite my inner prickly sensations of naughty-school-girl-hauled-before-the-headmistress to release their grip on my chest. I ask, and she tells. When her words run dry, I reflect back her belief that thinking and talking about Nana makes the pain linger. 'I wonder if maybe, just maybe, different people have different ways of being with loss,' I suggest. 'For some, moving swiftly on works. For others, this feels like the person they loved has been wiped out, erased, deleted. They need to express their love and loss—and sometimes this is easier through art.'*

*We both see his eyes fill with tears at the truth of this for him. Her eyes well too and she reaches gently for his hand.*

A core intent of this soul-focus during the quakes was emotional limberness. I use the term 'limberness' in preference to the more accepted word 'regulation' which, to my ear, evokes regimentation and does not embrace the fluid organicity of my process. I also rather like the idea that limberness helps us to endure liminality. Healthy souls are limber—they can respond intentionally to strong feelings without seizing reactive control. This proactive flexibility enables us to engage and withdraw as required for growth and defence (Kass & Trantham, 2014). Those who haven't experienced early secure attachment and/or have experienced traumatic loss may have this ability to self-compose compromised. Wounded souls often struggle with emotional shifts, imagination is injured and limberness stutters. Fortunately, adults and children can re/cultivate earned internal composure and soul-wellbeing (Seigel, 1999). A soul-focussed relationship-based therapeutic process can help clients become limber enough to ride the emotional teeter-totters triggered by their grapples with grief.

*She's a small, wild-haired personification of chaos. Each session she dashes to the arts materials and, gathering armfuls of paints/pipe cleaners/collage/glitter/coloured clay, she erupts into unfettered explosive creation. Then she dances/stories/sings/enacts these into vibrant life, enrolling me in ingenious ways. Her mum tells me that our un-boundaried play helps her—she's generally calmer, more able to self-soothe and the shrieking nightmares don't grip every night as they used to.*

*But I feel something else is thrumming for attention . . .*

*Today she's at her most feral yet and sand from the tray is flying. Tracking what this evokes in my being, I feel into myself and encounter the scurrying-ants of my own anxiety and inadequacy. I gently nudge these aside . . . and there it is: sorrow, deep blue with sharp silver prickles. As she pauses dramatically, hands full of sand raised above the tray, I seize my moment, 'I've this strange feeling in my heart . . .'*

*She freezes, slippy sand softly trickling through her little fingers.*

*I feel so sad, my heart's crying . . . I wonder if your heart feels this too?*

*The room is so quiet, so very very quiet. Her spine tightens. Her hands grip. Then she drops the sand and turns to me a little face crumpled by anguish.*

*Her story comes in sobs. I make this sense of it: Grandad died last year. She didn't really get it but saw all the adults pretending everything was okay. But yesterday her old dog was taken to the vet and didn't come home. She suddenly knows about death and the not-coming-backness of it all. She's deeply sad . . . and deeply worried for them. Are they scared and lonely?*

*I wonder aloud if she'd like to make some art to help them feel safer. From clay, we craft Grandad and Kessa. She gifts them with feathery soul-wings. Then we build them a glorious multicoloured and glittery 'spirit house' which she equips with food, water and soft beds. She sweetly sings them a lullaby and I'm filled with tears. We hold hands quietly for a while. I've never seen her so still. I've never felt her so deeply.*

Creative processes that involved mindful-flow seemed to help clients re/cultivate their emotional limberness. The healing state of focussed-absorption called 'flow' by Csikszentmihalyi (1990) can be reached through mindfulness—the "direct, pre-symbolic experience of the lived moment" (Avstreih, 2014, p. 186). Mindful practices encourage the artist/client/therapist to allow the image to emerge rather than attempting a predetermined outcome. This invites inner states to be externalised and explored, providing access to the eye—the part of us that can observe the storm as it is. This inner space may become known

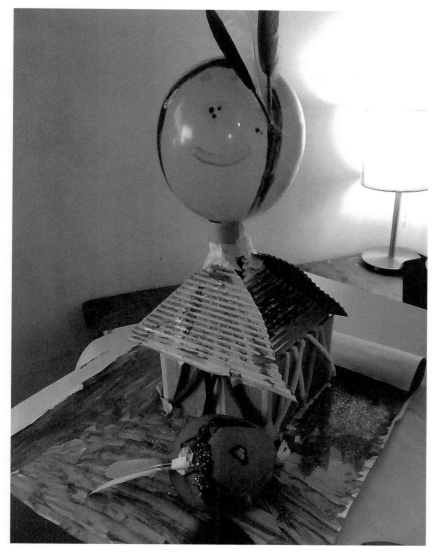

*Figure 31.5* Spirit House (Client-M, July 2011)

as a secure nourishing home (Avstreih, 2014; Rappaport, 2014a) and befriending this inner-witness facilitates the simultaneous ability to be within and outside the experience.

> *I'm intrigued by a symbol created by several clients. These clients didn't know each other, so their creative congruence—in drawings, paintings, worked into clay, etched into the damp sand of the tray, and built with pipe-cleaners, cardboard and papier-mâché—is compelling.*
>
> *I've recreated this shape in clay and now it's dry: a wedge, a three-dimensional triangle all corners and sharp angles and edges. I drop-into the felt-sense it evokes and feel my dead mother's presence whisper down my spine. Together we ponder this symbolic shape as it sits on my open hand.*
>
> *It's so contracted. So compact. My fingers close about it and I find I'm squeezing tight as I tap into my grief, my heart pounding and my breath shallow.*

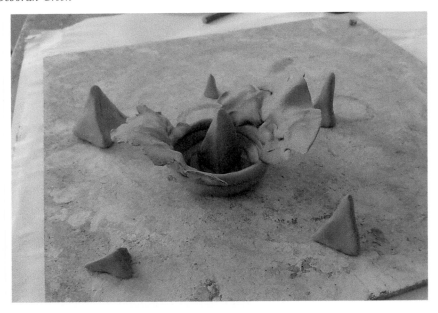

*Figure 31.6* Soul-Wings (Green, September 2013)

> *Suddenly I know this shape.*
> *I know because it bites into my palm and my fingers.*
> *I force myself to open my hand. Bloodless-lines are imprinted into the soft flesh.*
> *Grief makes me clench tight. I contort and control. I lose breath. I don't bend. But this wedge cannot be held so forcefully without harming me. I need to unclench, to let it rest gently on my palm. I need to let the air move around its edges and sharp planes.*
> *I breathe into this idea and ask the wedge for a way forward. I feel drawn to work further with clay. I let my hands lead, giving over to my haptic sense, and find I'm making a nest/bowl to hold the triangle.*
> *This vessel grows wings.*
> *I sit back in pleasure, loose-limbed and open-handed. I've created space and companionship, a feeling of safety and gentle-holding, with the nest . . . and I've opened this even further with the soul-wings as symbolic invitation to flutter into newness.*

## Liminality, Soul and Communitas

We heal and thrive most effectively when socially connected (House, Landis, & Umberson, 1988) as 'being-with-others' is how we are 'restored to ourselves and thereby transformed' (Levine, 2009, p. 45). Attachment and relationship development are thus core to therapeutic healing (Bowlby, 1988; Rogers, 1980). Clients seem able to cope with high levels of disruptive grief when we forge relationships that are authentic, in-the-moment, collaborative, embodied, emotionally responsive and suggest that new forms of both art- and soul-making are possible (Levine, 2009). When clients and I engaged in communal tasks with full attention, we often entered the flow-state in which action and awareness merged, the self became irrelevant and we experienced 'unity, seamless unity' (E. Turner, 2004, p. 99; Waller & Sibbett, 2008). This seamless unity, named 'communitas' by Turner

(1969), is healing, richly charged with feeling and 'has something magical about it' (E. Turner, 2004, pp. 98, 99).

*I emerge sweaty and spent from a deep difficult session with a troubled client. I write my session notes, attempting to describe and make sense of our delicate intricate interplay of poetic action and soulful emotion. Very little and a huge amount happened simultaneously—he spoke and I listened, I was moved by what he said and I reflected this to him. I encouraged movement and witnessed him dance, was deeply moved again and so responded with my own dance. We shared by mirroring each other's movements and then sat in quietness, seemingly both feeling a special communion, like something mysterious and new was being breathed into life through our combined efforts. We didn't try to analyse or find solutions, rather we honoured the deep hurt and paid respect to the strength in him to hold this pain and still engage in the act of living.*

*While this communitas, this sacred intimacy, may struggle to happen without the arts, I also know it certainly couldn't happen without the relationship my clients and I forge to wrap around and enable our imagical art-making.*

*The communion we build and rebuild is a healing thing in and of itself.*

*This fluidly flexible yet consistent connection pays homage to the vital primary-bond shared between infant and caregiver—coined as 'secure attachment' by Bowlby (1988). So, what does a therapeutic relationship modelled on secure attachment consist of? In my work, this takes the form of intersubjectivity. I'm moved by my clients and offer affective feedback (Levine, 2009; Stechler, 2000). I'm with Damasio (1994) who identified how vitally important emotional reciprocity is to our mental health—we feel our concrete reality, our meaningfulness and value, when we have an affective effect on others.*

*My foremost relationship-role is to emulate Winnicott's (1977) good-enough-mother, a mother who's well attuned but not suffocatingly so, who knows response-ability is grown through*

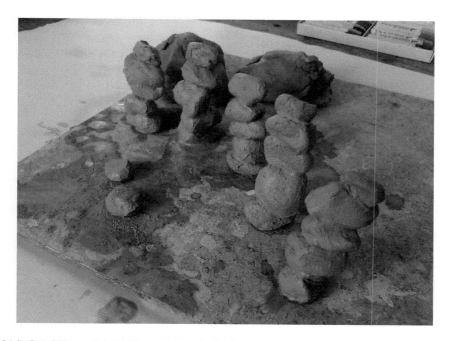

*Figure 31.7* Grief-Upon-Grief (Client-T, March 2012)

*rupture-and-repair, through trial-and-error, that living involves risk-and-reward, grunt-and-grit-and-glory, and that pain-and-joy are all part of the dance. I mentally check my sessions against this soul-sense of a healthy nurturing relationship that moves ultimately towards a courageous and trustful separation-and-individuation. This soul-sense is the velvet of a safe space, a magical connection, the spreading imagical wings of containment, dyadic communitas made manifest.*

According to Edith Turner (2004), communitas 'breaks into society' via the edges of structures during marginality, from beneath structures during inferiority and through crevices opened in structures during liminality—including times of major disaster which can place people in liminal 'mid-transition'. My clients and I, as earthquake-disaster neophytes, experienced quake-induced enduring liminality, as well as marginality and inferiority as the rest of the nation lost interest in our plight and we began to feel economically and emotionally burdensome. Just as those bereaved often find that society tends to tolerate a limited mourning period before beginning to give strong indicators that it's now time to move on, our encounters with those outside Canterbury showed increasing signs of intolerance towards our ongoing quake-struggles. While further complicating our grief, this layered liminality/marginality/inferiority invited deeper relational possibilities by opening opportunities for the soul-based attunement of communitas. Upon entering the liminal stage of ritual, everyday status-roles and rules fall away, allowing neophytes to form bonds that are "undifferentiated, egalitarian, direct, extant, nonrational, existential" (E. Turner, 2004, p. 98). Yet while these bonds eliminate divisiveness they simultaneously maintain multiplicity—identities are not merged and each person's gifts are fully alive, along with those of every other person (E. Turner, 2004) resonant with my multiplicit sense-of-soul.

The term 'communitas' commonly refers to group communitas (E. Turner, 2004), a form that often occurred between participants within my arts therapy groups. In addition, I've recognised and named three further manifestations of communitas that infused my soul-based work. Dyadic communitas allowed individual clients and I to find each other in seamless and often wordless ways. Using this dyadic connection, I could model and nurture the capacity for internal communitas—encouraging wretchedly sorrowing, angry, accusing, avoidant, fearful fragments-of-self to find profound connections and acceptances within the whole multiplicit self. Cultivating this internal acceptance also often held hands with transpersonal communitas which forged continuing bonds between the bereaved and the deceased. This oscillating and cyclical relationship between internal and transpersonal communitas resonated with ways in which grief, loss and restoration are often inter-braided as people experience deep sorrow while

*But most of all,*
*I think my grapples in the garden opened me to see how inviting into the Circle-of-Me those*
*I've lost but still love in strong, complicated and not-so-pure ways,*
*    deepens me.*
*I feel now,*
*a dropping-down-into myself,*
*into a mystery,*
*a concurrent descent into and rising up of richly textured thick-feelings,*

*a knowing that I'm more than any current imagining of myself, I'm not merely floating and buffeted, I'm connected to something.*

*Maybe it's something beyond me.*

*Maybe it's something created by my imagining.*

*Maybe it's both.*

*Maybe the privilege of working alongside Zulu and Xhosa traditional healers in Africa, where the ancestors were ever-present, opened me to these wonderings.*

*Maybe living in New Zealand now, a similar co-presence within the Māori worldview of those who have gone before, has opened me further.*

*Maybe these numinous knowings tangle the linearity of my Western upbringing that seeks to hurry my lost ones into the past.*

*But there's no maybe about how crazily delicious this all is, this delicate yet robust paper-chain of me's and we's looping across space-and-place. So, I thank you, Mom, Dad, m—real or imaginary—for this deepening concertina of me.*

simultaneously reorganising their lives (Stroebe & Schut in Neimeyer, 2014; Walter & McCoyd, 2009).

The porosity of communitas enables souls to cross thresholds and connect with each other and with the dead in 'a vast interchange of spirit personality' (E. Turner, 2004, p. 99). What I have called transpersonal communitas voices the possibility of an ongoing healthy relationship with the deceased (Klass, Silverman, & Nickman, 2014; Neimeyer, Klass, & Dennis, 2014). In rejecting the Freudian perspective of a maladaptive connection which needs to be relinquished, continuing bonds become a celebration (Root & Exline, 2014) that strengthens "a sense of connection with what is not lost" while creating "new meaning and purpose for those who carry forward the stories of the deceased" (Hedtke, 2014, p. 12). Throughout this chapter, I've recounted how, in my wild garden, I leaned into this way of being with those I've lost. During the quakes, when appropriate I invited contemplation of this option with clients . . . and several found great solace by inviting their loved ones back into their lives.

*We've been working through layer-upon-layer of loss and grief. Finally finding the courage to flee her emotionally abusive partner, the quakes have dragged ragged claws through her quest to rebuild—her dignity, self-respect, marriage, home, and large parts of her city lie in raw tatters.*

*In a previous session, she soothed her deep bitter tears with the beginnings of self-care, making herself a comforting bed and pillow from clay. On impulse, I responded with a small Stonehenge guarded by a snake. We decided this was encouraging her to invite a sense of the sacred and magical back into her grey world—and she moved her clay-bed into the centre of the Stonehenge where the snake took up a protective position on her pillow.*

*Today she begins with tears. I invite her to drop-inside herself. She takes the snake with her as companion, talking quietly to me as she journeys within. She heads straight to her heart. She and the snake sit quietly, patiently with her heart, welcoming, warm, accepting of what may come. The snake begins moving. It coils itself around her sad heart, right around until it's holding its tail in its mouth. Her heart beats deeply, trustingly.*

*Then it lifts . . . and beneath her heart lies the baby she aborted in order to survive her violent and manipulative marriage.*

*She arches with guilt, sorrow and loss for this small, barely formed scrap of being. The baby is a thin red outline and, as she watches, the snake joins her and wraps about the baby, again taking its tail in its mouth but this time its lithe body forms the infinity symbol. In response to my soft question, she suggests this shows that past, present and future are connected, that the stronger woman she is now can travel back to comfort the scared broken woman she was then.*

*'And what about the baby?' I ask. She tilts her head, eyes closed. She's listening. 'Jasmine?' she finally says. 'Yes, Jasmine,' I say, the new name like a sun-warmed pebble on my tongue. She smiles slightly and says it again, 'Jasmine. I can comfort Jasmine too. She's been very lost and lonely . . . '*

*I offer her sandtray or paint. She chooses paint. She dampens the page and uses her fingers. Immediately a rich image arrives—a red form splitting in two arcs. She's pleased. She swiftly adds green and yellow and a black boundary—'to contain it a bit.' My body is warmed by the new fluidity I'm sensing in her, my lungs open, my heart lifts. I reflect this to her and she laughs. 'Yip—that's me you're getting loud and clear.'*

*We tack the image to the wall and stand before it, she with her hands still red and green and yellow and tipped with black, wearing her paint like a badge of honour. We commune with the image, inviting it to share its gifts. She sees a phoenix, Jesus, birds in flight. A garden with abundance, a blue blue sky.*

*I encourage her to embody these feelings—the sacred, the rebirth, the flight. She crouches low, tightly holding herself and breathing deeply. Out come wings, slowly and purposefully, and she rises powerfully to stand, wings raised, magnificent. I mirror this glorious sequence back to her and tears fill our eyes. We commune, holding this moment.*

*Then we turn the image upside down and now she feels roots and speaks of simple gentle things that can allow her space and nourishment—time in her garden, walks, noticing the sky. These invite her to nurture herself in small doable ways that won't devour too much time or energy.*

*Again, she moves this—taking the same sequence and reversing it. She begins with her arms high, her body proud, then she folds gently into herself and curls to the floor breathing deeply— but this floor-pose is no longer tight and defeated, it's contained and protective.*

*She holds this for some time and I wait, breathing into her pause, wondering what is arriving.*

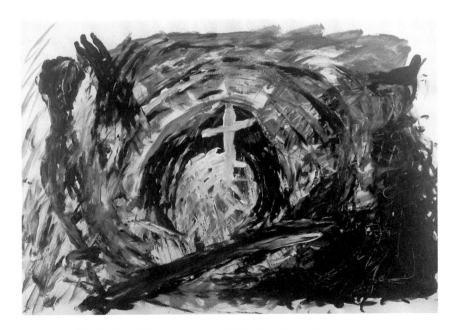

*Figure 31.8* Finding You-in-Me (Client-J, August 2011) (See Plate 4)

*Slowly with a deep building hum that I take into my own body and amplify, she again stands. But this time her arms are not rising. Rather she has them across her heart. She comes to her full height on strong legs and is gently cradling her lost baby against her heart.*

*She gazes down with deep love, tears softly falling, falling. I imagine, quite clearly, a small face gazing trustingly up at her.*

Soul-based and communitas-infused arts therapy offered many benefits to my grief work during the Canterbury earthquakes. This way of working paved a route to the healing state of flow while allowing clients to feel deeply supported through the most wretched moments of their sadness. It welcomed all emotional responses, even the taboo. It allowed us to express and transform the unspeakable, often without needing to find words. It invited self-compassion and -acceptance of internal fragments. It offered new and unexpected re/connections with those loved and lost. And it helped us to hold, honour and bless our sorrow and loss.

## References

Avstreih, Z. (2014). Authentic movement and mindfulness: Embodied awareness and the healing nature of the expressive arts. In L. Rappaport (Ed.), *Mindfulness and the arts therapies: Theory and practice* (pp. 182–192). London, UK: Jessica Kingsley Publishers.

Bowlby, J. (1988). *A secure base: Parent-child attachment and healthy human development.* London, UK: Routledge.

*Canterbury Quake Live.* (2017). Retrieved from www.canterburyquakelive.co.nz/

Csikszentmihalyi, M. (1990). *Flow: The psychology of optimal experience.* New York, NY: Harper and Row.

Damasio, A. (1994). *Descartes' error: Emotion, reason, and the human brain.* New York, NY: Putnam Publishing.

Gendlin, E. T. (1997). *Conference on after postmodernism: University of Chicago.* Retrieved from www.focusing.org/apm.htm

Green, D. (2012). Clearing a space. *Australia and New Zealand Journal of Arts Therapy, 7*(1), 42–51.

Green, D. (2016). *Quake destruction/arts creation: Arts therapy and the Canterbury earthquakes* (Unpublished doctoral thesis). University of Auckland, New Zealand.

Halprin, D. (2003). *The expressive body in life, art and therapy: Working with movement, metaphor and meaning.* London, UK: Jessica Kingsley.

Hart, J. (2012). Moving through loss: Addressing grief in our patients. *Alternative and Complementary Therapies, 18*(3), 145–147.

Hedtke, L. (2014). Creating stories of hope: A narrative approach to illness, death and grief. *Australian and New Zealand Journal of Family Therapy, 35*(1), 4–19.

Hillman, J. (1983). *InterViews: Conversations with Laura Pozzo on psychology, biography, love, soul, the gods, animals, dreams, imagination, work, cities, and the state of the culture.* Woodstock, CT: Spring Publications.

House, J. S., Landis, K. R., & Umberson, D. (1988). Social relationships and health. *Science, 241*(4865), 540–545.

Kass, J. D., & Trantham, S. M. (2014). Perspectives from clinical neuroscience: Mindfulness and the therapeutic use of the arts. In L. Rappaport (Ed.), *Mindfulness and the arts therapies: Theory and practice* (pp. 288–315). London, UK: Jessica Kingsley Publishers.

Klass, P., Silverman, D. R., & Nickman, S. L. (Ed) (1996). *Continuing bonds: New understandings of grief.* New York, NY: Routledge.

Leavy, P. (2013). *Fiction as research practice: Short stories, novellas, and novels* (Developing qualitative inquiry) [Kindle Edition]. Left Coast Press.

Levine, S. K. (2009). *Trauma, tragedy, therapy: The arts and human suffering.* London, UK: Jessica Kingsley Publishers.

Merriam-Webster. (2017). *Dictionary: élan vital.* Retrieved from www.merriam-webster.com/dictionary/%C3%A9lan%20vital

McNiff, S. (1998). *Art based research.* Boston, MA: Shambhala Publications.

McNiff. S. (2004). *Arts heals: How creativity cures the soul.* Boston, MA: Shambhala Publications.

McNiff, S. (Ed.) (2013). *Art as research: Opportunities and challenges.* Chicago, IL: Intellect Publishers.

McSaveney, E. (2014). *Historic earthquakes—The 2011 Christchurch earthquake and other recent earthquakes.* Retrieved from www.TeAra.govt.nz/en/historic-earthquakes/page-13

Neimeyer, R. A. (2014). The changing face of grief: Contemporary directions in theory, research, and practice. *Progress in Palliative Care, 22*(3), 125–130.

Neimeyer, R. A., Klass, D., & Dennis, M. R. (2014). A social constructionist account of grief: Loss and the narration of meaning. *Death Studies, 38*(8), 485–498.

NZETC. (2016). *The Maori as he was: A brief account of Māori life as it was in pre-European days: Spiritual concepts of the Māori.* Victoria University of Wellington. Retrieved on 26 August 2017, from http://nzetc.victoria.ac.nz/tm/scholarly/tei-BesMaor-c4-3.html

Rappaport, L. (2014a). Focusing-orientated arts therapy: Cultivating mindfulness and compassion, and accessing inner wisdom. In L. Rappaport (Ed.), *Mindfulness and the arts therapies: Theory and practice* (pp. 193–207). London, UK: Jessica Kingsley Publishers.

Rogers, C. (1980). *A way of being.* Boston, MA: Houghton Mifflin.

Rogers, J. E. (Ed.) (2011). *The art of grief.* New York, NY: Routledge.

Root, B. L., & Exline, J. J. (2014). The role of continuing bonds in coping with grief: Overview and future directions. *Death Studies, 38*(1), 1–8.

Seigel, D. (1999). *The developing mind.* New York, NY: Guilford Press.

Stechler, G. (2000). Louis W. Sander and the question of affective presence. *Infant Mental Health Journal, 21*(1–2), 75–84.

Turner, E. (2004). Communitas, rites of. In F. A. Salamone (Ed.), *Encyclopedia of religious rites, rituals, and festivals* (pp. 97–101). New York, NY: Routledge. Retrieved from http://cw.routledge.com/ref/religionandsociety/rites/communitas.pdf

Turner, V. W. (1969). *The ritual process: Structure and antistructure.* Chicago, IL: Aldine.

Waller, D., & Sibbett, C. H. (Eds.) (2008). *Art therapy and cancer care.* Seoul, South Korea: KakJiSa Publisher/OUP.

Walter, C. A., McCoyd, J. L., & Walter, P. C. A. (2009). *Grief and loss across the lifespan: A biopsychosocial perspective.* New York, NY: Springer Publishing Company, LLC.

Winnicott, D. W. (1977). *Playing and reality.* London, UK: Tavistock.

# 32  Snapshot of Practice

## Notes on Palliative Care Art Therapy in Singapore

*Hilary Rapp*

### About Me

I am an art therapist currently working in open studio settings with a UK mental health charity and people with multiple sclerosis; these greatly influence my own art. For twenty years I lived and worked in Asia, with past experience as a nurse in oncology and palliative care followed by humanitarian work with refugees which led to training in art therapy at LASALLE in Singapore. The international perspective to this training gave me some experience in relating across cultures.

### About the Context in Which I Work

People from China, Malaysia and India formed Singapore society initially. A former British colony, the working language is English; however, within families myriad dialects and customs are evident. The younger generations seldom learn dialects, resulting in a gulf in spoken communication between the elderly and their grandchildren. Over 80% of people live in supported housing, usually compact high-rise apartments sometimes home to an extended family; there is no welfare state. Singapore and Asia in general is traditionally a collective society, putting the needs of the community before individual and personal development. Emphasis is placed on humility and filial responsibility; these alongside religious tolerance are considered paramount to social harmony. These parameters have implications if exploring family dynamics and locus of control. Colonial history and hierarchy can also transfer into the therapeutic relationship in negative ways (Essame, 2012).

The hospice movement in Singapore is growing and diversifying to encompass the needs of people of many faiths in this small nation. General healthcare is sophisticated but costly, and stigma still surrounds mental health, sometimes resulting in a reluctance to seek professional help and a tendency towards somatization of emotional distress. Eastern spirituality does not make a distinction in mind-body experience; centering instead on a sense of inter-connectedness where imbalance might cause illness. This is sometimes expressed as *qi* or energy and the notion of *yin*—heaven or light and *yang*—earth or heaviness. Asian people accept a sense of strength gained through adversity (Chan et al, 2006).

Reticence about speaking of illness and dying stems from the belief that it may hasten or summon death, and the patient will lose hope. Families sometimes withhold the prognosis from their relatives. There are two important and somewhat contrasting festivals linked to death in Singapore: The Hungry Ghosts, where souls of the dead are appeased by burning offerings and Qingming, a tomb-sweeping day when ancestors are honoured. Art is revered and still considered the domain of a gifted few; in the written language of characters Chinese people often defer to professional calligraphers. Within the art therapy there is much to consider and not assume about symbols, colours, artefacts and their cultural meaning.

## Summary of Research Study and Findings

Art therapy was a new psychological approach in Singapore and I was interested to know more about its potential in end-of-life care in this cultural context. My research approach was further refined by reviewing the previous studies outlined by Wood et al (2011). Together with my supervisor from the Department of Palliative Medicine we formulated a small pilot study to look at its effect on anxiety and cancer-related fatigue (CRF). CRF is defined as generalized weakness and diminished concentration where healthy emotional reactivity is altered (Mitchell & Berger, 2006).

There were twelve adult participants of Chinese, Malay or Indian heritage whose average age was 41, and I was therapist and researcher. Doctors referred patients to the study on the basis of: social isolation, withdrawal from communication, anxiety about prognosis, family tension, low self-worth, history of mental illness, suspected depression. I thought it might be difficult to maintain contact with patients with hospital visits alone so for continuity the art therapy (AT) sessions were offered weekly, in a peripatetic manner at the place of care: hospital, hospice or at home according to the wishes of participants.

I chose The Creative Journey (Luzzatto & Gabriel, 2000) as the art therapy model adapted to a maximum of six sessions with an ending review. To expand the range of art materials a session using clay was added to the programme with a theme relating to obstacles or burden. I applied an existential phenomenological approach with reflective distance within the art therapy. The Hospital Anxiety-Depression Scale (HADS) (Snaith & Zigmond, 1994) and Brief Fatigue Inventory (BFI) (MD Anderson Centre, 1997) were quantitative measures at the beginning, midpoint and end of therapy.

Looking firstly at the assessment measures, I found initial levels of anxiety to be higher than for depression and overall patients' level of anxiety appeared to be reduced through the process of art making. Fatigue was less apparent by the midpoint of therapy although some people still reported feeling tired at the end of a session. This was described as a different exhaustion, of having achieved something or due to increased mental activity. I found the assessments acted as a lead, setting the intention of the work and providing phrases for complex emotions, but that measurements were not always congruent with the person's affect or artwork.

There were forty-eight pieces of artwork to consider—a large number of which comprised embodied images suggestive of active imagination (Jung, 1964; Schaverien, 1999). The images often contained multiple meanings and this capacity to hold contradiction and ambiguity enabled the person to explore their emotions symbolically. For example, the question of whether we were looking at sunrise or sunset and anticipation of what there *might be* after life or of what there *might not* be. Parallels emerged between some of those with higher scores and a negative transference from the images that contained less potential for transformation. In contrast, aspects of resolution or change in perspective were noticed in the images from some people with lower scores.

I found working in the home gave me further insight and context to the person in a life. The Creative Journey (Luzzatto & Gabriel, 2000) provided a framework so that changes in location did not adversely affect the therapeutic alliance.

## How My Research Has Informed My Art Therapy Practice/ Understanding

I undertook a small study to look at the potential of art therapy in Singapore as an aspect of palliative care and whether there might be measurable effects on anxiety and cancer-related fatigue. As such there were limitations; I was the sole art therapist, from a different culture than the participants and unable to share their language of choice when express-ing emotional experience. The lack of a randomized control group means we cannot draw accurate conclusions about the assessment measures. Nonetheless, I found the assessment process complemented the therapy and was useful in adding another dimension to the art works.

Themes emerged from the body of artwork and during the sessions, suggesting creative expression can awaken curiosity and have an energizing effect. I learned more about the qualities of art materials—collage offered structure and safety in the beginning, clay later on accessed shifts in affect and symbolic expression in ways that resonated with the Expres-sive Therapies Continuum (Kagin & Lusebrink, 1978). Managing the pace of work as therapy progressed was important; mindful that time was in essence limited. An adequate conclusion to each session was paramount. Working at home gave me a sense of family interactions where it seemed a shift in the locus of control and satisfaction with their art enabled the patient to reintegrate aspects of themselves, their heritage and engage with others more openly. This brought to mind the potential of shared sessions at home, the value of open studio for those who are isolated as well as the role these art works might play in bereavement support.

Significant to my work as an art therapist in the UK is the sense of context and relevance that the research process fostered. I now appreciate to a greater extent the diversity of experience at the end of life and the importance of noticing my counter transference to offer more appropriate interventions and support.

## One Idea That Shapes My Work

The inadequacy of words when relating to people who are in physical and emotional distress in hospital prompted me to seek other means of communication and to realise the potential of creative expression which led to training in art therapy. Whilst working in Asia I became more aware of somatization, where unaddressed fear or depression can manifest itself in unexplained physical symptoms (Freud, 1994). It began to make sense that someone experiencing intractable pain at the end of life despite the best analgesics might have something important to resolve from a relational perspective before relief could be achieved. Neuroscience has demonstrated that emotional trauma can leave tis-sue damaged in the brain. Van der Kolk (2014) also explains the ways our complex body systems can be altered by distressing emotional events. This understanding has led me to listen more intently to what is said about the body and to notice how this appears in myriad symbolic ways in the artwork. If there is one idea or a word for what has shaped my work it might be 'inclusiveness'—considering the person and their art entirely. As the art therapist I am not excluded from this effect; any one of us may somatise when our exter-nal and internal experiences become overwhelming and defeat our usual ways of coping (McDougall, 1989).

## Acknowledgement

With gratitude to Professor Cynthia Goh who supported and supervised my art therapy work in Singapore.

## References

Chan, C.L., Ho, R.T., Fu, W. & Chow, A.Y. (2006). Turning Curses into Blessings: An Eastern Approach to Psychosocial Oncology. *Journal of Psychosocial Oncology*, 24 (4). The Haworth Press, Inc.

Essame, C. (2012). in *Art Therapy in Asia: To the bone or wrapped in silk.* Chapter 6. Eds. Kalmanowitz, D. & Potash, J. London & Philadelphia: Jessica Kingsley Publishers, pp. 93–94.

Freud, S. (1994). *The Interpretation of Dreams.* New York: Modern Library.

Jung, C.G. (1964). *Man and His Symbols.* London: Random House.

Kagin, S.L. & Lusebrink, V.B. (1978). The Expressive Therapies Continuum. *Art Psychotherapy,* 5, pp. 170–180. Oxford: Pergamon Press.

Luzzatto, P. & Gabriel, G. (2000). The Creative Journey: A Model for Short-term Group Art Therapy with Post-treatment Cancer Patients. *Journal of the American Art Therapy Association,* 17 (4), pp. 265–269.

McDougall, J. (1989). *Theatres of the Body: A Psychoanalytical Approach to Psychosomatic Illness.* London: Free Association Books.

Mitchell, S.A. & Berger, A.M. (2006). Cancer-Related Fatigue: The Evidence out There for Assessment and Management. *Palliative and Supportive Care: Cancer Journal,* pp. 374–387.

Schaverien, J. (1999). *The Revealing Image: Analytical Art Psychotherapy in Theory and Practice.* London & Philadelphia: Jessica Kingsley Publishers Ltd.

Snaith, R.P. & Zignand, A.S. (1994). The Hospital Anxiety-Depression Scale. *Acta Psyciatrica Scandinavica,* 67, pp. 361–370. London: Muncksgaard International Publishing Ltd./Copenhagen & GL Assessment Ltd.

The University of Texas M.D. Anderson Cancer Center. (1997). *Brief Fatigue Inventory.*

Van der Kolk, B. (2014). *The Body Keeps the Score.* Allen Lane: Penguin Books.

Wood, M.J.M., Molassiotis, A. & Payne, S. (2011). What Research Evidence Is There for the Use of Art Therapy in the Management of Symptoms in Adults with Cancer? A Systematic Review. *Psycho-Oncology,* 20 (2), pp. 135–145.

# 33 Healing Wounds—Meeting Māori at End of Life

*Jennie Halliday*

## Introduction

Hospice care in Aotearoa/New Zealand is provided free to all people with a life limiting illness. The majority of medical care is government funded with social and family care funded by individual hospices. People may self refer though most are referred through medical personnel or agencies. With seemingly minimal barriers to the referral process we could hope that hospice service is accessible to all, however recent studies indicate there is often a gap for Māori, our indigenous people, at end of life due to a lack of cultural understanding (Moeke-Maxwell et al, 2014; Slater et al, 2015) and this is consistent with the experience of many indigenous peoples (Duggleby et al, 2015).

For Māori this disconnect is curious when, as Slater et al (2015) point out, Dame Cicely Saunders' "Total Pain" philosophy of hospice care resonates well with New Zealand's best known Māori model of health, Te Whare Tapa Whā (Durie, 1985). This model compares four sides of a house to different aspects of the person necessary for health. These are: taha wairua (spiritual), taha hinengaro (mental), taha tinana (physical) and taha whānau (family), (Durie, 1994). The gap in service for Māori requires that we look to our history of colonisation which has resulted in ongoing disparities in the health and mental health of Māori in comparison to Pākeha (New Zealanders of European descent), (Durie, 1994, 2001; Kumar and Oakley Browne, 2008; Ministry of Health, 2017). These disparities reflect poorly on upholding a commitment to equality and shared power signed into law 176 years ago.

## Our Treaty

The Treaty of Waitangi (Te Tiriti o Waitangi) was signed between Māori and British representatives of the Crown in 1840. As a nation we continue to struggle with we how we live the Treaty both collectively and individually. Lack of consistency in application and understanding of how the Treaty affects practice remains a contemporary problem within institutions (Durie, 2011).

New Zealand arts therapists are called on to acknowledge the Treaty in their work. ANZATA (Association for Arts Therapy in Australia, New Zealand and Singapore), includes this in their code of ethics:

> Arts therapists shall seek to be informed about the significance of respecting, understanding and the meanings of indigenous cultures in their work. This includes the meaning and implications of the Treaty of Waitangi and the principles of protection, participation and partnership with Maori people of New Zealand.
>
> (www.anzata.org, 2016).

What this means for the practice of arts therapists in New Zealand is not expanded on in arts therapy literature. While the Treaty relates to relationships between the Crown and Māori, I have an interest in how the principles could inform individual therapeutic relationships between Pākeha and Māori thereby in fulfilling our Treaty responsibilities. The arts therapies are uniquely positioned to do this in a culture with important ancestral legacy in the creative arts (Mead, 2016) and current practice across many forms.

> Creative arts therapy processes offer junctures for exploration of traditional knowledge, which in turn supports self-reflection, self-expression and self-realisation.
>
> (Turner, 2006, p. 60)

## Working Bi-Culturally

While this chapter is not a formal research project, I acknowledge the literature on culturally appropriate research, particularly that of Smith (1999) who states it must be Māori who benefit, not subject to re-colonisation by becoming objects of research. With a deficit of literature about arts therapies with Māori it is my hope that first and foremost Māori will benefit, particularly those in palliative care, where the reach is poor. Above all, this writing is offered in the hopes our field does not contribute to what Tolich (2002) coined "Pākeha paralysis" and that we are better informed by those who have contributed to the field of Māori research in order to come to our work with clarity about what it means to be Pākeha in postcolonial New Zealand with a Treaty we are called on to honour.

What follows is one account in the field of art therapy from New Zealand. It is the story of a Pākeha art therapist and a Māori client who met in a hospice service, which afforded a unique opportunity to acknowledge imbalances of power and invite new ways of being. The account is offered in the hope it will not be too long before there are more and this will begin a conversation about end of life care for our Tangata Whenua, people of the land, and the efficacy of art therapy in providing that care.

## Background

Matua M* came into hospice care after being released from prison as a result of unexplained falls and an eventual diagnosis of Motor Neuron Disease (MND). He had just moved into our area and the specialist palliative nurse who referred him to me was concerned that some challenging psycho-social needs had not been met in his previous location. She queried whether his history of incarceration and Māori ethnicity were factors in this along with his current presentation. Matua M was struggling with his anger, usually directed at staff and residents of his new care facility. On a few occasions his emotional burden had resulted in self harm creating some concern about suicidal intent.

I was told Matua M had matters he wished to resolve regarding the relationship with his mother. Specifically, he had a desire to be told by her that she loved him. An initial social, emotional, and spiritual assessment as part of admission to hospice care stated Matua M had insight about childhood deprivation, grief from the suicide of a brother, and loss of identity as a former gang leader. With this information I scheduled a home visit to introduce art therapy as part of hospice care.

* This partial pseudonym and how it came to be is addressed later in the chapter.

## Beginnings

Our first meeting was in an open area where other residents of the rehabilitation house were mostly involved in watching TV. We had sole use of the dining room table with our backs to the others which afforded some privacy and was acceptable to Matua M. When working in community settings the need to establish relationships with multiple people in addition to the client can be challenging. However, it can also be useful in challenging assumptions about power when we arrive at a space we do not "own". While Matua M was still new to this home it was his home more than mine. Recognition of myself as "other" when making hospice home visits helps disrupt unconscious enactments of power. In this situation I hoped my outsider status might result in a therapeutic alliance less influenced by our history of colonialism. Regretfully recent studies show "colonial—and colonising—encounters are only too common" (Moeke-Maxwell, 2012, p. 150) in the mental health field.

Matua M's recent release from prison was also on my mind as I approached this first meeting to introduce myself and art therapy to him. As art therapists we can offer a clean slate, literally and figuratively to our clients. The therapy begins with an opportunity to enter the creation process by making something new. I introduced art therapy as a practice that is able to be client led, with the therapist alongside. I elaborated describing the process as one in which the client works in their own way making images, or marks that hold meaning for them that we make sense of together. Matua M was open to embarking on an image and his first request was for a ruler. At that time I did not carry rulers in my art bag. I was uncomfortable with materials associated with notions of right and wrong, referencing some kind of non-existent precision in work that is often about self acceptance and tolerating imperfection. But a deeper problem had presented itself in relation to this Pākeha woman who arrived with words about choice for this Māori man that her actions were now poised to betray. For me this recalled our history of colonisation and the many betrayals of the Māori people.

Durie (2001) tells us interactions with Māori can be guided by knowledge of practices observed on marae, the ceremonial land and buildings belonging to Māori of the local area. This is an important place of belonging (Mead, 2016) and visitors must adhere to formal protocols if respect is to be afforded the hosts. The welcoming ceremony, pōwhiri, moves from sacred, tapu, towards a more informal balance between visitors and hosts so they may enjoy their time together informally. Achieving this balance, noa, is important for good relationships between parties. The visitor's understanding that it may take them time to discover what is required to maintain the balance of tapu and noa (Durie, 2001) has implications for therapeutic encounters between Māori and Pākeha.

This protocol was helpful to understand where my concerns arose as a visitor in this first meeting and the instinct I followed not wishing to offend nor overpower. I responded to the request for a ruler saying, "You know how Māori know Pākeha make promises and then go back on them? That's what I'm going to do, but I'm going to say why". This felt somewhat clumsy and blunt but I had not been prepared for the challenge I experienced with the request.

> In Māori protocol, if one party (tapu) overpowers another party (tapu) it signals a negative form of noa (freedom from restrictions), in that the person is rendered powerless, such as happens to slaves and prisoners.
>
> (Drury, 2007, p. 14)

Keenly aware of Matua M's prison history I hoped that at least naming the momentary power imbalance might counter potential damage of the therapeutic alliance we were just beginning to build. I went on to acknowledge that in fact, in spite of my words, I was changing the rules. To explain why I spoke with Matua M about notions of precision and accuracy, associations we have with something like a ruler and the importance in this work of valuing our own marks or lines. He then drew the lines that form the white area in the centre of his image (Figure 33.1) freehand. I commented that the lines looked like Rangi (sky father) and Papa (earth mother) from the Māori creation story, and in this instance, the central focus of Tino Rangitiratanga, the national Māori flag. Matua M looked at me, perhaps surprised at my recognition. He continued. As I sat alongside this man I silently celebrated the power of this image, identification with a symbol of autonomy, self determination and Māori independence. This felt like a rich template for future work and a clear signal that I was being taken at my word—that this process was his.

The literature on working with Māori cautions against making assumptions about how connected, or not, the person may be to their cultural heritage (Hirini, 1997; Durie, 2001). In art therapy the information can come freely, without prompts or verbal inquiry. Matua M's identification with his culture had been clearly communicated. Identification with the struggle for independence through his image was symbolically charged given his recent release from prison as a result of his MND. MND, sometimes known as ALS (amyotrophic lateral sclerosis), is a progressive disease that attacks the muscles used for walking, speaking, breathing, and swallowing.

At one point Matua M had written out the words "Tino Rangitiratanga" on the bottom portion of the page before going over the top of the words with black to complete the image of the flag (Figure 33.2). At the end of our time I wondered aloud if he had felt the need to cover up aspects of himself throughout his lifetime. Something important was

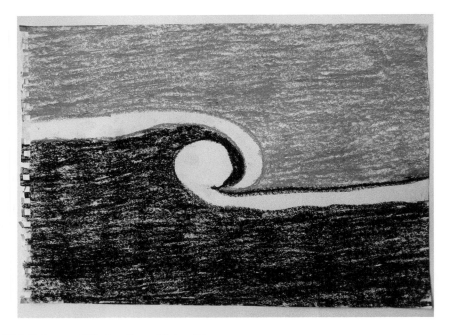

*Figure 33.1* Koha, an Offering From Matua M

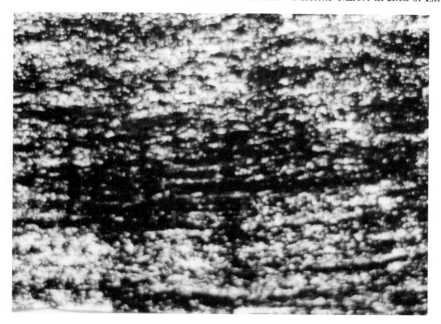

*Figure 33.2* What Lies Beneath

being communicated and it could be acknowledged and reflected back at the outset of our relationship. McKenna and Woods (2012) describe this as follows:

> what is being looked at collaboratively and seen are the levels of new meaning examined for the client and therapist alike.
>
> (p. 36)

At the conclusion of this first session Matua M placed his hands over the image and began a prayer, karakia, in Te Reo Māori (Māori language). I do not speak Te Reo, however I understood the act of blessing and began to wonder if I was going to be gifted the image. This gave rise to further concern about another potential cultural clash. The custom of koha, gifting, is the means by which visitors on the marae can acknowledge the host and forge bonds between the two parties (Durie, 2001; Mead, 2016). The hospice I work at has a policy that no personal gifts can be accepted, and this was my first test. The mana of my client was once again in jeopardy. Mana, defined as power, authority or prestige (Barlow, 1991), can build up over time with acknowledgement of achievement increasing respect (Mead, 2016). Rejection of this gift would be counter to the therapeutic process we had just begun.

I managed to explain that while I could not personally accept this gift I could do so on behalf of hospice and display the image in our art therapy room with the hope it may encourage others to see it. At that time a deeper cultural understanding and calmer disposition would have reduced the level of panic I was experiencing. A gift to the hospice community, over its individual representative, me, is very much in keeping with the custom of koha and Māori collectivism. The knowledge this koha was going to our art room, known as the Taonga room, honoured the gift further. Taonga is the Māori word for treasure, a highly valued object. Matua M was very happy with this idea and we parted ways with a plan to meet weekly.

## Forming a Partnership

By our second meeting I had negotiated a separate, private space to work in at the residential facility with the manager who had established a supportive and trusting relationship with Matua M. This was important as his family, whānau, were quite absent from his day to day life. I talked with Matua M about the advantage of good communication between the manager and myself with regard to his psychological needs. My proposal to debrief after our sessions carrying information that he and I had agreed on was accepted.

Moving to a dedicated space was helpful to our work. We had privacy and now that Matua M's speech function was being affected by his MND I was finding it difficult to understand him where there was extraneous noise. The room we met in was apart from the main building and had a ramp for wheelchair access. In these first few weeks working together we established a ritual in which I often verbalised our partnership. Together we loaded up the art supplies, most of them on Matua M's lap carefully secured under the armrests of his wheelchair. At his request I would push him to the bottom of a ramp and then ask for his help to propel the wheels as I pushed. A small thing perhaps, but calling attention each week to our partnership, and the necessity for it to reach our destination, became a symbolic foundation for the therapy.

Matua M told me about his whakairo, traditional wood carving, and we acknowledged his sadness at no longer being able to use his carving tools because of "his disease" as he always referred to it. He let me know he had a plan for something he wanted to make. In a stunning test of the partnership I named as we navigated the ramp together Matua M dictated a list of materials he required. The list had four items: Tracing paper, eraser, scissors, and a ruler. By the following week I had a special woven flax bag which became known as Matua M's contraband. This pleased him greatly and we laughed together about his victory.

For the next two weeks I sat across from Matua M holding one end of the ruler as he painstakingly measured out equal lines at the top and bottom of a very large sheet of

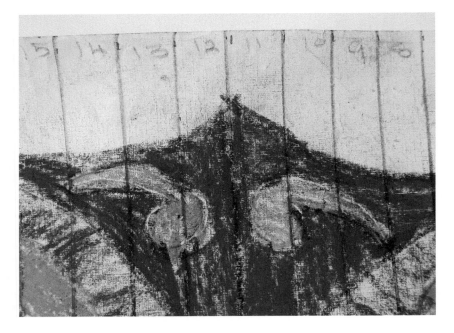

*Figure 33.3* Matua M Makes His Mark

paper (Figure 33.3). I wanted him to know that I would assist whenever he needed it, and asked for it, otherwise I would not encroach on his process. I also wanted him to know this was out of respect, not lack of empathy. In palliative settings I have often observed carers acting on behalf of patients without consulting the person first. Research with Māori at the end of life found that racism was sometimes a factor in the loss of independence, or rangitiratanga (Moeke-Maxwell et al, 2014). Art therapy offers a means by which agency can be experienced and rangitiratanga upheld.

Matua M worked very slowly with laboured breath making his marks on the paper, the many smudges testament to his struggle with compromised physical function, testing his psychological capacity to tolerate the loss. His resilience was greater than mine initially. The temptation to feel frustrated on his behalf was strong, more about me than him. As is often the case in this work, I was learning from the client. I had to get out of my own way and be clear about my transference in order to keep Matua M's needs central.

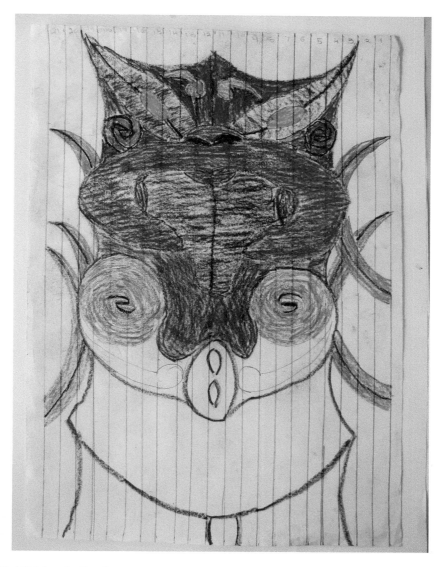

*Figure 33.4* Taking the Lead

## Weaving Together—Partnership Enacted

For many weeks we worked across the table from one another on this weaving (Figure 33.5). I experienced it as a dance of sorts—Matua M leading the way folding his strip of paper, me following. Each row we completed was a reminder that peaceful co-existence was possible. On one occasion he asked if I would teach my other students how to do this. I told him I was sad to hear him speak of himself as my student. This is not how I thought of him, and I encouraged him to see that in fact he was teaching me. Matua M was experiencing a new way of being and it was continuing to change him. The old habits of controlling others learnt in his biological and then gang family were absent in this work. The manager of his supported living facility was also noticing a positive change in his habitual anger, and the difficulty he had regulating it in his day to day life.

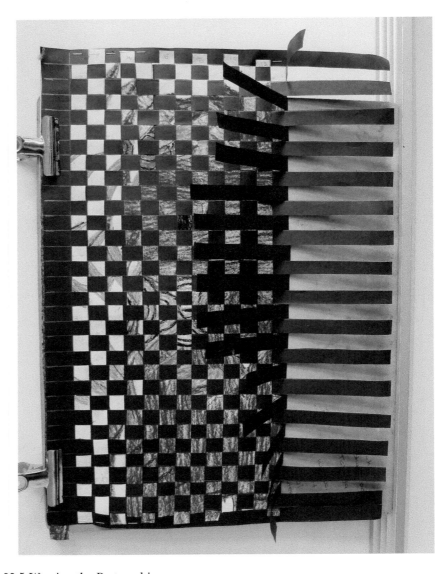

*Figure 33.5* Weaving the Partnership

Much of our time together was spent in silence after some initial conversation about events of the prior week: hospital admissions, rare visits from family, his Rātana faith. Silent though this relationship often was, the ability to trust that an other could be there for him on a consistent basis was one part of the work. Sitting alongside him in silent support, holding, and protecting a space for his creative and emotional expression was another.

At the end of each session I would hold up the image at a distance for Matua M to view. I often do this with clients so we can think about perspective and how things look different at a distance. The pride he experienced each time I did this was written across his face, and sometimes accompanied with words, such as "mean". One week Matua M offered to hold the image for me to view, something no other client has ever done before or since. I was moved by this experience and this demonstration of his thoughtfulness. Much like the actual image that was emerging from week to week a new self-image was forming. Matua M's early adaptation controlling others through his gang position was shifting and he was starting to give in addition to receiving. This symbol of our partnership was enacted at the end of each session in the weeks that followed as I held the work for him and then he for me.

## Protection—Equality and Respect

One of the great challenges for the person in palliative care is the environment in which medical interventions, medications, pressured schedules of medical staff and carers prevail. It can be difficult to protect privacy and the therapeutic space on behalf of the patient. On one occasion a nurse came to administer drugs to Matua M in the room where we worked. While I was thinking about how to later negotiate future interruptions with staff his shirt was lifted, without consultation, and he was fed through what is known as a peg in his abdomen. I had never experienced this before and felt very conflicted. Did I stay or go as this very personal interaction took place? I addressed Matua M and said I would be outside so he could have some privacy. After the nurse left, we talked about making the space private in future, a conversation I repeated with the nursing staff after our session. I expressed sadness to Matua M that he had not been asked about whether he minded others in the room while his stomach was exposed. Though he said he didn't mind and appeared to think he had no agency in the matter, he thanked me for respecting him as we left the room that day.

In some small way I felt this encounter threatened the third Treaty principle of protection—positive intervention to ensure equality for Māori, especially in the area of health (Durie, 1994). The concept of protection applied to individual relationships between Pākeha and Māori is difficult. The word itself could connote weak and strong parties with notions of heroic intercession. This would be the worst kind of misinterpretation in a bi-cultural therapeutic relationship, and an antithesis to the values inherent in rangitiratanga, independence, and respect. In the encounter described above, the actions of those caring for Matua M did not afford protection of his rights. In reflecting this back to him and negotiating for time dedicated to his psychological wellbeing, without intrusion, I can only hope my advocacy was understood as an act of solidarity not that of a saviour.

The day the weaving was completed Matua M said, "I'm in love with it". In art therapy, where the image acts as a form of self-portrait, hearing these words signalled further momentous change and a growing ability to love himself through loving his creation. Further acknowledgement of the partnership experienced in our work was given when he said, "Good working with you", and finally, "Thank you for the work". For the first time Matua M held the work for me to look at before I did so for him. I found this profoundly moving and felt we had reached a therapeutic milestone with this act.

## Whanaungatanga—Building Relationship

Matua M was now working alone with paint on canvas continuing with visual expression that celebrated his Māori culture (Figures 33.6 and 33.7). Our therapeutic dance continued. There were tests that I could be sufficient to his need. These came in the form of requests for particular paint colours over a number of weeks. Each week I faithfully produced them only to be told the requested colour was no longer required. Eventually I began to gently tease Matua M about this, and as a way of symbolically meeting the need I bought a large container of spare tubes of paint for him to keep while he needed them. As each new request for another item came we negotiated over what would be removed from the box having agreed that what was contained in the box was sufficient from week to week.

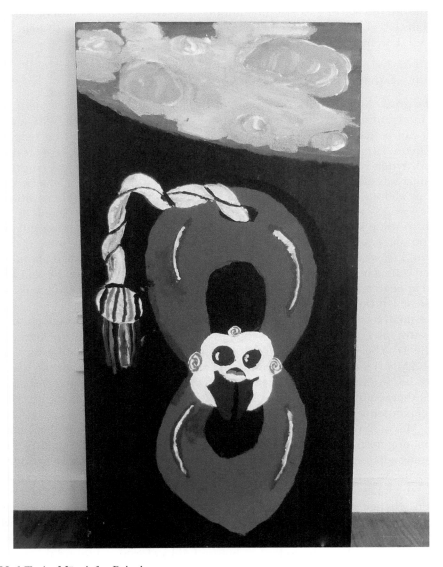

*Figure 33.6* Te Ao Māori, 1st Painting

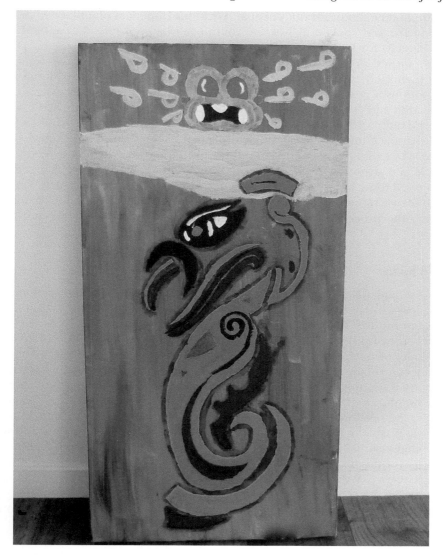

*Figure 33.7* Te Ao Māori, 2nd Painting

Over the following weeks and months of working together we spoke of many things, though not often at length. Matua M's power struggles within the house often threatened his psychological healing. Over and over we spoke of creation vs. destruction and reflected that his anger and its effect on his wairua, spirit, was decreasing. Sometimes the anger and disappointment about lack of support from his family was discussed and his sense of hopelessness that this could change. His love of Te Reo, the Māori language, and his desire to attend the Rātana church where it was spoken was expressed. His MND seemed secondary to the psychological journey he was on, though in any discussion about end of life and his loss of function Matua M expressed he was not fearful of death.

During this time the facility manager who had been a strong advocate for Matua M left. This loss created new challenges including difficulty with transport that meant church attendance was often not possible. With this came loss of a place where Te Reo could be heard and spoken. A hospice volunteer who spoke Te Reo agreed to make visits to Matua M for korero, conversation. When I told Matua M about this person he told me he wished to follow the protocols of a pōwhiri and "call her on" to his marae, which he identified as the room we worked in. On the appointed day Matua M called a welcome to us across the carpark from his wheelchair in front of our room. He was without a tribe and "stood" alone though this process established "a place for the feet to stand" (Mead, 2016, p. 48), acknowledging his birthright as Māori, and the right to stand in this space unchallenged. We approached as the volunteer acknowledged her visitor status by calling back. We made our way into the room where a speech was made by Matua M and answered by the volunteer. After waiata, songs, were exchanged by each of us we shared food, koha bought by the volunteer, and spent some time talking before taking our leave. Matua M's formal welcome to the volunteer increased his mana as host and though the process was somewhat unconventional it was a moving and heartfelt experience.

## Time and Space

Working with patients over a long period of time in our hospice is not usual, and this is becoming less so as pressures on service increase and admission criteria tighten. Almost one year after our first meeting Matua M disclosed he had been sexually abused by a family member from a very early age. His insight about this aspect of his life was striking—he was clear in his own mind that moving into leadership within his gang was the one way he had to keep control over others, blocking out reminders of a time when he was harmed by those supposed to protect him. That day I had the sense this is what we had always been working towards, another milestone made possible by the establishment of whanaunga-tanga. A trusted relationship, 12 months in the making, and for the first time in our work Matua M was unable to make eye contact as he told his story. "Allowing time and space to establish relationships" (Jones et al, 2006) is key in working with Māori. The time it took to build trust for this disclosure still surprises me and I feel grateful that it was available in our hospice service. We didn't speak about it much but eventually, in his own way, Matua M was able to make peace with what had happened to him and express forgiveness. In many ways this signalled the end of our work though completing our therapy sessions took a little longer for us to negotiate.

One of the great advantages I experience working in a hospice environment with a strong social care team and clinical manager, herself an art therapist, is the ability to navigate unconventional therapeutic conditions. Schaverien (2002) writes about disruption of the analytic frame when a client is diagnosed with a life limiting illness and what impact this has on conventional thoughts about boundary issues and how or whether the relationship progresses. She goes on to say,

> But there are no rules, and few guidelines, and it has to be a matter of judgment in each case.
>
> (p. 20)

And so it was with Matua M when I felt the need to formally close the therapy in order to offer experience of a positive completion and a joint acknowledgement of the healing journey. However, in the absence of family engagement and lack of connection to tribal groups it was felt I could offer ongoing support through less regular social visits.

## Participation Through Collaboration

Matua M had always had a strong desire for his story to be told if it would help others like him. He wanted his real name to be used in the telling. Seeking cultural advice on this writing resulted in the opinion that identification of Matua M had potential to cause hurt and pain for families and individuals affected by the crimes he had committed. Matua, a respectful form of address for an older man, similar to Mr., was suggested followed by the initial of his real name. An appropriate acknowledgement of the significant changes he had made in this work.

Maintaining a more informal relationship with Matua M in our post therapy visits meant I was able to report back after his story had been shared in various presentations. His usual query was about how it had been received. Both times I reported that people were saddened to hear of his early abuses of trust and what that had meant for him in the rest of his life. He was uplifted by the response and the sense that his participation meant other Māori might benefit from similar therapy. The uniqueness of the palliative care setting, and my ability to report back on the effects of his participation was a remarkable gift.

## Endings

While Matua M and I did not see much of one another in the last months of his life I learnt he was in hospital when trying to schedule a visit one day. Talking with hospital staff I found he had been in there for a number of weeks with no visitors and no thought by his supported living facility to notify hospice. Within a week I was back at hospital to wait with him while an ambulance came to bring him to our hospice inpatient unit. For an hour I stayed with him, listening to his reggae favourites on a small speaker I had bought with me, attending to his request to be fed ice chips. As I stood beside the bed feeding him I was reminded of the earlier test of my capacity to attend to his need with requests for different paint colours each week. We spoke little and enjoyed the music a lot. I let Matua M know I would see him when I returned to our hospice building later that day. As I left I asked if he would like to hongi now or later. He replied, "now and later". Hongi is the act of pressing noses together as a sign that visitors and hosts on a marae are united spiritually, even if differences exist (Durie, 2001). It was only the second or third time we had observed this practice.

Returning to hospice later that day, I spoke with our hospice Kaumātua, elder, himself a Rātana minister who we had asked to visit Matua M. We spoke briefly before he went to meet him and I summarised Matua M's passions describing them as the three R's—Reo, Rātana, and Reggae. On that day I was proud of our hospice's ability to attend to Matua M's cultural need in the absence of family as he prepared for death.

Before I left for the day I went to visit him. He was not his usual self and we worked through his concerns and worries about practical matters such as being able to reach the bell. I asked him if he was at peace within himself. He said he was. As I stood beside him for the second time that day I realised his bed was in the old art room, the room where his first image had been displayed until we moved to make way for our inpatient suite. When I told him this, and described its former location on the wall directly behind his head, a familiar smile spread across his face along with his favourite expression of approval, "Mean".

It was the end of my week and leaving that night meant it was likely I would not see Matua M again. Another advantage of long-term relationships with patients like Matua M where family were not present is that many of our hospice staff knew him well and were able to support him while he was with us. As I left we shared a final hongi. Farewells he had taught me that we usually exchanged were not.

> Ma te wā, goodbye for now,
> to which he would reply,
> Hei konei rā, see you next time.
> Matua M died peacefully the following day.

## Closing the Circle

Moeke-Maxwell (2015) speaks about Māori practice approaching death as, "preparing the wairua, the spirit, to travel to Te Arai and pass through that veil to the other side". It is my belief that Matua M's creative expression, and the therapeutic exchange that art therapy offered, facilitated a peaceful journey after a violent life. He gifted his story with the hope that others would be helped. In our conversations about this I had spoken about my hope that his story would provide a clearer understanding of ways Māori and Pākeha might work together to symbolically heal wounds, past, and present, personal.

As a Pākeha, there will always be gaps in my knowledge of Te Ao Māori, the Māori world. I have not been raised in the culture and am bereft of the many riches embedded deep within the stories, sayings, songs, and traditions. But this should not be a barrier to offering service. It is our Treaty obligation to find a way. In the end, "Our bicultural appropriateness will be judged moment by moment by our clients and all others with whom we interact" (Crocket, 2012, p. 64). But we need courage and more examples of the work as we grapple with what the Treaty means in the practice of art therapy. The profession is still growing in New Zealand and only a handful of hospices currently employ one. More are needed as is a greater understanding of the way Māori can benefit from a modality that offers psychological healing in a culturally respectful manner at end of life.

> Ki tau te rangimarie
> May peace settle upon you

## Acknowledgement

Thanks to Hospice West Auckland and Catherine Spence for creating the opportunity for this work. And to Dr. Tess Moeke-Maxwell (*Ngai Tai ki Umupuia, Ngāti Porou, Ngāti Pukeko, Ngāti Pākehā*), Nikki O'Connor (*Ngāti Porou and Te Ati Awa*), and Dr. Terence C. Halliday for their responses to it.

## References

www.anzata.org. (2016). *ANZATA Code of Ethics 2015*. [online] Available at: www.anzata.org/Resources/Files/3.Ethics/Ethics-CodeofEthics-2015 [Accessed 25 October 2016].

Barlow, C. (1991). *Tikanga whakaaro*. Auckland, N.Z.: Oxford University Press.

Crocket, A. (2012). Cultural safety: Towards postcolonial counselling practice? *British Journal of Guidance & Counselling*, 40(3), pp. 205–220.

Drury, N. (2007). A Pōwhiri Poutama approach to therapy. *New Zealand Journal of Counselling*, 27(1), pp. 9–20.

Duggleby, W., Kuchera, S., MacLeod, R., Holyoke, P., Scott, T., Holtslander, L., Letendre, A., Moeke-Maxwell, T., Burhansstipanov, L. and Chambers, T. (2015). Indigenous people's experiences at the end of life. *Palliative and Supportive Care*, 13(6), pp. 1721–1733.

Durie, M. (1985). A Maori perspective of health. *Social Science & Medicine*, 20(5), pp. 483–486.

Durie, M. (1994). *Whaiora*. 1st ed. Auckland, N.Z.: Oxford University Press.

Durie, M. (2001). *Mauri ora*. 1st ed. Auckland, N.Z.: Oxford University Press.

Durie, M. (2011). *Ngā tini whetū: Navigating Māori futures*. 1st ed. Wellington, N.Z.: Huia.

Hirini, P. (1997). Counselling Maori clients: He whakawhiti nga whakaaro i te tangata whaiora Maori. *New Zealand Journal of Psychology*, 26(2), pp. 13–18.

Jones, R., Crengle, S. and McCreanor, T. (2006). How tikanga guides and protects the research process: Insights from the hauora tāne project. *Social Policy Journal of New Zealand*, 29, pp. 60–77.

Kumar, S. and Oakley Browne, M. (2008). Usefulness of the construct of social network to explain mental health service utilization by the Maori population in New Zealand. *Transcultural Psychiatry*, 45(3), pp. 439–454.

McKenna, T. and Woods, D. (2012). Using psychotherapeutic arts to decolonise counselling for Indigenous peoples. *Asia Pacific Journal of Counselling and Psychotherapy*, 3(1), pp. 29–40.

Mead, S. (2016). *Tikanga Māori*. 2nd ed. Wellington, N.Z.: Huia.

Ministry of Health. *Annual Update of Key Results 2014/15: New Zealand Health Survey*. Wellington: Ministry of Health. [online] 16 February 2017.

Moeke-Maxwell, T. (2012). The face at the end of the road: Exploring Māori identities. *Ata: Journal of Psychotherapy Aotearoa New Zealand*, 16(2), pp. 149–163.

Moeke-Maxwell, T. (2015). Interviewed by Ryan, K. Maori palliative care stories become nursing resource. *Nine to Noon*. (11 June 2015) 9:37am Radio New Zealand. [online] Available at: www.radionz.co.nz/national/programmes/ninetonoon/audio/201757984/maori-palliative-care-stories-become-nursing-resource [Accessed 6th July 2015].

Moeke-Maxwell, T., Nikora, L.W. and Te Awekotuku, N. (2014). End-of-life care and Māori whānau resilience. *Mai Journal*, 3(2), pp. 140–152.

Schaverien, J. (2002). *The Dying Patient in Psychotherapy*. Basingstoke, Hampshire: Palgrave Macmillan, p. 20.

Slater, T., Matheson, A., Ellison-Loschmann, L., Davies, C., Earp, R., Gellatly, K. and Holdaway, M. (2015). Exploring Māori cancer patients', their families', community and hospice views of hospice care. *International Journal of Palliative Nursing*, 21(9), pp. 439–445.

Smith, L. (1999). *Decolonizing Methodologies*. London: Zed Books.

Tolich, M. (2002). Pākeha "paralysis": Cultural safety for those researching the general population of Aotearoa. *Social Policy Journal of New Zealand*, 19, pp. 164–178.

Turner, S. (2006). *Māori Worldviews and Art as Therapy*. MAAT Dissertation, Whitecliffe College of Art & Design.

# 34 Art Therapy's Contribution to Alleviating the HIV Burden in South Africa

*Hayley Berman and Nataly Woollett*

South Africa carries one of the world's most prevalent burdens of disease, HIV. Living surrounded by so much illness and death and against an historical backdrop of violence and poverty, many young people have had multiple exposures to trauma and bereavement with little opportunity to grieve and recover. One of the many tragedies in South Africa is a deficit of parental figures to provide containment, safety and a space for processing complex trauma and complicated grief. At present there are insufficient therapeutic resources to meet the depth and breadth of need. Many of the existing psychosocial practitioners, while facilitating courageous and extraordinary projects, have inadequate training and are often traumatised themselves.

We are two art psychotherapists; one having worked within a community art therapy centre, the other in the public health system. We will outline the psychosocial context in which many young South Africans are raised and describe an experiential art therapy group with HIV counsellors with the primary objective of becoming 'surrogate parents'. This enabled their capacity to work more effectively and creatively with groups, increasing their propensity for empathy, being able to receive emotional support, as well as encouraging group cohesion with increased productivity.

## Introduction

### Mental Health and HIV

Mental health needs of children and adolescents globally do not get the attention and resources required, but are severely underserved in low and middle-income countries (LMICs) such as South Africa (Cortina et al, 2012; Patel et al, 2007). Mental disorders account for a large proportion of disease burden and mortality in young people in all societies, but especially so for youth in LMICs as a result of scarce resources and strong associations with social determinants of health, such as poor attachment, poverty, food insecurity, violence, poor access to education and healthcare etc. (Patel et al, 2007). The HIV pandemic has increasingly brought attention to the unmet mental health needs of children and adolescents. In 2012 it was estimated that there were approximately 369 000 adolescents under the age of 14 years and 720 000 15 to 24 year olds living with HIV in South Africa (Shisana et al, 2014).

### Orphanhood

Around 15 million children in sub-Saharan Africa have lost one or both parents to the AIDS epidemic, including 2.5 million in South Africa (UNICEF, 2013). In South Africa, the overall level of orphanhood in 2012 among those 0–18 years of age and younger was

16.9% (maternal, 4.4%; paternal, 9.3%; double, 3.2%) (Shisana, 2014). Many adverse outcomes of being orphaned have been reported, including loss of effective guidance and supervision, inconsistent care, psychological distress and poor mental health, loss of educational opportunities, impoverishment, increased sexual vulnerability and high rates of risk taking (Lowenthal, 2014). Studies from African countries have found that compared with non-orphans, children and young people who have lost at least one parent to AIDS have more unmet basic living needs and more psychological problems including negative mood and pessimism (Remien & Mellins, 2007). They are often exploited by new caregivers and have to survive with limited resources (Remien & Mellins, 2007). In addition, being orphaned as a result of HIV/AIDS has more severe consequences than being orphaned as a result of non-AIDS related death (Cluver et al, 2011). Cluver et al (2011) report that children and adolescents orphaned by AIDS were 117% more likely to be suffering from post-traumatic stress disorder than children and adolescents whose parents were alive, and also 67% more likely than children and adolescents orphaned by other causes, including homicide, suicide and cancer.

### Bereavement and Grief

One of the key risks for poor mental health, especially among orphans, is bereavement (Cluver et al, 2012; Willis et al, 2014). Research indicates that most bereaved children and adolescents will show resilience in adjusting to loss, however, certain factors may influence their ability to grieve. How children comprehend and understand the reality and complexity of death depends on many factors including; the child's level of cognitive development, the nature of his/her relationship with the person who died, the specific manner of the death, resilience, quality of subsequent care and social support (Webb, 2003; Wood et al, 2006). After a major death, a child's immediate social environment either facilitates or inhibits his/her ability to engage in adaptive grief processes and achieve key developmental tasks (Li et al, 2008).

Cross-cultural research on natural grieving processes suggests that most humans need to recognise their grief and be able to express it directly in order to resolve their loss (Li et al, 2008). This can become formidable in contexts such as South Africa where there is a culture of silence around death and grieving when it comes to children and adolescents (Wood et al, 2006). In many instances, children and adolescents are not told that their parent has died, or are informed of events with euphemisms such as the parent has 'gone away'. It is also quite typical for adults to whisper in the child's ear while they are sleeping regarding death of a family member and these events are discouraged to be discussed again thereafter (Daniel et al, 2007). Oftentimes, although intended to be protective, children and adolescents are excluded from cultural rituals, such as funerals, that would aid in their grieving and legitimise their role in participating in community practices (Daniel et al, 2007). AIDS-related bereavement is likely to be especially complicated and difficult to accommodate, largely as a result of HIV related stigma and its latent denial (Wood et al, 2006). The denial inherent in this silence and its formulation over time and through development leads to poor understanding of perinatally infected (i.e. those infected vertically at birth) children and adolescent's own HIV disease and reinforces stigma around HIV with costs to mental health functioning (Daniel et al, 2007; Woollett et al, 2016). Profound and multiple losses, often unrecognised and unmourned, can lead to complications in the ability to grieve. Doka (1989) defined the concept of 'disenfranchised grief' as the grief people experience when they incur a loss that is not or cannot be openly acknowledged, publicly mourned or socially supported (cited in Crenshaw, 2005).

## Resilience

There is little doubt that HIV leads to experiences of anxiety and depression in children and adolescents, and a 'pathologising' focus may serve as a significant contributing factor, in highlighting the hardship experienced by children and adolescents. However, in contrast, Masten (2001) coined the term 'ordinary magic' to refer to resilience as something nurtured by everyday resources, common to individuals, families, communities and cultures. These conventional roots of resilience suggest that resilience is not rare and that active steps can be taken to develop and sustain resilience among young people who are placed at risk by ordinary and extraordinary hardship. There is evidence to suggest that resilience is present in the lives of many children and adolescents living in circumstances of extreme adversity and HIV (Woollett et al, 2016). Recent traumatology research attributes fostering resilience to multiple sources, including individual, family, community, culture—it is contextual, cultural, epigenetic and relational (Southwick et al, 2014).

## The Power and Potential of Image-Making in Relation to an Other

There are considerable challenges to implementing mental health interventions at a public healthcare level in South Africa that need to be thoroughly addressed for optimum impact. These include lack of skilled mental health professionals available to intervene and the need to utilise and upskill lay counsellors to meet the demand ethically with targeted training and consistent expert supervision (Ventevogel, 2014; Mendenhall et al, 2014). Addressing mental healthcare in children and adolescents has the potential to improve HIV treatment and prevention; however, with poor resources of specialised mental health providers to facilitate care, the emotional needs of patients are largely untreated. Psychologists and psychiatrists are in short supply with 0.28 psychiatrists and 0.32 psychologists per 100,000 population working in the public health sector (Lund et al, 2010).

It seems prudent that not only are more creative arts therapists needed to provide appropriate support for children and adolescents in the public health sector in South Africa, but also that task-sharing, whereby non-mental health specialists provide mental health services under supervision of specialists, may be the most feasible way to deliver inexpensive, effective mental health services in primary care (Mendenhall et al, 2014). Increased skills in the use of non-verbal methods of working in conjunction with experiential and theoretical psychodynamic input are required and are easily transferable. The counsellors we worked with were open to this way of engaging patients and did not require prior qualifications other than HIV counselling and testing training.

Non-verbal means of working with children and adolescents have been proven to be effective for the treatment of bereavement and post-traumatic stress disorder (PTSD) (Webb, 2003; Goodman et al, 2009). Research indicates the meaningful contribution of neuroscience to understanding the importance of the use of images and 'action-oriented' interventions in working with those who experience trauma, the precursor to PTSD (van der Kolk, 2007).

Trauma, the emotional response to a terrible event underscored by fear, helplessness or horror, demonstrates long-term effects. In particular, it interferes with declarative memory, or conscious recall of the event, whilst implicit memory, emotional responses, and sensorimotor sensations related to the experience remain intact (van der Kolk, 2007). The images and experiences are stored in incoherent, disorganised and fragmented ways, often indescribable in words. Non-verbal methods offer a simplified mode of communication when direct verbal access to trauma-related experiences are not possible or advisable. These methods facilitate recall of memories, enabling them to be processed and for the artist to have control over this process (Buk, 2009). The creative product serves as a container for the affect, aiding in emotional regulation. Creating art uses both sensory and emotional stimuli, thus making the artistic process a beneficial vehicle to access and integrate memories (Lusebrink, 2004). The act of creating offers the opportunity to externalise and make meaning associated with painful experience.

There also needs to be overt recognition of the power dynamic latent between adult counsellors and child/adolescent participants and managed ethically. Contextually, obedience to and respect for adults are values that are strongly emphasised so that young people seldom speak up or voice their opinions to adults (Clacherty & Donald, 2007). Practices that utilise non-verbal methods, such as image-making, are particularly ethical as they offer children and adolescents active participation in the therapeutic process, authenticating their voice through their engagement, offering more developmentally appropriate means of accessing information, diminishing stress in the child/adolescent-adult interaction and providing a more comfortable method of engagement than language (Clacherty & Donald, 2007; Willis et al, 2014). The therapeutic relationship, the creative process and the work in a group promotes integrated relationships, integration in the brain and ultimately a path towards emotional and physical health (Siegel, 2017).

## Community Art Counsellors—Lefika La Phodiso's Model

Lefika La Phodiso (meaning 'rock of holding or healing' and referred from now as Lefika) is Africa's first psychoanalytically informed community art counselling centre. Established in 1994, its core mission is to respond to the deficit of mental health resources in South Africa. Applied psychoanalytic thinking informs the model of practice. The notion of 'cryptonomy', has been useful in looking for ways to help unlock the inaccessible 'mental graves' that disrupt symbolisation and integration. These 'mental graves' refer to the locked up or put away parts of ourselves—seemingly dead and unavailable for use (Abraham et al, 1994). This is particularly relevant when exploring the multiple levels of trauma, and trans-generational secrets and myths that permeate South African society. It is also relevant to the specific denialism on a governmental level in relation to HIV/AIDS and the stigma associated with disclosure, resulting in the embedded secretive encasement of the disease.

## Case Study

In 2008 an HIV/AIDS public health organisation approached Lefika to run a two-day training course with their HIV lay counsellors in order to enable them to work more effectively with groups. The objective was to expand their current reach of clients through group work, and support them in the work they were currently doing. These counsellors face the day-to-day challenges of coping with the physical and emotional needs of affected and infected individuals, families and communities in public health clinics. Their duties include pre- and post-test counselling, prevention of mother-to-child transmission counselling, HIV disclosure and adherence counselling for groups of adolescents. Many were outreach workers linked to the hospital setting but visiting patients in their homes in more rural communities, thus largely unsupported and unavailable for supervision. They were regarded as 'volunteer' counsellors, many without qualifications, some illiterate and paid a stipend (below a living wage) for doing this important work.

All the participants consented to the process being documented and pseudonyms have been used.

There were 18 counsellors (all women) ranging from ages twenty to sixty, with high expectations. The group expectations were very concrete including: a certificate, wanting to play and have fun and acquisition of new skills. Reflexive space was felt by most to be boring, exhausting (many fell asleep) and not productive. The catered food felt insufficient and not 'good enough' revealing enormous emotional hunger and dissatisfaction. Their feelings of being taken from, without getting anything back (failed cases, dead clients) was projected onto me as facilitator. It was as if asking them to explore their feelings or thoughts was experienced as theft. Both the group and I were fragile and defensive.

In response to the group state of mind, they were invited to tear up wads of old newspaper, as an outlet to physically and verbally express their frustration and rage. This process in itself was a vehicle for a release and simultaneously offered an opportunity to transform the chaos and mess into something more productive. There was some discussion about creating something from the fragments as a group, or engaging with the debris on an individual level. Predictably, the group chose individual engagement; they were not able to be a group yet. Some participants created figures, many created bunches of flowers—usually referring to a funeral ritual. Some of the mess was left on the floor which came to represent those patients who could not be helped, those that refused to take their medication and died.

One group member created a fist of power, and painted it red. Someone in the group noticed the 'red fist' and said it was (not looked like) a placenta. She said it was the afterbirth, 'bloody and ugly'. Other group members laughed, not able to respond empathically. The person who created it felt attacked and misunderstood. It was interesting that the attack was directed at the 'placenta', the most primordial container. There seemed to be a constant to-ing and fro-ing, between life and death forces. I commented on the striking sense of an absence of empathy, patience or respect for one another. I interpreted that they were probably so overwhelmed, exhausted and full of other's stories and tragedies as well as their own, that there did not seem to be any more space to have empathy for their colleagues.

The following day, after having some space, distance and having recognised the very fragile space they inhabited, I came back with some anxiety and a greater sense of empathy for their enacted struggle. I reflected my experience of them as functioning within a protective and defensive realm. I spoke about the usefulness of the group as a microcosm, providing a mirror of their external worlds. They were invited to create an image of the moment or experience that led them to choosing to do this work as HIV counsellors. They were given a significant amount of time and space to create an image and then to share their images in pairs, allowing them to develop trust and really listen to one another and have space and time for personal reflections. When they returned to the large group, many chose to share their stories within the container of a collective witness. This process elicited profound emotion and sadness.

Most shared very personal and tragic histories. The encrypted secrets so tightly held inside finally had room to breathe, be witnessed and heard. There was room to cry, to be sad and connect with the multiple disappointments and losses. Many disclosed their HIV status and spoke of the shame of illiteracy and not having had access to information about HIV and AIDS. This gap in their own experience propelled them into this work—to repair the damage. This process felt like a huge breakthrough, as if the unbearable pain that they were so carefully defending against the previous day was given room to 'be'. The complex paradox of having held these secrets in the context of their work which primarily involves encouraging their clients to disclose their HIV status and go onto treatment, exacerbated the potential impact of 'unlocking' their 'mental graves'. We reflected about the significant movement from sleepiness, boredom, disruption, anger, and sadness to joy in such a short space of time and the capacity and resilience of the group to survive some of the unbearable feelings. There was evidence of a capacity to mourn and grieve, which seemed unavailable for thought or experience earlier in the group process.

## Extended Group Work With HIV Counsellors

Almost a year later, Lefika received some funding to work within the HIV/AIDS sector and approached the head of psychosocial services (co-author Nataly Woollett) to continue with this group. She was enthusiastic, as the clinics were facing many changes and the counsellors were under attack from clinic management. The adherence groups for adolescents that the counsellors were facilitating had poor attendance and the adherence statistics had dropped dramatically, and the counsellors were blamed for this problem. Counsellors were made to feel responsible and therefore felt like failures. In responding to this pressure, counsellors had abandoned the structure of support/counselling groups, and shifted the adherence groups to more outcome-based, didactic, HIV education groups.

The group met for an intensive 4 days of training with monthly full day workshops to integrate and present their applied practice. Some went on to complete the full Community Art Counselling training at Lefika over 18 months.

## The Working Group

Over time, with different interventions and surviving the projections, attacks and pain, the group formed sufficient trust enabling the use of the group dynamics as an object to learn and grow from. The image-making process became an important vehicle to communicate complexities. Lizzy risked sharing her diagnosis of a brain tumour with the group and traced her hand proudly, 'with this hand I can do anything!' The quality of the images and reflections indicated an increased capacity for curiosity as well as an increased capacity to hold loss and reflect on the 'other'. In acknowledging this shift, it became possible to be transparent about the group process and evolution since the previous year. Memories shared included feelings of mistrust and anxiety. Lettie remembered, 'I was very angry, I felt I couldn't exist'. Several group members expected to be told how to run a group, not how to be in a group. Experiential learning was unfamiliar and felt to be a waste of time. Their responses mirrored the developmental phase of the group at the stage of dependence.

> The group's dependence can vary from expectations that the conductor provide practical solutions, to views of the conductor as an omnipotent and omniscient figure, who is the source of strength and gratification.
>
> (Nitsun, 1989, p. 252)

The group was able to acknowledge their initial defensive acting out behaviour. We were able to reflect on the experience of a working group capable of entering sustained moments of integration as opposed to the early phases of a group that exuded 'un-integration' and fragmentation (Winnicott, 1976, p. 44). Using objects and/or art materials assisted to gradually detach from the dependence of the mother, as a transitional bridge learning to be independent yet relational. Particularly within the context of the HIV epidemic, the image provides evidence of existence and offers valuable opportunities for active witnessing of one another's experiences. The image can function as memory that may preclude repression or foreclosure. Making developmental links to the process enabled each group member to begin to apply their experience to working with their clients in the clinics.

The group was invited to engage with clay to explore early childhood connections of a significant relationship that had felt held and connected. Many group members allowed the clay to determine what emerged, and trusted the material to elicit form rather than predetermining it. Phumi spoke profoundly of the messiness of the clay and the resistance with which she engaged with it. She compared the clay to HIV+ children at the clinic who are malnourished, dirty, have sores and whom she did not want to touch. As time went on, she came to know the clay and what it could do and made the analogy of getting to know these children and coming to respect their individual qualities and being able to play with them and be available to them. She spoke of the transformation of the children once they were on antiretrovirals (ARVs) as being able to play and relate. She said, 'I felt a bond with the clay eventually as I do with the children'. Interestingly, the following week, the clay had cracked which she associated with the fragility of the children (and by extension, those parts of herself). One group member said, 'it is when we know what we know and can't bear to think we know it'. This is not only a manifestation of the 'unthought known' (Bollas, 1987), but also the things that are known yet never articulated, so prevalent in South African society. The stigma of HIV and AIDS and the added myths of needing to protect children from the truth make for a very uncomfortable psychic position to be in.

## Death in the Room

Group members spoke of multiple losses of patients, colleagues and family members and expressed how little emotional support they had to manage it all. Sibongile spoke of an HIV+ four year old who was raped and not on treatment. She sobbed about her own experience of rape. Zandi created a black 'doek' [head cloth] usually worn to signify that someone has died. She reflected on making it beautiful, and embellishing it with buttons and beads respecting those who have died, while acknowledging that through death something beautiful that holds memory can be internalised.

We reflected on the group process, the silence, the sadness and the capacity to sit in the depths of emotion without having to escape the pain of it. Through experience we were able to weave in the learning of applied thinking within their workplace. The weaving of ritual, memorial, making images and playing—the activities of doing enabled by 'things' in the environment—allowed something to be worked through. Perhaps the combination of doing and thinking, promotes a 'deeper' and potentially more sustainable outcome. They could see the possibility of moving away from their didactic approach of providing solutions, to being able to sit in the unknown space and survive it. We could explore the current situation of being able to trust what had emerged without limitation, and consider the quality of silence and the holding capacity of the group.

## Applied Thinking and Practice

In preparation to end the group, stories filled the space describing moments of engagement with clients using their new art counselling skills and increased capacity for empathy. Phumi shared something about her shift in approach and attributed it to her time at Lefika: 'A child was diagnosed HIV+, usually the nurse tells the child and starts medication without consulting or counselling the child, nor mother. I intervened, and spoke discretely with the mother empowering her to tell her child with my support and we used drawing to help the child express her feelings about it'.

Counsellors seemed to be able to provide a more compassionate and considered approach to the needs of the client and the situation. They used the term 'containment' to describe an added capacity of patience, and 'holding' to describe an increased capacity for empathy. Ntuli reflected a situation of a mother who came into the clinic and found out her child was HIV+. The client sat and cried with the counsellor. When she had finished crying she said, 'thank you, I could not do this at home' and left the room. This example alluded to the capacity to provide a safe space, tissues and a glass of water and instead of feeling helpless and useless she felt 'good-enough'.

There was an increased consciousness and theoretical understanding of what trauma, bereavement and the 'unthought known' bring that elicit a compensatory or reparative mode of being. They could understand how their fear of conflict or discomfort propels them to engage their defence mechanisms and carefully structure and determine the outcomes. We were able to reflect about ways of facilitating a group, allowing space for the unknown and for a more open approach to a group's natural evolution.

## Consolidation of Their Journey

The group exhibited their work and provided witness to one another's journey. Ntuli said; 'The group gives you the courage to learn to be safe. When I missed a session I felt like a baby missing a feed, I was very thirsty. The group provides nourishment'. They had acquired a new space to think and be thought about.

Zandi carried on working on her 'doek' and added a key that she sewed onto it; 'it is a symbol of opening any door in my life'. She gathered found objects and seeds from within the studio and outside, symbolic of planting seeds for the future. The images embodied the contradictions and struggles, hope and hopelessness, resilience and foreclosure.

Some overall reflections seemed to capture the precariousness of life and the importance of Winnicott's notion of 'going on being' (Winnicott, 1956) and the reliability of an environment. The participants expressed surprise and gratitude for the fact that they could leave their art work in the studio between training days and would return to find them still there. The therapeutic space could hold and take care of their internal worlds, and the images provided visual evidence of the shifting narratives in their lives; 'I talked about things that were difficult to talk about and the world didn't end'. The reflections indicated that something of the importance to 'speak one's mind' had been internalised, sharing in a group as a possibility of something that could always be available to them revealing the importance of survival and resilience.

## Conclusion

Cultural silence does not help children, adolescents or adults deal with loss and bereavement; it increases isolation and undermines a sense of security (Daniel et al, 2007). Breaching cultural silence may be seen as a protective factor enhancing resilience (ibid).

As evidenced in this chapter, creating, sharing, documenting and remembering signifi-cant people in their lives whom they had lost was a critical element of their life story. This facilitates a parallel process with the child and adolescent patients they treat in the pub-lic health system. The authors strongly advocate that with the provision of sensitive and appropriate training for carers, gains can be felt on a greater scale with less reactivity and destruction and more mindful reflection and containment.

This chapter particularly highlights the struggle inherent in the attempt to provide sustainable pockets of care in response to the HIV/AIDS epidemic. The epidemic itself on many levels precludes making sense of, and straddles living with, death and invest-ing in life continuously. While the authors have been aware of their search for hope and resilience to keep believing and engaging in the work, they have also become aware of the constant negotiation from illusion to unbearable disillusionment and despair. There seems to be a continual vacillation of understanding and not under-standing, of myth and 'reality', of denial and enactment, moments of hope and often immense hopelessness. Therefore, Donald Winnicott's belief that illusion is absolutely necessary for healthy development holds true in such a context. 'You can only accept being disillusioned, if you have been illusioned' (Green quoting Winnicott in Kohon, 1999, p. 30).

The orphans, guardians and counsellors in this case material reveal the continuums of hope and despair and the capacity and failure to hold and be held. As practitioners, we need to embrace the complexity, beauty and transformational potential of this work. The invitation is to attune to and make overt the multiple layers of engagement. There are pro-found internal connections, inter-connections between individuals, between the images made and the reflections, within a group and the broader psychosocial sphere inhabited by complexity of the HIV/AIDS epidemic. The richness of these layers of relational spaces facilitate opportunities for physiological changes in the brain, in the quality of empathic connections and thus the expansive potential of preventative and palliative social cohe-sion and well being.

'*Thanks for the caring for our children and their caregivers and thanks for the caring of ourselves*' (lay counsellor after training).

## References

Abraham, N., Torok, M. and Rand, N.T., 1994. *The shell and the kernel: Renewals of psychoanalysis* (Vol. 1). Chicago, IL: University of Chicago Press.

Bollas, C., 1987. *The shadow of the object: Psychoanalysis of the unthought known.* London: Free Associa-tion Books.

Buk, A., 2009. The mirror neuron system and embodied simulation: Clinical implications for art therapists working with trauma survivors. *The Arts in Psychotherapy, 36*(2), pp. 61–74.

Clacherty, G. and Donald, D., 2007. Child participation in research: Reflections on ethical chal-lenges in the southern African context. *African Journal of AIDS Research, 6*(2), pp. 147–156.

Cluver, L.D., Orkin, M., Boyes, M., Gardner, F. and Meinck, F., 2011. Transactional sex amongst AIDS-orphaned and AIDS-affected adolescents predicted by abuse and extreme poverty. *JAIDS Journal of Acquired Immune Deficiency Syndromes, 58*(3), pp. 336–343.

Cluver, L.D., Orkin, M., Gardner, F. and Boyes, M.E., 2012. Persisting mental health problems among AIDS-orphaned children in South Africa. *Journal of Child Psychology and Psychiatry, 53*(4), pp. 363–370.

Cortina, M.A., Sodha, A., Fazel, M. and Ramchandani, P.G., 2012. Prevalence of child mental health problems in sub-Saharan Africa: A systematic review. *Archives of Pediatrics & Adolescent Medicine, 166*(3), pp. 276–281.

Crenshaw, D.A., 2005. Clinical tools to facilitate treatment of childhood traumatic grief. *OMEGA-Journal of Death and Dying, 51*(3), pp. 239–255.

Daniel, M., Malinga Apila, H., Bjø rgo, R. and Therese Lie, G., 2007. Breaching cultural silence: Enhancing resilience among Ugandan orphans. *African Journal of AIDS Research*, 6(2), pp. 109–120.

Goodman, R.F., Chapman, L.M. and Gantt, L., 2009. Creative arts therapies for children. In Foa, E.B., Keane, T.M., Friedman, M.J. and Cohen, J.A. (Eds.), *Effective Treatments for PTSD: Practical Guidelines from the International Society for Traumatic Stress Studies*, 2nd Ed. (pp. 491–507). New York: Guildford Press.

Kohon, G., 1999. *The dead mother. The work of Andre Green*. London: Routledge.

Li, X., Naar-King, S., Barnett, D., Stanton, B., Fang, X. and Thurston, C., 2008. A developmental psychopathology framework of the psychosocial needs of children orphaned by HIV. *Journal of the Association of Nurses in AIDS Care*, 19(2), pp. 147–157.

Lowenthal, E.D., Bakeera-Kitaka, S., Marukutira, T., Chapman, J., Goldrath, K. and Ferrand, R.A., 2014. Perinatally acquired HIV infection in adolescents from sub-Saharan Africa: A review of emerging challenges. *The Lancet Infectious Diseases*, 14(7), pp. 627–639.

Lund, C., Kleintjes, S., Kakuma, R., Flisher, A.J. and MHaPP Research Programme Consortium, 2010. Public sector mental health systems in South Africa: Inter-provincial comparisons and policy implications. *Social Psychiatry and Psychiatric Epidemiology*, 45(3), pp. 393–404.

Lusebrink, V.B., 2004. Art therapy and the brain: An attempt to understand the underlying processes of art expression in therapy. *Art Therapy*, 21(3), pp. 125–135.

Masten, A.S., 2001. Ordinary magic: Resilience processes in development. *American Psychologist*, 56(3), p. 227.

Mendenhall, E., De Silva, M.J., Hanlon, C., Petersen, I., Shidhaye, R., Jordans, M., Luitel, N., Ssebunnya, J., Fekadu, A., Patel, V. and Tomlinson, M., 2014. Acceptability and feasibility of using non-specialist health workers to deliver mental health care: Stakeholder perceptions from the PRIME district sites in Ethiopia, India, Nepal, South Africa, and Uganda. *Social Science & Medicine*, 118, pp. 33–42.

Nitsun, M., 1989. Early development: Linking the individual and the group. *Group Analysis*, 22(3), pp. 249–260.

Patel, V., Flisher, A.J., Hetrick, S. and McGorry, P., 2007. Mental health of young people: A global public-health challenge. *The Lancet*, 369(9569), pp. 1302–1313.

Remien, R.H. and Mellins, C.A., 2007. *Long-term psychosocial challenges for people living with HIV: Let's not forget the individual in our global response to the pandemic*. AIDS, 21(suppl 5), 55–63.

Shisana, O., Rehle, T., Simbayi, L.C., Zuma, K., Jooste, S., Zungu, N., Labadarios, D. and Onoya, D., 2014. *South African national HIV prevalence, incidence and behaviour survey, 2012*. Cape Town, HSRC Press.

Siegel, D.J., 2017. The integration of attachment, mindfulness, and neuroscience. In Gojman-de-Millan, S., Herreman, C. and Sroufe, L.A. (Eds.), *Attachment Across Clinical and Cultural Perspectives: A Relational Psychoanalytic Approach*. London: Routledge.

Southwick, S.M., Bonanno, G.A., Masten, A.S., Panter-Brick, C. and Yehuda, R., 2014. Resilience definitions, theory, and challenges: Interdisciplinary perspectives. *European Journal of Psychotraumatology*, 5.

UNICEF, 2013. *Towards an AIDS-free generation: Children and AIDS: Sixth stocktaking report*. New York: UNICEF.

Van der Kolk, B.A., 2007. The body keeps the score: Approaches to the psychobiology of post-traumatic stress disorder. In van der Kolk, B.A., McFarlane, A.C. and Weisath, L. (Eds.), *Traumatic Stress: The Effects of Overwhelming Experience on Mind, Body and Society* (pp. 214–241). New York: Guildford Press.

Ventevogel, P., 2014. Integration of mental health into primary healthcare in low-income countries: Avoiding medicalization. *International Review of Psychiatry*, 26(6), 669–679.

Webb, N.B., 2003. Play and expressive therapies to help bereaved children: Individual, family, and group treatment. *Smith College Studies in Social Work*, 73(3), pp. 405–422.

Willis, N., Frewin, L., Miller, A., Dziwa, C., Mavhu, W. and Cowan, F., 2014. "My story"—HIV positive adolescents tell their story through film. *Children and Youth Services Review*, 45, pp. 129–136.

Winnicott, D.W., 1956. *Through Paediatrics to Psycho-analysis: Collected Papers*. New York: Brunner/Mazel.Winnicott, D.W., 1976. *The Maturational Processes and the Facilitating Environment*. London: The Hogarth Press.

Wood, K., Chase, E. and Aggleton, P., 2006. "Telling the truth is the best thing": Teenage orphans' experiences of parental AIDS-related illness and bereavement in Zimbabwe. *Social Science & Medicine, 63*(7), pp. 1923–1933.

Woollett, N., Cluver, L., Hatcher, A.M. and Brahmbhatt, H., 2016. "To be HIV positive is not the end of the world": Resilience among perinatally infected HIV positive adolescents in Johannesburg. *Children and Youth Services Review, 70,* pp. 269–275.

# 35 Narratives East West—Art Therapy in a Hospice in Northern India

## A Patchwork of Cross-Cultural Encounters

*Lara Cooke, Mari Ebbitt and Eloïse Raab*

## Introduction

The aim of this chapter is to present our combined experience of providing art therapy to terminally ill cancer patients in a hospice in Rishikesh, Northern India. Central to this subject, we look at what India and the West can learn from each other in the current field of hospice and palliative care. We will begin by describing the hospice where this work took place and include a brief overview of the current landscape of palliative care in India. We will then compare the role of art in Indian culture in contrast to the West, with a focus on Rishikesh. We will look at the complexities involved in relation to the cultural context of the work and reflect upon the challenges we faced in our attempt to provide a culturally sensitive art therapy service. This will include a critical reflection on our own cultural conditioning from the perspective of being white and Western. Finally, we will include examples of how we approached interweaving both Eastern and Western narratives within our work. This is presented in the form of three short sections: the first describes a partnership project between St Christopher's Hospice in London and Ganga Prem Hospice in Rishikesh; the second presents the work we underwent when providing art therapy during home visits; and the third includes two vignettes that detail the power and impact of art-making during bereavement events held at the hospice.

The identities of those in the case material have been withheld to protect confidentiality. Consent has been granted for the imagery used within this chapter.

## The Hospice

Ganga Prem Hospice (GPH) is in the Indian state of Uttarakhand in Northern India. It is situated between Rishikesh and Haridwar, at the foot of the Himalayas by the Ganga River Bank. The hospice building was inaugurated in March 2017, however, much of the palliative care service is still provided through their home care programme and in various clinics in Uttarakhand. The hospice describes itself as a spiritually oriented, non-profit hospice for terminally ill cancer patients. The staff are a mix of Indian palliative care specialists, Western physicians and therapists who volunteer. The hospice service is funded by donations from charitable trusts and NGOs.

We are three art therapists who trained and work in London. The link with the hospice was initially made in 2016 through an art therapy project at St Christopher's hospice in London where one of us is based. St. Christopher's hospice is located in South London, England and was founded in 1967 by Cicely Saunders, whose work is considered to be the basis of modern hospice philosophy.

At the time, the hospice was developing its psychosocial model of care offered to patients, welcoming an array of Eastern and Western therapeutic and holistic interventions. This led to the initial visit to the hospice in February 2017 where both 1:1 and group art therapy with patients, carers and the bereaved was introduced. The project continued in January 2018 when two other art therapists joined the team; their work followed a similar pattern.

In Britain, hospices are largely secular and open to all. Despite this, the majority are rooted in a Christian ethos, evidently marked by their Saint names. Therefore, we were interested in how the spiritually oriented model of Ganga Prem hospice differed from the hospice model we know. At times, our Western art therapy training can feel inappropriate and ethnocentric when working with a diverse mix of cultures in Britain, so our motivations for working in Rishikesh stemmed from a desire to gain a greater insight into new ways of working cross-culturally within the field of hospice and palliative care. Our intentions were not to instil or indoctrinate a Western art therapy model into an Indian hospice context, for this would perhaps echo a power relation of India's colonial past. Khosla et al (2012) advocate, 'India has the potential to lead the way and enlighten others rather than being subservient to those countries that enjoy resource wealth' (p. 154). Instead, our motivations stemmed from desire to form a relationship with the hospice rooted in reciprocity, allowing for sharing, observing and thinking about different ways of working. Kapitan (2015) posits: 'The greatest potential benefit of cross-cultural art therapy is the opportunity to learn from one another and deepen awareness of how we are positioned interdependently as global citizens' (p. 110).

## The Current Landscape of Palliative Care in India

Palliative care is a relatively new concept to India, emerging in the mid-1980s. The current provision of services is deficient and hugely disproportionate geographically where it is evident that there is greater provision in the South than the North (McDermott et al, 2008, p. 586). Uttarakhand is one of the nineteen states in India that have no provision for palliative care. There is no national palliative care policy and government funding is scarce and inconsistent. Furthermore, medical insurance does not play a substantial role in providing hospice or palliative care (p. 587). This being said, efficient services are evolving through non-governmental organisations and in public and private hospitals and hospices.

McDermott et al (2008) propose that successful models exist for the development of affordable, sustainable community-based palliative care services, which have 'arisen from adapting Western models of hospice and palliative care for implementation in the Indian cultural context' (p. 583). However, Indian authors Khosla et al (2012) highlight the problem with educating Indian palliative care practitioners in the West and contend that theory does not coincide with practice (p. 154). Similarly, Kumar posits, 'the Western hospice system in its entirety is not practical in India. For cultural, economic and social reasons, India needs a system adapted to the Indian scenario' (1996, p. 293). We will later explore some of the challenges that we encountered working specifically as art therapists within this cross-cultural framework and question whether it was ethical to practice Western modes of working with end of life within an Indian cultural context.

The main adaptations of the traditional Western model of hospice and palliative care that we observed at the hospice were that most of the care was community and home care based, valuing family and community over the individual. Additionally, much more importance was placed on spiritual care than in the West.

For a palliative care service to fit the Indian social and cultural milieu it primarily needs to be economical. Expensive clinical inpatient units won't accommodate a million people nor would they fit with a cultural standpoint where people generally prefer to live and die at home. In contrast to the West, Rajagopal (2001) contends that the family structure in India is a strong point in their favour, supporting the notion of cheaper home-based services, where relatives are 'empowered in the care of the patient' (p. 66).

Much of the current palliative care literature in India focuses on the development of palliative care community-based home care schemes such as the Neighbourhood Network of Palliative Care (NNPC) formed in 2001 in Kerala. The NNPC offers medical, psychosocial and spiritual support using volunteers from the local community who are trained to identify problems of the chronically ill in their area and to intervene effectively with active support from a network of trained professionals (Kumar et al, 2005).

It is no surprise that with the imposition of austerity on the NHS in Britain, that many chief hospices in London are now starting similar schemes to offer psychosocial support. Compassionate Neighbours is one example which was set up to replicate the NNPC scheme in India. It emphasises the shared responsibility of society and community for public health, 'a free community-led project for anyone living with a chronic, long-term or terminal illness, or who is 85+ and experiencing loneliness or social isolation' (Compassionate Neighbours, 2018).

We were fortunate enough to be working alongside some of the leading professionals in the region who were shaping this landscape of palliative care. While travelling to home visits we would speak with specialist palliative care doctors and were able to have some of these discussions first hand, exploring what interventions were appropriate for this context. This went on to inform and influence how we approached the art therapy work.

## Indian Art and Ritual

It was our initial concern that the art therapy space would feel too foreign, of no use and that there would be a reluctance to make art. To avoid this ethnocentric bias, we had to immerse ourselves in the social, political, economic and cultural forces at hand (Talwar, 2010) and engage in a process of critical reflection. Having said this, we also thought about the therapeutic aspect of art-making imbued in ritual, one that has been embedded in Indian culture for years. We wondered if our initial assumptions and concerns stemmed from a culture of art therapy in the West that has become increasingly evidence-based so it can be demonstrated as an efficient and cost-effective provision. Accordingly, a huge amount of the art therapy in palliative care literature focuses on affirming the benefits and the efficacy of art therapy (Connell, 1992; Falk, 2005; Sibbett, 2005; Luzzatto, 1998; Malchiodi, 2013; Wood et al, 2013). However, we were now working in a culture that very much believed in the healing nature of the arts; with less focus on effectiveness, we were able to rethink our initial concerns and trust in the art-making process.

Singh (2012) writes about the therapeutic, holistic and spiritual underpinning of art in India and refers to the Hindu text *Chitrasutra* of the *Vishnudharmottara Purana*. Singh contends that it is the oldest treatise on art in India which specifies:

> The aim of painting [is] one of communicating an emotion and causing particular spiritual states of mind. . . . Painting cleanses the mind and curbs anxiety, augments future good [and] causes the greatest delight.
>
> (2012, p. 192)

Singh describes how Indian art and culture advocate the view that the pursuit of art-making across all disciplines is therapeutic, 'creating a sound mind in a sound body' (p. 195). Furthermore, referring to the Chitrasutra, she illustrates how art is embodied throughout Indian culture, a colourful combination of a love of naturalism adorning and ornamenting all surfaces and spaces, ' . . . to mud, stone, metal, cloth, paper and even the human body, through applying paint, tattoos, henna and other herbal pastes' (p. 192).

It felt crucial to recognise how art-making was understood in India in comparison to the West. In India the relationship between art, ritual and spirituality is to some extent more cohesive than in the West. Perhaps Western cultures have become more secular, and it could be said that rituals that once guided communities have with time faded.

We also considered the significance of the city of Rishikesh itself, rather than India as a whole. Rishikesh is a notorious hub for yoga, meditation and spiritual healing, attracting many Westerners. In 1968, the infamous English rock band The Beatles travelled to Rishikesh to take part in a meditation training course in a local Ashram. Unsurprisingly, their visit added to the city's reputation as one of India's most sacred and spiritual places.

## Being White in Rishikesh: A Critical Reflection

Literature that addresses working cross-culturally in art therapy often highlights the importance of recognising how deeply the profession is embedded within a Western perspective (Kapitan, 2015; Hocoy, 2002; Kalmanowitz and Lloyd, 2005). Consequently, one of the growing concerns when introducing art therapy to another culture is that power imbalances between therapist and clients are re-enacted through unconsciously providing a commodified Western art therapy model (Kapitan, 2015). Hocoy (2002) explains that 'the most central issue concerns the potential for art therapy to perpetuate Western cultural imperialism' (p. 141). In tackling this, several art therapists emphasise the importance of self-reflexivity, cultural sensitivity and awareness of ethnocentric biases (Hocoy, 2002; Kapitan, 2015; Kalmanowitz and Lloyd, 2005; Skaife, 2013).

Given the historical context of India—ruled by the British Raj for almost a century before gaining independence in 1947—we were aware that our whiteness, education and language embodied that of the coloniser. We knew that our skin colour was privileged in society and we questioned the assumptions on which theory and technique in art therapy are based. This awareness however did not prepare us for navigating the culture internalised within ourselves, nor did it provide us with practical advice for dealing with our own guilt of the colonial.

Central to this subject of guilt was our exposure to a particular context where we observed, at times, that 'being white' in Rishikesh provoked a more common 'Western saviour complex' in us as we began to question like Horton (2013) whether 'global health' remains a neo-colonial venture that attempts to 'civilise' others. Were our intentions undermining pre-existing cultural healing practices and competency? Was our presence reinforcing Western cultural imperialism? As 'white Westerners', offering art therapy in a poor socioeconomic setting, this critical 'neo-colonial' lens led us to reflect closely on our own motivations, purposes and practice.

Roy (1999) describes the therapist needing to be "empty' enough to continue to learn from the client, and allow new information to make a difference' (p. 127). He goes on to explain that 'curiosity is a fundamental cornerstone to the practice of culturally sensitive therapy' (p. 127). When confronted by the reality of working cross-culturally and how best to navigate our deeply embedded biases, we did feel that we were 'empty' enough; not having our 'safety net' of theories and concepts to fall back on as many of them did not feel appropriate or relevant. We had to turn this 'emptiness' from a negative into a positive and take it as an opportunity to learn from the client and the local community, from a position of curiosity. This opened a space where we could build trust and where we were able to connect on a human level.

## Narratives East West

In July 2016, an initial partnership project began with an art therapy group at St Christopher's Hospice in London. The project was called 'Narratives East West'. It was an open group that was made up of patients and bereaved persons. Members of the group explored their experiences of loss by making a patchwork quilt. Every pocket patch was made individually and inside was embedded artwork, poetry and relics.

The group spoke about how loss and grief in the West was a difficult subject to discuss. They felt it had become more private and less of a shared communal experience in today's Western society. In January 2017, their patchwork quilt was passed on to GPH in exchange for a quilt made by an art therapy group which we ran in Rishikesh (Figure 35.1). Narratives were shared and translated from English to Hindi and vice versa. Their artwork explored personal losses as well as uniting people globally through a sharing of narratives, where they were able to think about mourning death as universal—a condition that unites us. However, it felt important not to think about the specific narratives as universals, as each were embedded in their own specific cultural contexts. Kapitan (2015) explains, 'Whether one's focus is interpersonal or societal, a risk of harm arises when art therapy assumes universality and remains unexamined for ethnocentric bias' (p. 104). The artwork enabled a flow of autonomy, an organic patchwork stitching together a kaleidoscope of cultural perspectives whilst unobtrusively embodying personal feelings of loss.

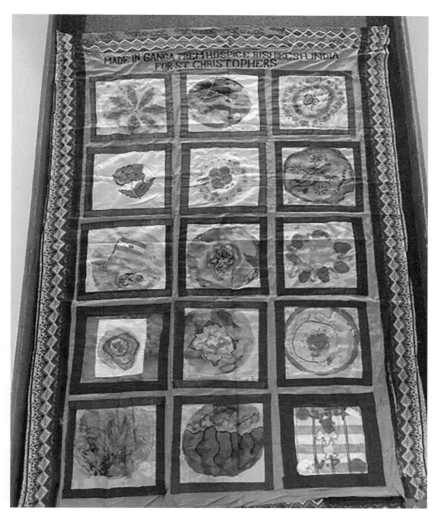

*Figure 35.1* Ganga Prem Hospice Patchwork Quilt

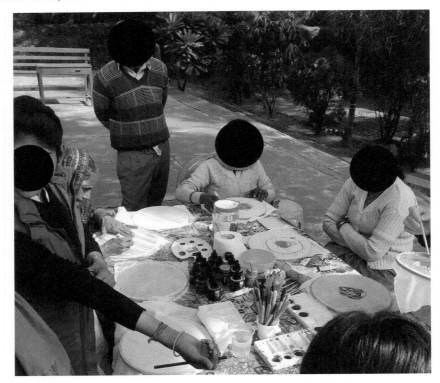

*Figure 35.2* Art Therapy Group in Rishikesh

The art therapy group in the hospice in Rishikesh was made up of five women and one man, both patients and bereaved members who lived in rural areas of the community (Figure 35.2). Most had come as they felt isolated and wanted a space to share their losses with others experiencing the same. The art materials were laid out and the group were invited to make a patch. We offered materials which were familiar, offcuts of local saree fabrics and silk, embroidery materials and fabric paint. One lady worked on a face flannel which had belonged to her husband, embroidering his initials and the Hindu god Ganesh into the fabric. Ganesh is known as the god of wisdom and art, and the remover of obstacles. This experience seemed meaningful for her, as she spoke about what she had made with another lady.

Most of the artwork embodied symbols and motifs which had a religio-spiritual and symbolic significance, such as the lotus leaf. According to Hindu philosophy, human beings ought to live like a lotus flower, unaffected by the muddy waters in which they grow. It felt important to familiarise ourselves with some of this symbolism to understand what was being communicated.

## Home Visits

As stated earlier, the majority of the work that the hospice carries out is home care, attending to patients and families within their home environment. Almost daily, visits were carried out by the hospice which was a lengthy affair, with three cities to cover within the Uttarakhand region: Haridwar, Dehradun and Rishikesh. Separate vehicles would leave from the centre of Rishikesh in the morning, transporting a doctor, nurses and often a translator and western therapist or volunteer (a range of skills were provided as a result of this, from psychological therapies to complementary therapies).

At times, the quantity of staff would mean it was a struggle to fit in the home of the patient, leading us to question whether our presence was helpful or perhaps unnecessary and intrusive. When initially meeting the families, it was at this point that we really felt like outsiders when our 'foreignness' was most prominent. It was down to the trusting relationship that the staff had built with the families that enabled us to be welcomed into the lives of the people we were working with. We were able to offer patients weekly sessions; however, the schedule and rota of the home visits changed on a daily basis which led to little consistency. This would mean that we weren't able to arrange set times, days or length of sessions—a fundamental part of the practice ingrained within us.

As much as possible, when providing therapy in the West, we would aim to provide the client with privacy, confidentiality and a safe space. Our understanding and reasoning for this had to be revised. The whole family would often be present at these visits, information would be delivered in front of them and decisions would be made as a collective. This was also the case for therapy sessions and it was difficult for the individuals we were working with to understand why privacy and space to themselves could be beneficial. Referring to working with people from Aboriginal communities, Connolly and King (2017) speak of a 'communal identity':

> Therapists from Western cultures have to suspend their concept of individualised identity. (. . .) Attitudes to the concept of boundaries and connection are modified: I am not 'me' in a Western sense—I am me as part of something bigger.
>
> (p. 64)

Although Connolly and King are working specifically with Aboriginal people, we felt this was relatable to working with many families from the community we were based in. The individual, within *their* family was a crucial part of their identity and very quickly, the significance of their role and their purpose within the family would arise within the session. For many of the women we worked with, their role as a mother and wife was a significant part of their identity. Many of the men were the main breadwinners, financially supporting a large extended family. We weren't just working with the individual; we were working with the individual within the family.

As we immersed ourselves deeper in the therapy work, it felt as if we were integrating ourselves deeper within the families and the community. This was crucial in order to build trust and to be of support. We had to adapt our understanding to what a therapy 'session' was and instead would have therapeutic visits, involving cups of chai, sharing of food with the family and scrolling through photos albums in which we often encountered photographs of family weddings. After a time, the children in the families would start to address us as 'Didi', which translates as 'older sister' or 'cousin'. We began to realise the significance of being incorporated into the family, where only then could emotional and therapeutic support be provided. When working with death in this community, most of the time was spent celebrating the life of the patients and the families they were part of.

'Home' was a central and recurring theme in many patient's artworks. We were struck by how often the same colourful drawing of a house would reappear; often surrounded by mountains, sunshine and the river Ganga (Figure 35.3). There was a sense of pride in these images as they illustrated the importance of home and how intrinsically linked a home can be to one's sense of identity. We were reminded of Papadopoulos (2002) who describes 'home' as a type of container that provides 'the basic psychological processes which facilitate early human development', such as feelings of continuity, constancy, stability, familiarity, confidence and warmth (p. 5–19). The sense of belonging and safety

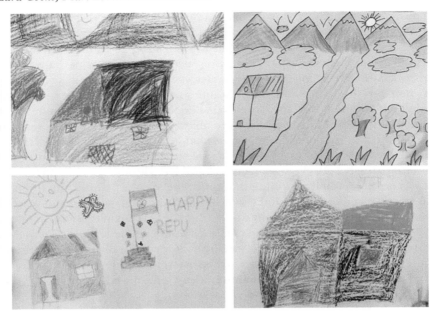

*Figure 35.3* Artwork of Four Different Patients

that these homes represented (both in their physical state and in the images made) were often palpable, leaving us to question whether the fear of leaving home, either through dying or being moved to the hospice, was also being expressed.

## Ganga Prem Celebrates Lives

### Vignette 1

The hospice invited us to provide an art therapy space for a bereavement day where they invited relatives and the local community to celebrate the lives of their loved ones who had died. The social event aimed to unite people who were going through the pain of losing a loved one through music and art.

The event was planned by both Western and Indian hospice staff at the hospice and echoed some of the community engagement work that takes place in British hospices. Such work includes inviting the local community into the hospice environment to take part in the arts with the aim of reducing any fear relating to illness and death. It also provides a supportive space for the bereaved to come together, to share their experiences, lessening feelings of isolation.

At the time the hospice building was not finished and so it took place outside of their current cancer clinic, a concrete open-air space amidst the bustling sounds and commotion of the city but enclosed by the surrounding buildings. Moon (2002) advocates the importance of being a 'mobile therapist' by responding to and making use of chance and circumstance in any environment to create a space for art therapy. Furthermore, she envisions the practice of a traditional studio model of art therapy to be achievable anywhere, even in the most unlikely places. When setting up our art therapy space we were reminded of Moon's description of 'a studio smacked down, dead centre, in the middle of life' (p. 71). A stark contrast to the art therapy studio in the hospice garden in London, sheltered and contained amongst primroses and ponds, analogous to Moon's description of the idealised studio, 'a sanctuary set a part from the rest of life' (ibid).

Our thinking around the art therapy space was informed by Kalmanowitz and Lloyd's (2005) notion of the 'portable studio' based on the premise that the internal structure we carry within us as art therapists can enable work to take place in a range of settings.

> Central [to this internal structure] is a belief in the individual as possessing internal resources rooted in experience, resilience and culture rather than being a powerless victim for whom the therapist alone holds the solutions.
>
> (Kalmanowitz and Lloyd, 2005, p. 108)

Essentially, our focus kept returning to the fundamental importance of holding and enabling a safe space for art-making to take place. Staff at the hospice came up with the image of a tree of remembrance, which was created on a large sheet of fabric. During the bereavement day, people placed photos of the deceased around the tree. Following this they were invited to draw or write a personal message to their loved one on a fabric leaf; there was little direction given and most people became engrossed in the art-making. There was also the opportunity to light Diya oil lamps, creating rangoli art (Figure 35.4) and decorating the tree with flowers, which are an intrinsic part of Hindu worship and rituals. The artwork felt alive as it grew and changed shape, like an organic installation sculpture. It felt important to include art practices and rituals which were familiar to those involved: those that had spiritual significance but also allow for a space to create artwork using materials which weren't so much associated with religious ritual. One man who was grieving his brother expressed his gratitude for the therapeutic space and said 'they had never had this experience before'. He voiced his sadness in his struggle to carry on with his life as it were before, sharing his drawing of his brother.

Where the relationship between ritual and art-making in Rishikesh is often embedded in religious intent, we wondered if holding a space which was not intended entirely for religious purposes allowed for him to express his grief more openly. There was a strong sense of unity and togetherness, aided through the music and artwork. The session ended with a group meditation facilitated by the hospice's spiritual advisor.

### *Vignette 2*

On our return to the hospice the following year, the new building was complete which is where the second bereavement event was held (Figure 35.5). Its location was of great contrast to the space the event was held in the previous year, physically settled in the heart of Rishikesh. Literally and metaphorically, the new building was distant from the community; its remote location is situated in a rural village outside of Rishikesh town. Travelling there involved many transport changes, including an auto rickshaw and a safari-like jeep which took us through jungle land. Daylight hours were safer due to the risk of jungle animals roaming around. The journey was onerous, highlighting to us the significance of the exhausting journeys some of our patients were experiencing.

The building itself felt clinical and bare, significantly different to many of the patients' homes we visited, which were full of energy and spirit and bursting with family members. When we first arrived, less than a handful of patients inhabited the building. We often witnessed the struggle many of the staff faced when trying to persuade patients to stay in the hospice when coming close to death. They continuously expressed their need to have their family around, to be at home and integrated in

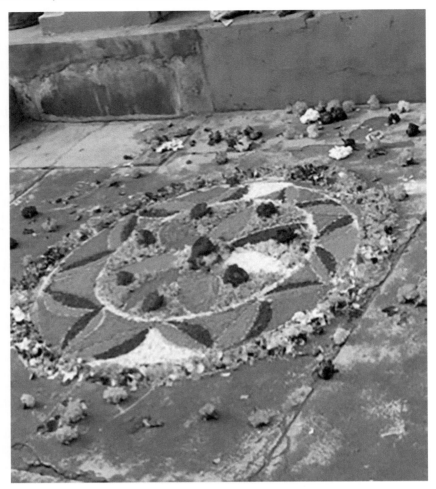

*Figure 35.4* Rangoli Art (See Plate 5)

the community. Staff at the hospice were desperate to break down some of the barriers that were preventing patients and the community from accessing the new hospice
building. They hoped that this event would bridge the gap between the new building
and the community.

As stated earlier, Rishikesh is a renowned spiritual city. It is one of three cities, alongside
Haridwar and Varanasi, where the devotional ritual Ganga Aarti is performed towards the
holy river, The Ganges. The river threads throughout India and is often referred to by
the local community as 'Mother Ganges' or the 'Divine Mother'. The ceremony is held at
sunset every day, and lamps and candles are placed in small boats filled with flowers and
are lit and 'offered' to the Goddess Mother Ganga, seeking blessing, purifying all who
touch, bathe or drink the water. The light and glow from the fire brings life to the water,
like a vein pumping blood into the heart of Rishikesh. Locals often referred to the ritual
as the 'remover of pain'. The Aarti ceremony is commonly facilitated by Hindu priests;
however, there is no named or determined form of 'God' that this ceremony is performed
for, making it universal and accessible to all, transcending the boundaries of language
and culture.

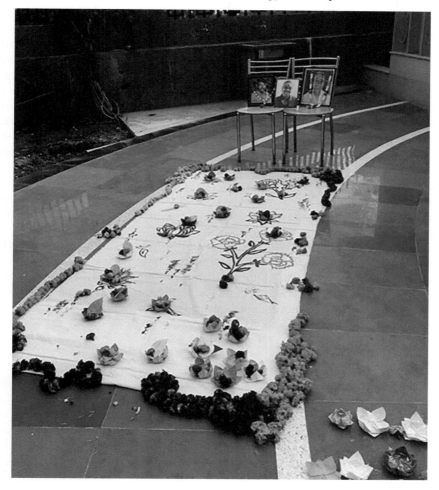

*Figure 35.5* Art Installation Decorated by Patients and Bereaved Families

Much of the imagery in the artwork created by individual patients and bereaved family members in art therapy depicts the beauty that Rishikesh had to offer. It was clear that their hometown was extremely meaningful for them. We wanted to facilitate a space for the bereavement event that was connected and inspired by the rituals from the Ganga Aarti ceremony, despite being geographically disconnected. We created a water-like mural, with floating flowers on a large piece of fabric representing the River Ganga. This was placed beside the spiritual temple in the garden of the hospice building while music played by local musicians energised the space. Beside the mural was a table set up with a variety of locally sourced art materials including pens, inks, paints and traditional patterned paper. We also created petal-like segments, and small paper flower boats, symbolising the flowers offered in the Aarti ceremony. We invited bereaved family members, staff and other community members to place a flower boat onto the water. They included messages to loved ones, names of those who had passed away or they simply just lit a candle and placed a boat onto the water, in memory. Photos of some of these individuals surrounded the 'water', reminding us of the lives they had lived and the impact they had on those around us. Some people wanted to share stories, some simply wanted someone to acknowledge how meaningful and profound their relationship with the deceased was.

Often, and particularly during this event, we struggled to communicate verbally with many of the people we were working with. We were initially concerned that the language barrier may have been an issue. However, staff members introduced us and explained what the event was for and the lack of shared language seemed to have no negative impact on our relationship with the attendees. Instead, the art-making took precedence and communication manifested in a non-verbal way. We were reminded of how a relationship forms between a mother and infant, a universal relationship, 'conveyed by manner, facial expression, gesture, or posture [. . .] ' to cite Bateman et al (2010, p. 99), the therapeutic relationship is built from the same foundation (ibid).

Staff, many of who had also lost loved ones, participated in this experience and towards the end of the event, we decided to take part ourselves and placed our own flowers onto the water. It felt important for us to participate in the experience, metaphorically integrating ourselves into the hospice and the community.

As the sun set onto the temple in the garden and the candles flickered together, we were united in an experience that did transcend all boundaries, reminding us of our experience of Ganga Aarti. It brought life to the hospice building, which now held energy, hope, strength, power and spirit, akin to what we felt in the family homes we had visited. The barriers between the community and the new hospice building began to dissolve as experiences of loss and love were shared, something faced by all of us.

## Conclusion

Within any hospice context, we are accustomed to the reality that physical illness does not stay within the prescribed boundaries (Schaverien, 2002) and often, we must be adaptable with the physical spaces in which we work. The therapeutic frame becomes something that is held in the space between us and the client, instead of being constructed externally. This was even more pertinent when working in Rishikesh because as Westerners it became crucial to embrace the cultural spaces and contexts in which we worked, instead of denying the fabric of our cultural environs through restrictive boundaries. In our endeavour to engage with our cultural framework, we found enabling spaces to create installation art, which became infused in ritual, particularly useful. Moon (2002) explains that the use of installation art in art therapy puts emphasis 'on relationship to the surrounding environment and relationship to the people who inhabit the space' (p. 98).

Using ritual in our art therapy practice has since influenced our work back in Britain. In 2017, during a patient art exhibition held at St Christopher's Hospice, we held an interactive installation ritual in the hospice garden, inviting the local community in to engage with art materials in response to the hospice environment. Some of the materials included rangoli powders, candles, a box of donated broken jewellery and relics from patients. The process outcome was named Galaxy.

Wasilewska (2013) explains that the process of art-making can be associated with specific rituals, 'that are deeply rooted in ourselves and our cultural traditions' (p. 198). Where rituals can be understood to 'reflect and reinforce belief' (ibid), it feels important to question what part they can play in art therapy when thinking about matters of spirituality at end-of-life in a Western hospice and palliative care setting. Bell (2012) explains spirituality as a process of meaning making, 'the affirmation of individual and collective values and beliefs' (p. 229), thus using more rituals in our art therapy practice could further help clients to reach a place of self-realisation and acceptance.

The current field of hospice and palliative care in India and the West have much to learn from each other. It is crucial for each system to remain indigenous to its cultural backcloth, however, to respond to the ebb and flow of globalisation, it is equally important to interweave and stitch together a patchwork of cross-cultural encounters within the field in order to inform our own practice.

# References

Bateman, A., Brown, B. and Pedder, J. (2010). *Introduction to Psychotherapy: An Outline of Psychodynamic Principles and Practice*. East Sussex and New York: Routledge.

Bell, S. (2012). 'Art Therapy and Spirituality', *Journal for the Study of Spirituality*, 1 (2), pp. 215–223.

Compassionate Neighbours. (2018). *About Compassionate Neighbours*. [online] Available from: http://compassionateneighbours.org/about-compassionate-neighbours/ [Accessed 31 May 2018]

Connell, C. (1992). 'Art Therapy as Part of a Palliative Care Programme', *Palliative Medicine*, 6, pp. 18–25.

Conolly, C. and King, J. (2017). 'Art therapy with an aboriginal child', in Meyerowitz-Katz, J. and Reddick, D. (eds.) *Art Therapy in the Early Years: Therapeutic Interventions with Infants, Toddlers and Their Families*. Abingdon, Oxon; and New York: Routledge, pp. 60–73.

Falk, B. (2005). 'Fear of annihilation: Defensive strategies used within art therapy groups and organizations for cancer patients', in Waller, D. and Sibbett, C. (eds.) *Art Therapy and Cancer Care*. New York: Open University Press, pp. 172–184.

Hocoy, D. (2002). 'Cross-cultural Issues in Art Therapy', *Art Therapy*, 19 (4), pp. 141–145.

Horton, R. (2013). 'Offline: Is Global Health Neocolonialist?' *The Lancet*, 382 (9906), pp. 1690.

Kalmanowitz, D. and Lloyd, B. (2005). 'Inside the portable studio: Art therapy in the former Yugoslavia 1994–2002', in Kalmanowitz, D. and Lloyd, B. (eds.) *Art Therapy and Political Violence: With Art, Without Illusion*. London and New York: Routledge, pp. 106–125.

Kapitan, L. (2015). 'Social Action in Practice: Shifting the Ethnocentric Lens in Cross-Cultural Art Therapy Encounters', *Art Therapy*, 23 (3), pp. 104–111.

Khosla, D., Patel, F. D. and Sharma, S. C. (2012). 'Palliative Care in India: Current Progress and Future Needs', *Indian Journal of Palliative Care*, 3, pp. 149–154.

Kumar, S. and Numpeli, M. (2005). 'Neighborhood Network in Palliative Care', *Indian Journal of Palliative Care*, 11, pp. 6–9.

Kumar, S. and Rajagopal, M. R. (1996). 'Palliative Care in Kerala: Problems at Presentation in 440 Patients with Advanced Cancer in a South Indian State', *Palliative Medicine*, 10, pp. 293–298.

Luzzatto, P. (1998). 'From psychiatry to psycho-ontology: Personal reflections on the use of art therapy with cancer patients', in Pratt, M. and Wood, M. J. M. (eds.) *Art Therapy in Palliative Care: The Creative Response*. East Sussex: Routledge, pp. 169–175.

Malchiodi, C. A. (2013). *Art Therapy and Health Care*. London: The Guilford Press.

McDermott, E., Selman, L., Wright, M. and Clark, D. (2008). 'Hospice and Palliative Care Development in India: A Multimethod Review of Services and Experiences', *Journal of Pain Symptom Manage*, 35, pp. 583–593.

Moon, C. M. (2002). *Studio Art Therapy: Cultivating the Artist Identity in the Art Therapist*. London: Jessica Kingsley Publishers.

Papadopoulos, R. K. (ed.) (2002). *Therapeutic Care for Refugees: No Place like Home*. London and New York: Karnac.

Rajagopal, M. R. (2001). 'The Challenges of Palliative Care in India', *National Medical Journal of India*, 14, pp. 65–67.

Roy, R. (1999). 'Culturally sensitive therapy: Accents, approaches and tools', in Campbell, J., Liebmann, M., Brooks, F., Jones, J. and Ward, C. (eds.) *Art Therapy, Race and Culture*. London: Jessica Kingsley Publishers, pp. 117–134.

Schaverien, J. (2002). *The Dying Patient in Psychotherapy: Desire, Dreams and Individuation*. Basingstoke: Palgrave: Macmillan.

Sibbett, C. (2005). 'Liminal embodiment: Embodied and sensory experience in cancer care and art therapy', in Waller, D. and Sibbett, C. (eds.) *Art Therapy and Cancer Care*. Berkshire: Open University Press, pp. 50–81.

Singh, S. S. (2012). 'The arts: A unique mantra for healing', in Kalmanowitz, D., Potash, J. S. and Chan, S. M. (eds.) *Art Therapy in Asia: To the Bone or Wrapped in Silk*. London and Philadelphia: Jessica Kingsley Publishers, pp. 190–195.

Skaife, S. (2013). 'Black and White: Applying Derrida to Contradictory Experiences in an Art Therapy Group for Victims of Torture', *Group Analysis*, 46 (3), pp. 256–271.

Talwar, S. (2010). 'An Intercultural Framework for Race, Class, Gender, and Sexuality in Art Therapy', *Art Therapy: Journal of the American Art Therapy Association*, 27 (1), pp. 11–17.

Wasilewska, E. (2013). 'Viewpoints: Ritual and Art Making', *Art Therapy Journal of the American Art Therapy Association*, 9 (4), pp. 198–200.

Wood, M. J. M., Low, M., Molassiotis, A. and Tookman, A. (2013). 'Art Therapy's Contribution to the Psychological Care of Adults with Cancer: A Survey of Therapists and Service Users in the UK', *International Journal of Art Therapy*, 18 (2), pp. 42–53.

# Glossary

**Bilateral Art Therapy** An approach developed for the treatment of trauma related disorders, integrating art therapy theories and practices as well as theories and practices developed by Eye Movement Desensitization and Reprocessing (EMDR) (Tripp, 2007).

**Candlelighters Simcoe** Candlelighters Simcoe is a not-for-profit organization that provides programs and services for young cancer patients residing in Simcoe County and surrounding areas and to their friends and family. Candlelighters Simcoe was established in 1990 by the parent of a childhood cancer patient.
Information available at: www.candlelighterssimcoe.ca

**Community Art Counsellors** A new category of professionals trained by Lefika la Phodiso in Johannesburg, South Africa. The training was developed by Hayley Burman, art psychotherapist, to help close the gap between resources available versus resources needed within South African communities. The trained community workers acquire skills and experiences in art therapy, to then be transferred to those they work with among the communities of their focus. More information on Lefika la Phodiso available at: https://lefikalaphodiso.co.za

**Community Engagement Arts** An empowering two-way process allowing communities to utilize the arts as a tool for social, emotional, cultural, and even economical community growth.

**Disenfranchised Grief** Disenfranchised grief occurs most often when a person feels they do not have the right to grieve; when a person feels there is something instinctually wrong with their grief; or when a person feels judged for issues related to their grief.

**Ethnographic Imagination** Paul Willis (2000), a sociologist and ethnographer, emphasized that when learning about cultures and communities it is essential to experience the aesthetics, non-verbal meanings, and objects of the people.

**Graphic Narrative** The "graphic narrative" is an art-based element of the intensive trauma therapy approach developed by Linda Gantt and Lou Tinnin (2007, 2009). The client is asked to create a series of images, used as a way to visually tell their story.

**Healing Circle** The use of healing circles, where people sit together in a circular formation, have been used by indigenous people for centuries and today healing circles are used in the field of mental health as a way of providing group support for people who are dealing with various issues including grief and trauma.

**Hodgkin Lymphoma (Hodgkin Disease)/Non-Hodgkin Lymphoma** Hodgkin lymphoma and non-Hodgkin lymphoma differ depending on the type of cells they affect in the body. Both forms of lymphoma are cancers that start in the cells, which affects the body's immune system.

**Hypoxic Ischemic Encephalopathy (HIE)** is a type of brain damage that occurs when an infant's brain does not receive enough oxygen and blood. It is a dangerous condition that requires immediate medical intervention.

**Immersive Visual Analysis** An art and sensory-based method of visual thinking that extends 'response art' into art-making-as-research to thematically analyze audio recorded narrative and visual data.

**Juvenile Batten Disease** A group of rare diseases caused by a genetic mutation, which affects an individual's vision and can cause seizures, dementia, and abnormal movements.

**LGBTQ** Lesbian, gay, bisexual, transgender, questioning, queer

**Meitheal** Meitheal is the Irish tradition whereby neighbours came together socially, for example sharing songs, stories, dancing, poems, dancing at the crossroads or assisting with various important life tasks.

**Mortality Salience** Awareness of one's own inevitable death.

**Motor Neuron Disease (MND) (also known as Amyotrophic Lateral Sclerosis—ALS)** A group of progressive neurological disorders that destroy motor neurons; leading to difficulty in voluntary muscle activity such as speaking, walking, breathing, and swallowing.

**Neuroblastoma** A malignant tumor composed of neuroblasts, most commonly in the adrenal gland. It is a form of cancer that starts in certain types of very primitive nerve cells found in an embryo or fetus.

**Osteosarcoma** Osteosarcoma is a malignant tumor of the bone in which there is a proliferation of osteoblasts. It is the most common type of cancer that develops in bone.

**Process-Focused Method of "Thinking in the Act"** Erin Manning and Brian Massumi are theorists who explored the connection between the creative processes and thinking; illustrating that, according to their explorations, art and thought are intertwined. Erin Manning and Brian Massumi (2014, p. II).

**Sensorimotor Psychotherapy** An approach which incorporates sensory experiencing with cognitive and emotional processing. More information is available at: www.sensorimotorpsychotherapy.org

**TBI** Traumatic Brain Injury, which may occur after a direct blow to the head, a puncture wound, or violent shaking and can cause temporary or permanent impairment of cognitive, psychosocial, or physical functioning.

**'Third Hand'** The art therapist becomes like a 'third hand' for the client, allowing art to be created by the therapist as envisioned by the client and holding true to that which the client hopes to convey (Edith Kramer, 1986).

**Whakairo** Māori traditional wood carving.

# References

Gantt, L. & Tinnin, L. W. 2007, 'Intensive trauma therapy of PTSD and dissociation: An outcome study,' *The Arts in Psychotherapy*, vol. 34, no. 1, pp. 69–80.

Gantt, L. & Tinnin, L. W. 2009, 'Support for a neurological view of trauma with implications for art therapy,' *The Arts in Psychotherapy*, vol. 36, no. 1, pp. 148–158.

Kramer, E. 1986, 'The art therapist's third hand: Reflections on art, art therapy, and society at large,' *American Journal of Art Therapy*, vol. 24, no. 3, pp. 71–86.

Manning, E. & Massumi, B. 2014, *Thought in the act*, University of Minnesota Press, Minneapolis, MN.

Tripp, T. 2007, 'A short term therapy approach to processing trauma: Art therapy and bilateral stimulation,' *Art Therapy*, vol. 24, no. 4, pp. 176–183.

Willis, P. 2000, *The ethnographic imagination*, Polity Press, Cambridge, MA.

# Appendix: Art Therapy Associations Worldwide

Art therapy associations from around the world help to support the profession of art therapy and the professionals practicing within the field. They offer professional, educational, and research opportunities; the associations help to advocate for the use of art therapy within the broader realms of mental, medical, and psychosocial health; and they help to ensure that the practice of art therapy is held up to a professional standard.

AUSTRALIA, NEW ZEALAND AND ASIA
Australian, New Zealand and Asian Creative Arts Therapies Association (ANZACATA)

BELGIUM
Belgian Art Therapy Association

BRAZIL
Brazilian Union of Art Therapy Associations

BULGARIA
Bulgarian Association for Art Therapy

CANADA
Canadian Art Therapy Association
Ontario Art Therapy Association
British Columbia Art Therapy Association
Association Des Art Therapeutes Du Quebec

CARIBBEAN
Caribbean Art Therapy Association

CHILE
Chilean Art Therapy Association

CHINA
Hong Kong Association of Art Therapists

COLUMBIA
Colombian Art Therapy Association

CROATIA
Croatian Art Therapy Association (Hrvatska Udruga Art Terapije—HART)

CYPRUS
Cyprus Art Therapy Association

CZECH REPUBLIC
Czech Art Therapy Association

DENMARK
Association for Integrative Art Therapy, formerly Association of Art Therapists

ESTONIA
Estonian Creative Arts Therapies Association

EUROPE
European Consortium for Arts Therapies
European Federation Art Therapy

FINLAND
Finnish Art Therapy Association

FRANCE
French Federation of Art Therapists

GREECE
Art and Psychotherapy Center

GERMANY
Germany Association of Art Therapy

HUNGARY
Hungarian Art Therapy Association

ICELAND
Icelandic Art Therapy Association

INDIA
Art Therapy India

ITALY
Professional Association of Italian Art Therapists (APIART)
Art Therapy Italiana

IRELAND
Irish Association of Creative Arts Therapists

NORTHERN IRELAND
Northern Ireland Group for Art as Therapy

ISRAEL
Israeli Association of Creative & Expressive Therapies

**KOREA**
Korean Art Therapy Association

**LATVIA**
Art Therapy Association

**LITHUANIA**
Lithuanian Art Therapy Association

**LUXEMBOURG**
Luxembourgish Association of Qualified Arts Therapists

**MALTA**
Creative Arts Therapies Society

**NETHERLANDS**
Federation Vaktherapeutische Occupations
Dutch Art Therapy Association

**NORWAY**
Art Therapy Association

**POLAND**
Polish Association of Art Therapists

**PUERTO RICO**
Puerto Rico Art Therapy Association

**ROMANIA**
Romanian Association for Expressive Therapies

**RUSSIA**
Russian Art Therapy Association

**SINGAPORE**
Art Therapists' Association Singapore

**SOUTH AFRICA**
South African National Arts Therapies Association (SANATA)

**SPAIN**
Spanish Federation of Professional Associations of Art Therapy
Spanish Association for Art Therapists

**SWEDEN**
Swedish National Association for Art Therapists

**SWITZERLAND**
Swiss Professional Association of Art Therapists

TAIWAN
Taiwan Art Therapy Association

TURKEY
Arts Psychotherapy Association

UKRAINE
Art-therapy Association

UNITED KINGDOM
British Association of Art Therapists

UNITED STATES
American Art Therapy Association
International Expressive Arts Therapies Association

## References

Global Art Therapy Resources. Available at: http://www.arttherapyalliance.org/GlobalArt TherapyResources.html (accessed 03/25/2019)

Maria Paula Guerrinha Arte-Psicoterapeuta. Available at: https://paulaguerrinha.com/global/art-therapy-associations ( accessed 03/25/2019)

# Contributors

**Emma Allen, HCPC registered art psychotherapist and Sandplay therapist,** (British and Irish Sandplay Society), works at Rampton Hospital, one of three high secure hospitals in the UK. She is a published author, clinical supervisor, forensic psychology lecturer at Nottingham Trent University, and is the founder of 'Forensic Sandplay Therapy'.

**Annalie Ashwell, HCPC registered art psychotherapist and clinical supervisor,** qualified as an art psychotherapist in 2012. She has developed and implemented arts therapy and wellbeing services within three adult hospices in and around London, and has worked in both children's and adult palliative care. Annalie specialises in participatory arts projects, co-production and curatorial practice, and is curator for an independent gallery supporting emerging national and international artists.

**Heidi Bardot, MA, ATR-BC, LCPAT,** is Director of the Art Therapy Graduate Program at The George Washington University in Washington, DC. She is a licensed, registered, board certified art therapist. Bardot has brought an international focus to GW Art Therapy through her creation of immersion diversity courses and service-learning programs in France, India, United Arab Emirates, South Africa, and Croatia and has assisted in creating a post-master's program in Croatia. In Lebanon she has collaborated with local organizations to work with refugees and to train relief workers in art techniques, self-care, and trauma. Bardot has published and presented nationally and internationally on war relief, trauma, resiliency, grief, ethics, and international education.

**Simon Bell, PhD, HCPC registered art therapist,** qualified as an art therapist in 1986 and has experience working in the fields of adult mental health, adults with learning disabilities, hospice and palliative care. He was awarded his PhD in 2008 focusing on art therapy, spirituality and palliative care. In 2016 he took up the post of Clinical Manager for a charity called Share Psychotherapy based in Sheffield, UK which offers medium to long-term psychotherapy for adults with mental health difficulties. He currently maintains his interest in working with physical illness, end of life care, spirituality and complex mental health needs, particularly trauma and dissociation.

**Hayley Berman, PhD** is a registered art psychotherapist HCPC(UK) and HPCSA (SA), practicing visual artist and engaged researcher interested in creating long—term psychosocial change. As Founding Director, she remains an active Board Member of Lefika la Phodiso, a Community Art Counselling and Training Institute.

Currently her role is Programme Leader for the MA in Art Therapy at University of Hertfordshire (UK).

**Amy Bucciarelli, MS, ATR-BC, LMHC** is faculty with the University of Florida's Center for Arts in Medicine. She is a board-certified art therapist and licensed mental health counselor with more than ten years of clinical art therapy practice experience focused on child and adolescent care within medical and mental health settings.

**Susan Carr, PhD** is currently Co-Editor in Chief for *The International Journal of Art Therapy*, and an art therapist in private practice with 12 years experience working in palliative care. Susan is also a writer and practicing artist, with her first book entitled *Portrait Therapy* published in September 2017 by Jessica Kingsley.

**Nadia Collette, PhD** is an art therapist in the Palliative Care Unit of Sant Pau Hospital (Barcelona, Spain), with a PhD in Psychology, Bachelor of Science in Medical Biology, Bachelor of Arts in Fine Arts, Master in Transdisciplinary Art Therapy and Human Development, Master in Integrative-relational Counseling for bereavement. Nadia coordinates the Research Group of the Spanish Professional Association of Art Therapists.

**Lara Cooke, HCPC Registered Art Psychotherapist,** has a BA in Fine Art and History of Art and went on to study a PGCE in secondary school Art and Design education. She taught for five years in inner London schools and then studied for her masters in Art Psychotherapy at Goldsmiths. Lara currently works as an art therapist at St Christopher's Hospice, as well as supervising students on their clinical placements. Her research interests focus on spirituality and art making. Lara has also undertaken research in Ganga Prem Hospice in India.

**Hannah Cridford, M(Des), MA, HCPC registered art psychotherapist,** was awarded the Corinne Burton Memorial Trust Scholarship, graduating from Goldsmiths College in 2013. Prior to qualifying as an art psychotherapist, Hannah developed community and participatory arts projects. Since qualifying she has specialized in palliative care, currently working with patients, their families and the bereaved in two adult hospices.

**Urania Dominguez MA, AT, CCLS** earned her masters in art therapy in Barcelona, Spain. She has worked in multicultural educational settings and specialized in cultural sensitivity within art therapy. Now in Puerto Rico, she has facilitated trainings for teachers regarding the creative process in the classroom and working with special needs children. Urania has since focused her work on pediatric cancer where she combines art therapy goals with child life goals to provide better psychosocial care.

**Mari Ebbitt, HCPC registered art psychotherapist,** currently works for Latimer Community Art Therapy, an organisation providing art therapy to the community impacted by the Grenfell Fire in West London. Within this context, and following a project carried out with Ganga Prem Hospice in India, she has further developed her knowledge of and interest in working with loss, grief and trauma. As well as this, Mari has continued to build on her experience working with adults within the homelessness sector, as well as acute mental health settings, both of which are of special interest to her.

**Aya Feldman** is an art therapist, psychotherapist, senior supervisor (YAHAT, Israel Society of Art Therapists), materials researcher, supervisor and lecturer. She is senior lecturer to M.A. students at the Art Therapy Department, Hamidrasha-Faculty of Arts, Beit Berl Academic College, Israel. Supervisor and lecturer at the Winnicotian Analytical Institute, graduate of the Lesley College Cambridge, a certified focusing trainer and an artist whose work has been displayed in exhibitions and other cultural spaces around the world. For more than 13 years has been running a private art psychotherapy clinic. She is part of a research group on the subject of materials, their analytical significance and how to present and work with them in the art therapists' studio, and participated in the search for ways to help patients make deeper emotional connections with their parents' with dementia.

**Shahar Gindi PhD** is a clinical psychologist, senior lecturer, specialist in autism, supervisor and researcher in parenting. A lecturer in the Art Therapy and Education departments of Hamidrasha-Faculty of Arts, Beit Berl Academic College, Israel and part of the group of researchers focusing on examining ways to help patients make deeper emotional connections with their parents' with dementia.

**Deborah Green PhD MEd MAAT(Clinical)** engaged in community theatre and HIV/AIDS/life skills education and counselling in South Africa before immigrating to Christchurch, New Zealand, where during and after the earthquakes she provided arts therapy for the quake-affected of all ages. She is currently senior Arts Therapy lecturer at Whitecliffe College of Arts & Design.

**David E. Gussak, PhD, ATR-BC**, Professor of Art Therapy and Chairperson of the Department of Art Education at Florida State University David has published and lectured widely on art therapy with forensic populations. He is the author of *Art on Trial: Art Therapy in Capital Murder Cases* and co-editor of the *Wiley Handbook of Art Therapy* with Dr. Marcia Rosal.

**Jennie Halliday, MFA, MAAT, AThr,** is a clinical arts therapist based in Auckland, New Zealand. and is a professional member of ANZACATA (The Australian, New Zealand and Asian Creative Arts Therapies Association). Jennie has worked as part of a clinical palliative care team in a hospice setting for 6 years providing arts therapy for patients and family members. Her private practice has a focus on complex trauma and abuse recovery with adolescents and adults. Jennie has contributed to two books on the arts therapies and continues to have a passion for presenting case work that exemplifies the power of the arts therapies as a clinical practice.

**Uwe Herrmann PG Dip AT, MA, PhD** Professor Herrmann developed the art therapy service at the State Training Institute for the Blind in Hanover, Germany, where he has practised for 27 years. Concurrently he has lectured on the MA Art Therapy Programme at Weissensee Academy of Art Berlin since 2000.

**Ofira Honig PhD**, Art Psychotherapist. senior supervisor (YAHAT, the Israel Society of Art Therapists). A senior lecturer, head of the Master program in Art Therapy and head of the Art Therapy Department at the HAMIDRASHA—Faculty of Arts at the Beit Berl Academic College, Israel. Supervisor at the Winnicotian Analytical Institute. Photographer and part of a research group on the subject of art materials, their analytical significance and how to present and work with them in the art therapists' studio. Participated in the search for ways to help patients make deeper emotional connections with their parents with dementia. For over 20 years Ofira has been running a private Art psychotherapy clinic, working with adolescents, adults, victims of terrorism, widows and orphans; and instructing clinical psychologists, social workers and youth investigators.

**Becky Jacobson LPC, ATR, LMT,** works with individuals, families, and groups addressing life transitions, grief and loss, trauma, pain and stress management, and overall health and well being through art therapy, psychotherapy, therapeutic massage, and other mind-body practices. Becky has worked in hospice, hospital, community-based, and private practice settings. She has worked internationally in the field of art therapy as well, focusing on youth empowerment. She has contributed to two IRB-approved studies and was chosen as a delegate at the Clinton Global Initiative University Conference.

**Gudrun Jones BA (Hons), Dip A.T, M.Phil, City & Guilds First Aid CBT,** Hywel Dda University Health Board. Gudrun obtained her degree in Textiles from West Surrey College of Art and Design, then qualified as an art therapist from Goldsmith College, University of London in 1989. Gudrun practices art therapy through the medium of Welsh and English. She has worked in oncology and palliative care in the health board since 1992.

**Jacqueline Jones, MEd, MA, ATR-BC**, is a creative arts therapist at the Invisible Wounds Center at Eglin Air Force Base, treating active duty service members recovering from traumatic brain injury and psychological health conditions. Previously, with support from the National Endowment for the Arts, she established the Creative Arts Therapies program at the Intrepid Spirit Center at Fort Belvoir Community Hospital after interning at the National Intrepid Center of Excellence.

**Lynda Kachurek** currently lives in Richmond, VA. Her husband, Patrick Kachurek, passed away in January 2015, and she attended mind-body art therapy as part of her grief support and recovery.

**Girija Kaimal, EdD, MA, ATR-BC** is research faculty in the PhD program in Creative Arts Therapies department at Drexel University. Her research focuses on the physiological and psychological outcomes of visual self expression on health and well-being. She teaches graduate courses in research methods and philosophies works on federally funded research on art therapy with military service members, patients with cancer and their caregivers as well as children and adults facing chronic stress and adversity. Her contributions in this book are based on a mixed methods study of caregivers of patients in home-hospice care.

**Karen Kelly, MA, BMUS, G.Dip,** Music Therapist. Karen has been working in Milford Care Centre, Ireland since 2007. She specializes in Specialist Palliative Care and Care of the Older Person and has previous experience in the areas of mental health, autism and supporting vulnerable families. Karen lectures and supervises students on clinical placement.

**Jean McCaw, MA, LCPAT, ATR-BC** is a licensed and board-certified art therapist and oncology therapist with over 30 years working with children, adolescents, adults and families coping with serious illness, terminal illness and end of life. Jean worked for 14 years in hospice and palliative care with children, adolescents and their families navigating terminal illness, grief and loss. She has worked in the pediatric oncology and adult oncology communities for the past 10 years with children, adolescents and adults navigating life transitions related to illness and treatment, end of life and bereavement. Jean has authored the book *Touching Grief—Frequently Asked Questions About Child and Adolescent Grief*, a resource for parents and caregivers who care for children and adolescents who are grieving.

**Claudia Mandler McKnight, BA, BEd, MA, DTATI, RP, RCATA** is a practicing artist, arts educator, and art therapist in Barrie, Ontario, Canada. A graduate of Queen's University at Kingston, the University of Toronto and the Toronto Art Therapy Institute, Claudia has been in private practice for over twenty years. Claudia is a registered member of the College of Registered Psychotherapists of Ontario, and the Canadian Art Therapy Association. Her clients range in age from 4 to 86. Claudia also teaches the postgraduate level course "Art Therapy, Spirituality, Grief and Loss" for the Toronto Art Therapy Institute, and provides clinical supervision for art therapists-in-training and graduate art therapists.

**Jennifer Newson McMahon, MA,** Advanced Art Therapy Studies–senior art therapist. Jennifer worked as an art therapist in palliative care and in mental health services for older adults for 16 years. Her background includes working as an SRN, a rape crisis counsellor and she is an accredited facilitator on the Advanced Communication Skills Training in Palliative Care programme.

**Rachel Mims, MS, ATR-BC, LPC-AT** served 10.5 years in the U.S. Army before earning her MS in art therapy at Florida State University. Rachel focuses on using art therapy to help veterans and their families improve their quality of life and in 2017 she founded a nonprofit called Veteran Art Therapy.

**Deirdre Ní Argáin BSc., MA** studied art therapy at Goldsmiths College London. On her return to Ireland she was a founder member and former chair of the Irish Association of Creative Arts Therapists. Over the past 25 years she has introduced art therapy to a number of palliative care settings in Ireland and currently works as senior art therapist with the Galway Hospice Foundation.

**Grace Ong AThR** is a registered art therapist from Singapore. She received her master's in art therapy from LASALLE College of the Arts. She spent her first 4 years as an art therapist at Assisi Hospice, helping to establish the art therapy service within the inpatient, day care and home care settings, specializing in grief and bereavement work. She is currently pursuing a diploma in Montessori for children between the ages of 3–6 at the Maria Montessori Institute in London to deepen her understanding of child development.

**Kayleigh Orr HCPC Registered Art Psychotherapist** developed the art therapy service for end of life children and young people and pre-and post-bereaved family members at Keech Hospice Care, UK. Kayleigh is a committee member of the British Association of Art Therapists' Special Interest Group: *Creative Response: Working with Loss*. Kayleigh also works part time as an art therapist for West London Mental Health Trust.

**Barbara Parker-Bell, PsyD, ATR-BC**, is currently director of art therapy at Florida State University and president of the Art Therapy Credential Board (ATCB). She has engaged in extensive academic and research exchanges with Tomsk State University in the Russian Federation, including a Fulbright Teaching and Research Scholarship in 2016–7.

**Sara Powell AThR** Sara is from the UK and is the founder of ATIC Dubai. She has an MA in Art Therapy from LASALLE Singapore. She is a registered member of the professional association for Creative Arts therapists in Australia, New Zealand and Asia (ANZACATA). Sara has over 9 years' experience and worked on numerous projects in collaboration with Government in Singapore and UAE. She specializes in women issues, child and adolescent related disorders.

**Lucy Pyart HCPC registered art psychotherapist** has a background in physiotherapy and completed her Masters in Art Psychotherapy, at the University of Roehampton. She now works as an art psychotherapist within a primary school setting and has an interest in art psychotherapy within the medical contexts.

**Eloïse Raab, HCPC registered art psychotherapist,** received her masters from Goldsmiths University. She works as an art therapist in a Central London based refugee centre and for Latimer Community Art Therapy, an organisation supporting the community impacted by the Grenfell Fire, since June 2017. As well as recent work for Ganga Prem Hospice in India, Eloïse continues to develop her practice in working with trauma and loss both in schools (primary and secondary) as well as supporting adults with eating disorders. Eloïse has a BA in Fine Art and works as an artist alongside her Art Therapy practice.

**Rachel Rahman FHEA, CPsychol, AFBPsS**, senior lecturer, Psychology Department Aberystwyth University. Rachel is a senior lecturer at Aberystwyth University, Wales, UK and the Director of the Centre for Excellence in Rural Health Research. Her current research explores the use of telemedicine and technology innovation in rural health and social care; with particular interest in chronic disease and palliative care.

**Hilary Rapp HCPC registered art psychotherapist** works in an open studio with a UK mental health charity, facilitates a group for people with multiple sclerosis and bereavement work. For 20 years Hilary lived and worked in Asia, with past experience as a nurse in oncology and palliative care followed by humanitarian work with refugees which led to her masters in Art Therapy at LASALLE in Singapore. She is a co-founder of the Art Therapists' Association, Singapore.

**Shlomit Rinat MA** art therapist, psychotherapist, senior supervisor (YAHAT, the Israel Society of Art Therapists), and researcher into the incorporation of emotional processes into the educational system. Supervisor and lecturer in the MA program of the Art Therapy Department, Hamidrasha—Faculty of Arts, Beit Berl Academic College, Israel. She has worked as a social worker for the last 20 years. She is also a published poet. She has also worked as a senior supervisor for the Education ministry and is part of a research group on the subject of materials, their analytical significance and how to present and work with them in the art therapists' studio, and has participated in the search for ways to help patients make deeper emotional connections with their parents' with dementia.

**Martine Robson, BA (Hons), PGCT HE** Fellow Associate lecturer Psychology Department Aberystwyth University.

**Stefania Romano** is an art therapist member of Professional Art Therapist Italian Association (A.P.I.ART), specialized in psycho-oncology at Regina Elena Institute (Rome). Since 2010 she has worked as an art therapist in the three hospices of Florence both with patients and staff. She is a professional counselor (licensed from SIPT—Italian Society of Therapeutic Psychosynthesis) and trainer in psychosynthesis for spiritual paths. She has focused her work on mental disabilities, palliative care and developing path. She also works with young students facing learning and emotional difficulties.

**Sarah Yazdian Rubin, LCAT, ATR-BC, CCLS** is a creative arts therapist and child life specialist. Sarah was the first art therapist to join the palliative care service at Mount Sinai Hospital in New York City where she established an annual creative arts journal (*The Loom*) created by patients and caregivers, and a memorial service geared towards children. Sarah received her master's in art therapy from New York University and is currently in private practice in Nashville, TN.

**Anastasia A. Stipek, PhD (Psychology)** is currently a teaching specialist and assistant professor at Tomsk State University, Russian Federation, where her responsibilities include the development of online courses. She is a practicing psychologist and art therapist. Her focus is on phenomenology, existential psychotherapy, psychology of creativity, vocation and authenticity.

**Todd Stonnell LPC, ATR-BC** currently practices as an art therapist in a residential substance abuse treatment center. He attempts to bring playfulness to each session, nurturing each person's resiliency and curiosity. He lives by the belief that each moment has the potential to be an awfully big adventure.

**Jody Thomson, PhD candidate,** has specialised in cancer and end of life art therapy for the last ten years, working with groups, individuals and families. She has designed and facilitated short and long-term art therapy programs for hospitals, community and charity organisations. Jody's research interests focus on poststructuralist, new materialist and post-human theorisation of art-making in art therapy, in the context of the therapist's experience of working with terminally diagnosed clients. Her work has been published and presented internationally.

**Meghan Treacy MA, BA, H.Dip**, Art Therapist. Meghan has been working in specialist palliative care and care of the older person in Milford Care Centre, Ireland since 2015. Meghan has worked in a variety of mental health settings, including working with survivors of abuse, domestic violence, ex-offenders and youth at risk of offending who present with challenging behaviour.

**Tally Tripp MA, MSW, LCSW, ATR-BC** is a registered and board-certified art therapist, licensed clinical social worker and certified trauma therapist working extensively with complex trauma, grief and loss in the Washington, D.C. area. In addition to her practice, Tally is an assistant professor of Art Therapy at the George Washington University where she is the director of the GW University Art Therapy Clinic, a training clinic that provides art therapy to the community and specializes in trauma treatment. Tally has lectured and presented numerous papers, workshops, and trainings both nationally and internationally and is the author of several articles and publications focusing on experiential approaches for the treatment of trauma

**Tatiana A. Vaulina, PhD (Psychology)**, is currently an associate professor of the Psychology Department of Tomsk State University, Russian Federation. She teaches and works as a Coordinator of International Projects of Psychology. She has been awarded two Fulbright Grants, one in 2008–2009 and another in 2014. She received a DAAD award in 2009–2010.

**Neasa Whelan MA, BA, G.Dip,** Senior Music Therapist. Neasa has worked in specialist palliative care and mental health services for older adults since 2001. Qualifications include: bachelor of arts in music, graduate diploma in music education and master of arts in music therapy. She is a visiting music therapy lecturer, supervisor of music therapy students on clinical placement and participates in research projects.

**Michèle J.M. Wood HCPC registered art psychotherapist, SFHEA.** Michèle has worked extensively as an art therapist since 1987 and is a Winston Churchill Fellow. Her expertise is palliative care, with a research interest in digital technology in art therapy. In addition to working as an art therapist in a London hospice, Michèle co-ordinates the British Association of Art Therapists' Special Interest Group *Creative Response: Working with Loss*, is a clinical supervisor, a Schwartz Round Facilitator and a Principal Teaching Fellow at the University of Roehampton, London.

**Nataly Woollett, PhD, ATR, RPT-S** is a South African therapist and researcher, trained in the fields of psychology, play therapy and art therapy. She is registered in the U.S. and South Africa and has practiced in multiple countries. She is committed to issues of social justice and the rights of vulnerable populations. Nataly's expertise is in trauma and bereavement; and the intersection of mental health, HIV and violence. She is a senior lecturer at the University of the Witwatersrand.

# Index

Note: Italicized page numbers indicate a figure on the corresponding page. Page numbers in bold indicate a table on the corresponding page.